Lung Cancer

in

-lioma

Lung Cancer and Mesothelioma

Howard A. Gutman

Comment or suggestions about the book are welcome and may be sent to howian@aol.com. For information about new treatments or developments, consult our newsletter at www.lungcancerbook andnewsletter.com

This book was printed in the United States of America.

To order additional copies of this book, contact:
Xlibris Corporation
1-888-795-4274
www.Xlibris.com
Orders@Xlibris.com
20167

616
.99424
G985x

JAN '06

Contents

DEDICATION

This book is dedicated to my father-in-law Frank Paden who had lung cancer and demonstrates that a man's smoking history bears no relationship to his contribution to society, importance to his family, and value as a person.

PREFACE

Lung cancer remains a difficult disease. The disease arises a number of years after initial exposure to a carcinogen with alteration to various growth factors, tumor suppressor genes, and other cellular components combining to create the changes we call cancer. At its earliest stages the tumor can be removed, but most are diagnosed when the cancer has advanced to lymph nodes or other organs. My goal is to help the patient and family member untangle the complexities of this disease, and direct you to areas for further research and questioning.

My book is an overview of lung cancer touching on a number of different topics. It is intended as a "middle book," more detailed than a general guide but easier to understand than a medical text. The goal is to provide some basic information about medical topics to help you understand the disease and its treatment.

I begin by discussing what cancer is and how the orderly process of cell reproduction goes awry. The first part of the book provides the groundwork for the remainder, with a discussion of cancer terminology, cell cycles, genes and lung cancer anatomy. These topics will help you understand the medicine behind your treatments. Each chapter is designed to be independent, and your first step might be to review the material on your type of cancer, such as stage 4 non-small cell lung cancer.

The middle chapters discuss different types of treatment, surgery, radiation, chemotherapy, gene therapy, their benefits and risks, and when they are utilized. Adding some background about cell structure and treatments, I then review non-small cell lung cancer devoting a chapter to each stage.

A cautionary note. I am not a doctor and in any event you should never base your treatment on information in a book. Lung cancer research is rapidly changing, protocols evolve, and physicians design treatments based upon your age, condition, and medical history. The book helps to provide the background to help you discuss treatments with your oncologist. Instead of asking basic questions about the disease, I hope you can focus your discussions on the specifics of your treatment.

The third part of the book discusses public policy, legal, and insurance questions associated with lung cancer. Should there be screening for smokers, when are doctors responsible if tumors are not timely diagnosed, what types of treatments are covered by insurance, and how should we improve treatment. While smoking continues to be the primary risk factor, diet, and occupational carcinogens like asbestos are discussed.

Keep a medical dictionary nearby and feel free to reread a chapter and keep other medical references nearby. I spent well over 2,500 hours writing this book, don't expect to completely understand some difficult topics in far less time.

Cautionary Note

Again this book is intended to be a general reference, not advice regarding specific treatment. No warranty is made as to the accuracy, completeness, or applicability of any of the material herein to a specific patient. The author is not a physician and all medical advice should be obtained from your physician

CHAPTER 1

WHAT IS CANCER?

1.0 WHY PATIENTS AND THEIR FAMILIES NEED A BASIC UNDERSTANDING OF LUNG CANCER

This book is designed to provide a detailed, but understandable, review of lung cancer. Specifically:

- By understanding the basics, you can direct your questioning to the details of your condition, rather than asking for general explanations about cancer and how it develops.
- Some decisions may not be made by the doctor alone. In many cases, there are experimental treatments. Knowing the medical basis for the treatment may help you make the decision of whether a particular clinical trial or other treatment is for you.
- Understanding what certain chemotherapy drugs are trying to do, and why certain side effects develop may help you to understand and deal with them.

1.01 Approach

As I worked on this book, a member of my family contracted cancer, and I realized firsthand the stress that diagnosis entails. Nonetheless, I have tried to discuss lung cancer in an analytical fashion, laying out the facts and science even where they may paint a difficult picture, believing that being educated can only help the patient and his family. This is designed to be a middle book, more detailed than a general book about cancer, easier to read than a medical text. My goal is to lay out the science of lung cancer in a thorough, comprehensive, but understandable fashion.

1.02 Limits

Some caveats. This book is not designed to provide medical advice regarding any individual's condition, and treatment alternatives may depend upon a number of individual factors. Cancer research is an evolving area, and some areas may have changed from the date of publication. There may be new studies and older ones may be reevaluated. Again, my goal is not to provide medical advice and you should make treatment determinations with the advice and guidance of your physician. My goal is to provide some basic information about lung cancer to make those consultations as meaningful and informative as possible.

1.1 COMMON CHARACTERISTICS OF CANCERS

1.11 Abnormal Growth

Cancer is a group of related diseases characterized by uncontrolled multiplication and disorganized growth of affected cells. Cancer is a significant disruption of the normal, orderly and regulated cycle of cell replication and division in the body. Cancers share three basic characteristics: unregulated growth, lack of cell differentiation, and the capacity to metastasize to neighboring tissues:

> "Cancer manifests itself as a population of cells that have lost their normal controls of growth and differentiation and are proliferating. In the first instance, these cells, derived initially from a normal cell, form a primary tumor (literally a swelling) . . . . {This} primary tumor comprises a population of cells which are said to be growth transformed—that is they have acquired a set of mutations to a set of genes which allow them to divide repeatedly in a way that normal cells cannot." Vile, (1) at 24.

1.12 Cell Division and Multiplication as a Normal Process

Cell division and replacement is a normal process in the body. Cells in some parts of our body are constantly growing like fingernails and hair.

In other areas, cells divide to replace dead or damaged cells, such as in the skin or the intestinal tract. While one characteristic of cancer cells is their propensity to divide and multiply, normal cells do that too:

> "Cells do all kinds of things, including divide into more cells: one cell can divide into two cells, each "offspring cell" can divide into two cells, and so on. Cell division occurs at various times and for various reasons: cells divide during the growth and development of the embryo and the fetus, for example, and when there is a need to repair an injury in the body, such as a scraped knee. Cells also divide in cancer—cancer occurs when they divide out of control." Coleman (2)

1.13 Why Cell Division is Necessary

Cell division occurs for various reasons in the normal person. First, many parts of the body are subjected to daily wear and tear that kills or damages cells, and cell division is the body's method of replacing these dead or damaged cells. Secondly cells may divide in order to perform certain tasks. When a germ enters our body, cells in the immune system divide and increase in number to kill the germ. Thirdly, cell division helps the body grow. Cell division is required for a child to increase in physical size and grow into adulthood.

Whether to replace old cells, perform specific functions, or help the body grow, cell division is usually a necessary and orderly process. Cell division is tightly regulated; with the cells signaled to divide only to perform specified functions. Normal tissue exists in a careful regulated balance of cellular division and cellular death. In contrast, cancerous tissue grows out of balance, resulting in an excess of cellular division.

Unregulated growth means a tumor grows without regard to the needs of the tissue or the normal controls for that cell or gene:

> "In the first stage, a normal cell undergoes an initial genetic change which partly releases it from the normally very stringent

controls imposed upon its growth potential; the daughter cells accumulate further genetic mutations which accentuate this loss of normal growth regulation, until a population of tumor cells emerge which no longer respond to normal signals preventing cell division and growth. The cells of the primary tumor are, therefore, said to be growth transformed. The genetic mutations which accumulate in these primary tumor cells are members of two classes of cellular genes, the proto-oncogenes and the tumor suppressor genes. These genes control the ability of cells to pass through the cell cycle and, hence, their ability to divide or, alternatively, to stop dividing and to undergo [differentiation]." Dermer, (3)

Cancer is generally not unique behavior in a cell, but normal behavior expressed to an extreme or in an incorrect context. Division and duplication of cells, movement of cells to damaged areas, are each characteristics of normal cells. Even metastasis, movement of cells to other organs may occur with healing of wounds, the development of a fetus, or attacking bacteria.

1.14 Unregulated Growth

To call the growth of cancer cells wholly unregulated or unpredictable is inaccurate. Tumors possess certain common characteristics and we can, to some extent, predict how they will behave. Some types of tumors grow and divide rapidly, like small cell cancer, while others grow slowly.

1.15 Classifying Tumors Based Upon Growth Characteristics

Physicians classify tumors primarily upon their capacity to grow and move to other organs (metastasis). There are two main categories of lung cancer: small cell (sclc) and non-small cell (nsclc). Small cell tumors grow rapidly but are susceptible to chemotherapy while non-small cell tumors grow more slowly. I will later explain the categorization scheme for lung cancer.

1.16 Differentiation

Not only do cells divide to replace damaged or dead cells, they also develop to assume their final form and function in the body, a process called differentiation. Normal cells are differentiated, that is constructed or organized for a specific purpose. When a cell changes from a normal to cancerous one, the cell often loses some or all of its ability to form normally functioning tissue structures. Cancer cells are classified from well-differentiated to poorly differentiated, with the degree of differentiation one indicator of how the cell has changed. Under a microscope, a pathologist can look at the cell, determine and categorize its differentiation.

1.161 Well-Differentiated and Poorly Differentiated Cells

Well-differentiated means relatively limited changes are seen in the cell. A well-differentiated cancer cell may assume an appearance that is somewhat similar to its original tissue, and even display some normal functions. Poorly differentiated means the original structure and function is almost entirely absent. The extent of differentiation of the cancer cell is somewhat correlated with the aggressiveness of the tumor; poorly differentiated tumors tend to be far more aggressive than well-differentiated tumors. While the extent of differentiation is one factor in evaluating the status of the patient, it has not become a critical factor. Instead the extent of metastasis, or movement to other tissues, has become the chief factor in determining the status of the tumor and the treatment which will be administered.

1.17 Metastasis

Probably the most serious danger in cancer development is the tendency of cancerous cells to metastasize, that is, invade neighboring structures, and transmit the cellular malfunctions to those cells:

"Whereas a benign tumor will expand in size as a consequence of cell division, it will not invade surrounding tissues nor will it shed cells that are capable of initiating tumor foci elsewhere in the body. A malignant tumor will, however, actively invade and destroy surrounding tissue and also give rise to cells which often spread to produce foci of tumor growth at distant sites." Vile, (1) at 101-102.

1.171 Analogies to Normal Cellular Behavior

Metastasis, the movement of cancer cells to normal organs and structures seems strange. However, the processes associated with metastasis are not unique to cancer cells and the ability of cells to travel to different areas of the body is a normal and necessary process to maintain health. For example, circulating white blood cells must be able to exit the blood through the capillaries and enter infected tissues in response to the injury. During early development of an embryo, cells that become the embryo's placenta must be able to invade the mother's womb to allow the developing embryo to attach and grow. Healing of a cut requires the movement of different types of cells to cover the wound and re-form skin and blood vessels. Each of these processes is tightly controlled such that the invasion is limited in time and space.

The body would likely repair the leg by replenishing cells and repairing damaged sources of blood supply. With a cancer, the body believes the area is damaged, so it connects with neighboring sources of blood and nourishment to replenish the damaged area. In truth, many cancers do reflect damage to DNA, but the remedy the body creates simply spreads the cancer, rather than repair the damage. Comparisons to the behavior of normal cells can be made:

> "It is also important to remember that expression of invasion promoter genes is not a purely pathological phenomenon seen only in cancer. Certain normal cell types demonstrate different elements of the phenotype as part of their usual functions. Thus, leukocytes resemble metastatic cells in many ways since they must leave the bone marrow and move, via the circulation, to specific sites elsewhere in the body where they must penetrate to sites of infection and inflammation. Similarly, embryonic cells must move between developing tissues in a way that can be likened to tumor cell invasion . . . . Therefore, expression of the invasive phenotype by cancer cells should be thought of more as the activation of normal cellular programmes in an inappropriate cellular context, than as the expression of completely novel phenotypes. In this way, it may be possible to understand how and why the genes of invasion are expressed so aberrantly in tumor cells and, therefore, to generate more mechanism-based and effective treatments." (1) Vile, at 24

1.172 Tumors Are Categorized Based Upon the Extent of Metastasis

Cancers are categorized based upon the extent of metastasis (as well as growth). Non-small cell lung cancers (the largest type of lung cancer) are classified from stage 1 to stage 4. Stage 1 tumors are limited to a defined area in a single part of the lung. Stage 4 means the tumor has metastasised to another organ, with stages 2 and 3 assessing the extent of movement to adjoining or distant lymph nodes. Stage one cancers are usually treated with surgical removal of the tumor, while stage four metastatic tumors treated with chemotherapy.

1.2 DIFFERENCES AMONG CANCERS

1.21 Cancer as a Group of Diseases

Cancers share the three traits of unregulated growth, loss of differentiation, and propensity to metastasize, though the extent of each trait may vary. Some cancers are highly metastatic meaning they move quickly to other parts of the body, while others move slowly over years or even decades. Most scientists believe that cancer is a group of related diseases with common characteristics, not a single disease. While cancers share certain characteristics there are significant differences among different cancers. Some skin cancers may be relatively harmless in their early stages, while others may be more serious especially in advanced stages.

1.22 Causes of Cancer

The causes of cancers vary. Diet plays a critical role in the development of colon cancer, but has a limited role in lung, and perhaps no role in skin cancer. Nutrition plays a role in many cancers, but does not affect others. Given that the factors which create cancers vary, not surprisingly the resulting tumors themselves vary. Cancers behave differently depending upon their type and the organ where they originate.

1.23 Differences in Behavior of Different Cancers by Organ

The behavior of cancers depends primarily upon their type and the organ where they originate. Some cancers spread or metastasize very quickly while others are slow-moving. For example, pancreatic cancer is a very serious form of cancer, while some forms of skin cancer are relatively innocuous.

1.24 Treatment is Organ-specific

Treatment is generally by organ; a skin cancer is treated differently than a prostate tumor. Clinical trials which test a particular drug may be limited to tumors in a particular organ, or at least results will be categorized by organ. Lung cancer is a solid tumor, unlike, for example, leukemia. There are some common traits among solid tumors and some of the same drugs are used for various types of solid tumors. Some drugs used for colon and breast cancer are used for lung.

1.25 Differences within the Same Organ

Since there can be different types of cancer in a particular organ, treatment within a particular organ can vary. As we see later, small cell lung cancer is treated differently than non-small cell.

1.26 Metastatic Cancer Cells Retain the Characteristics of the Original Organ

One writer explains:

> "Even though cancers enlarge, invade adjacent body parts, and travel to distant metastatic locations, they remain unchanged. The characteristics of human tumors, with rare exceptions, are fixed for the life of every tumor, regardless of where or when distant metastases of the tumor are found. In 1874, Dr. W. Moxon, an English pathologist, described rectum in liver, referring to rectal tumors that were growing in their original unchanged forms after metastasizing to the liver .... a prostate tumor that is

diagnosed early prostate specific antigen (PSA) was detected in
the blood will continue to produce PSA years later at a metastatic
site." Dermer, (3) at 46-47

Cancer is treated differently than non-small cell lung cancer. This
book is about lung cancer, or more specifically tumors which originate
in the lung. Thus, we may discuss metastasis to other organs, which
will still be treated as lung cancer in most respects.

1.3 RESERVED

1.4 HOW NORMAL CELLS CHANGE TO CANCER CELLS

1.41 Proto-Oncogenes and Oncogenes

Cancer cells are basically good cells gone bad and we can, with
some precision, identify those cells which can become cancers. These
are genes already involved with cell division and growth which are
called proto-oncogenes. "Mutations to a proto-oncogene alters its
structure and activates it to produce an oncogene. The protein product
of the oncogene is itself altered so that it can no longer be switched off
by normal cellular signals and its expression directs the cell to divide."
Vile, (1) 4-5

A proto-oncogene is a normal gene which performs certain growth
functions but when altered, can turn into a cancerous oncogene:

"The beginnings of cancer lay not in a wholesale rewiring of
the cell, but in a subtle alteration of a fistful of key genes among
the human quote of DNA. Under normal circumstances, such
genes play a vital, growth-related role in all or most tissues of the
body. In some tissues, the genes may set up the rounds of simple
division, helping skin cells to proliferate into a scab around a
wound, or allowing the immune system to send out a host of
antibodies to assail an invading pathogen . . . . Whatever their
assigned tasks, the genes that scientists have designated oncogenes
share a common characteristic: they are vulnerable to mutations.
And once mutated, the genes contribute to the birth of a

tumor . . . . , it's important to keep in mind that our cells possess oncogenes not because some nasty natural or supernatural force place them there to keep our population in check, but because the body requires the genes to grow." Angier, (4) at 5.

"An oncogene is a sequence of deoxyribonucleic acid (DNA) that has been altered or mutated from its original form, the proto-oncogene. Operating as a positive growth regulator, the proto-oncogene is involved in promoting the differentiation and proliferation of normal cells. A variety of proto-oncogenes are involved in different crucial steps of cell growth, and a change in the proto-oncogene's sequence or in the amount of protein it produces can interfere with its normal role in cellular regulation. Uncontrolled cell growth, or neoplastic transformation, can ensue, ultimately resulting in the formation of a cancerous tumor." Britannica (5) at 5. See excerpt in Cancer Medicine (15) for a more detailed summary.

It's somewhat like an eight year old boy playing baseball in the house, a normal activity performed in the wrong context where it can do substantial harm.

1.42 How Oncogenes are Categorized

We have identified a number of proto-oncogenes and oncogenes. The term oncogene derives from the Greek term onco, meaning mass, and cancer is a mass of abnormal tissue. Genes and oncogenes can first be identified by a specific location such as chromosome 17. Oncogenes are also given specific names, which are usually three letter abbreviations such as myc, erb, or P53. Sometimes a prefix will be added such as v, for virus, indicating that the oncogene is associated with a virus, or c, indicating that the oncogene is associated with a chromosome defect.

1.43 Two Types of Oncogenes: Growth and Tumor Suppressor Genes

At a basic level, two types of gene mutations combine to create a cancer. The first, is an abnormality of a gene involved with growth. An example is a gene that produces a protein that causes a growth-factor receptor on the cell's surface to be constantly on when in fact no growth factor is present. Thus the cell receives a constant message to divide.

The second type of gene which turns off the cell cycle and helps control cell growth is called a tumor suppressor gene. When the tumor suppressor gene malfunctions, the signal to the gene to stop duplicating is lost. Imagine a car. A car would travel when it wasn't supposed to if the accelerator was on (growth-factor gene) or if the brakes were not functioning, (tumor-suppressor gene):

> "To continue the analogy, ignition switches and accelerators (positive controls) start up the engines and get these processes moving, and brakes (negative controls) slow down or halt the processes when necessary. Like the cell cycle and apoptosis (cell death), the positive and negative controls comprise a series of modulations of protein activities through protein interactions and protein modifications." Griffiths (14)

Griffith's description gives us more insight into the carcinogenic process. It is not one growth gene and one tumor suppressor gene which combine to create cancer. Instead there are multiple growth genes, multiple tumor suppressor genes, and a system of cellular communication which malfunctions, part of which we understand and a part we do not. Targeting the particular offending gene to develop a cure, particularly with lung cancer, has been difficult.

1.44 How Do Cells Know When to Divide?

Cells divide or perform other functions in response to signals or stimuli from other cells. "Cells sense signals from both the outside environment and other cells and, in response, they regulate protein expression and function:

> "Although each cell carries an extraordinarily elaborate data bank in its genes, these genes cannot provide the cell with some very critical pieces of information. Genes cannot tell a cell where it is in the body, how it arrived there, or whether the body requires it to grow. Genes can only tell the cell how it should respond to

external signals, which must come from elsewhere—from other cells, nearby and distant. Each cell in the body relies on a host of other cells to tell it where it is, how it got there, and what it should be doing." Weinberg, (5) at 97

What types of signals does a cell receive:

"Signals can be a direct reaction to a stimulus, such as the secretion of insulin by pancreatic B cells in response to increases in blood glucose. Signal release can be triggered by the nervous system in response to either external or internal cues, as in the release of epinephrine by the adrenal glands in response to stress. Signals can also be continuous, such as those sent by the extracellular matrix. Usually, signaling molecules are stored in the cells and are released to provide communications with other cells under specific conditions." Devita (12)

Communication at the cellular level is called signal transduction. Cancer is really a signal transduction disease, in the sense that signals to replicate and perform other functions go awry, and cells are prompted to improperly replicate:

"The cell cycle is a highly ordered sequence of events that leads to cell growth and division. In normal cells, signaling pathways that detect signals from the cell exterior or interior tightly control the progression through the cell division cycle by regulating the activity of cell cycle control genes. In cancer cells, the deregulation of these signaling pathways or control genes can cause cells that are not dividing to enter the cell cycle and to begin to proliferate, leading to tumor formation." Osip (16)

1.5 GROWTH FACTORS AND RECEPTORS

1.51 A More Sophisticated Model of Cancer Development

The simplest model of cancer is a proto-oncogene creating growth, and a tumor-suppressor gene failing to stop it. Were cancer creation that simple, scientists might be able to isolate either gene and develop a vaccine or treatment. Indeed, scientists have come close to identifying the source of some simple cancers such as particular forms of leukemia and certain childhood tumors.

Unfortunately with lung cancer, the model is more complex, with an interrelationship of many different cells signaling one another; part of which we do not fully understand. "Our current state of knowledge of tumor suppressors shows a picture of complex interactions between multiple suppressor genes with oncogenes to generate the malignant state." Devita (12)

As an analogy, consider juvenile crime. We know that lack of education, family instability, educational difficulties, and gang affiliation are all connected with crime. However, we do not fully understand the relationship between each component in terms of causation, which factor is most important, which causes which, and where intervention would be most successful. There are many parts to cancer, particularly lung cancer, which has made the task of inhibiting cell duplication difficult. (In comparison, with a few tumors, we have been able to isolate the cancer-causing gene). Even today with 40 years of research, the most effective treatment for lung cancer is simply removal of the tumor in its early stages, a treatment which has been known for at least the last 50 years.

1.52 Growth Factors and Receptors

Another model of replication is the growth factor and receptor. A growth factor connects with a receptor on a cell to start a process of cell reproduction, something like putting a screw in a nut. Newer forms of cancer gene therapy seek to interfere with this process. The epidermal growth factor connects with its receptor as part of the lung cancer process. The new drug Iressa is an epidermal growth factor receptor inhibitor. That is, it attempts to prevent the epidermal growth factor from coming in contact with its receptor. Interestingly, the drug seems to have success with some patients but not with others. Thus, there appear to be different characteristics of lung cancers and perhaps different pathways among patients with the same disease. "Several signaling pathways" appear to be affected by the epidermal growth factor. Welch (13)

1.6 HOW GENES ARE DAMAGED AND BECOME ONCOGENES

1.61 Types of DNA Damage

A normal gene can be damaged in a variety of ways. Part of the gene can be lost (deletion), or a gene could be rearranged and ends up in the incorrect location (translocation). A gene may initially be defective or an outside product can cause damage. For some diseases, we can identify the genes which are damaged:

> "In Burkitt lymphoma, a malignancy of immature B cells, one characteristic feature is a chromosomal translocation about 80% of the time, a translocation between the long arms of chromosomes 8 and 14 are involved; less frequently, a translocation between the long arms of chromosomes 8 and 2 or chromosomes 8 and 22. All three translocations found in Burkitt lymphoma involve a specific position on chromosome 8 (8q24) that is occupied by the cellular proto-oncogene/oncogene, c-myc." Cancergenetics (8).

1.62 How Throat Cancer Occurs

Let us look at a model explaining the development of throat cancer:

> "Repeated exposures of high concentrations of alcohol were known to kill many of the cells lining the mouth and throat. The surviving cells in the tissues lining these cavities would then receive orders to grow and divide to replace their fallen comrades. These repeated rounds of growth and division would yield mutations in the DNA of these cells. Moreover, it seemed that DNA in the midst of replication was even more susceptible to damage from mutagens than DNA from nonproliferating cells. This explained why cigarette smoke, which contains dozens of different mutagens, and alcohol, which promotes cell proliferation, were a deadly combination. When used together, they generated as much as thirtyfold increase in risk of mouth and throat cancer." Weinberg, (6) at 59

1.63 Cancer Generally Involves Multiple Incidents of DNA Damage

While one instance of damage to the cell will usually not impair its form or function, the cell can be destabilized such that it becomes more susceptible to future damage. This is termed "genetic instability".

For example, the inactivation of certain DNA repair genes, may allow the buildup of genetic mistakes with each succeeding round of cell division. Inactivation of a tumor suppressor, may allow propagation of an occasional DNA copying mistake to the next cell division. Each event builds on itself.

1.64 Apoptosis

The body has a inherent protection against the development of cancer—apoptosis, or programmed cell death. Certain cells detect abnormalities and trigger cell death. This carefully regulated system prevents many cells with abnormalities from developing or dividing.

1.65 Time for Cancer to Develop

Since cancer requires the abnormal development of a growth factor, probably multiple defects in tumor suppressor genes, and the failure of the apoptosis system of cell death, we can surmise that cancer would take years if not decades to develop. Cancer increases with age, and most tumors are associated with a series of changes that occur over a period of 10 to 15 years or even longer.

1.66 Initiation Promotion Hypothesis

Many scientists see cancer development in different stages:

"The initiation stage is characterized by the conversion of a normal cell to an initiated cell in response to DNA damaging agents (genetic damage indicated by an X). The promotion stage is characterized by the transformation of an initiated cell into a population of preneoplastic cells, a result of alterations in gene expression and cell proliferation. The progression stage involves the transformation of the preneoplastic cells to a neoplastic cell population as a result of additional genetic alterations." Greenwald (13)

Greenwald suggests we stop seeing cancer as a defined event, for example the diagnosis of cancer. Instead, we would look to identify genetic damage and attempt to cure or correct it before it develops into a tumor. Some scientists call this chemoprevention using biomarkers to tell us which genes or cells have been damaged. "Acceptable biomarkers for cancer must be reliable (repeatable), highly sensitive and specific, quantitative, readily obtained by non-invasive methods, part of the causal pathway for disease, capable of being modulated by the chemopreventive agent, and have high predictive value for clinical disease." Greenwald (13). With the concept of biomarkers, we could identify damage in a smoker before a tumor has developed. Accepting the concept of biomarkers has been much easier than reaching agreement on a specific biomarker. Researchers in clinical trials are now taking various measurements to determine what changes confirm or presage the development and spread of disease.

1.7 HOW CANCER SPREADS

There are two basic ways that cancers metastasize, that is spread to other organs. The most common route is by channels that exist in every part of the body called lymph channels. Lymph channels are a fine network of vessels that carry the liquid portion of the blood from different parts of the body. Returning to the bloodstream, the lymph is filtered through lymph nodes and returns to a large lymph vessel near the heart. Given the flow of lymph to and from the lymph nodes, we can understand why the finding of cancerous cells in the lymph nodes will be critical. If the tumor has moved to a lymph node, its potential for dissemination throughout the body increases. A tumor which is detected and removed before a lymph node becomes cancerous has a far better prognosis than one which has infiltrated a nearby lymph node.

1.71 Regional and Other Lymph Nodes

In staging the patient, that is ascertaining his status, doctors consider whether the lymph nodes are cancerous, and where the cancerous nodes are located. The spread of a tumor to a lymph node located near the tumor, or a regional node, is less serious than the spread to one further away, indicating a greater spread of the tumor. A surgeon will generally obtain samples or biopsies from lymph nodes to ascertain the status of lymph nodes, and treatment will depend upon that assessment.

1.72 Blood Vessels

A tumor may also spread through the body through a blood vessel. There are various tests to ascertain the extent of cancer in the blood, however, blood vessels cannot be individually assessed as lymph nodes usually are.

REFERENCES

Following the format of many scientific journals, each reference is given a number. Most of the articles cited can be located in a medical library. Almost all the articles have abstracts, a short summary identifying the study's findings and conclusions, and these abstracts can be reviewed online on Medline.

Medline is the worldwide medical library compiled by the National Library of Science, a part of the National Institute of Health. A National Library of Medicine's search service provides access to over 10 million citations in Medline, PreMedline, and other related databases. For most journals, there is a charge to obtain the entire text, usually 10-15$ per article.

1. Vile, *Cancer Metastasis: From Mechanisms to Therapies* (Wiley & Sons 1995).
2. Coleman, *Understanding Cancer* (Johns Hopkins Press 1998).
3. Dermer, *The Immortal Cell* 46-47 (Avery Pub. Co. 1994).
4. Angier, *Natural Obsessions* 5 (Mariner Books 1999). www brittanica.com. (Cell Division and Growth).
5. Weinberg, *One Renegade Cell* (1998).
6. Lau, *Clinical and Molecular Prognostic Factors and Models for Non-Small cell Lung Cancer*, in Pass. Lung Cancer 604 (2001). www.cancergenetics.org. www.Brittainica.com (Cytokines). Brittanica online provides detailed but understanding information

for the general public on a number of specialized topics and is a good beginning for much research. www.growth-factor.net.

7. Greenwald, *Science, Medicine, and the Future, Cancer Chemoprevention*, BMJ 2002;324:714-718.

8. Devita, *Cancer, Principles and Practice of Oncology* (Lippincott, 2001).

9. Welch, *Erb B Expression and Drug Resistance in Cancer*, Signal, vol. 3, iss 3 (2002).

10. Griffith, *Modern Genetic Analysis* (1999).

CHAPTER 2

CANCER TERMINOLOGY

2.1 TREATMENT TERMINOLOGY

2.11 Primary Site

The organ where the cancer originates is called the primary site. Cancers retain characteristics based upon where they originate. Thus, a cancer which originated in the lung but metastasized to the breast would still be characterized and treated as a lung cancer. A lung tumor which metastasized to the bone would be called a lung cancer with metastasis, not bone cancer.

2.2 RESPONSES TO TREATMENT

Clinical trials measure a drug's impact in a number of ways to obtain information about the disease and its interaction with the drug. When you review the results of a clinical trial, you can usually check complete response, partial responses, and disease stabilization or time of disease progression.

2.21 Complete Response

Complete response is the elimination of any evidence of cancer, as seen from a particular test, such as an X-ray or CT Scan. A complete response is unfortunately not always a cure. There may be microscopic cancerous cells which cannot be detected by the Ct Scan or x-ray and cancer can reappear. Nonetheless the percentage of complete responses is an important indicator of the effectiveness of a treatment.

2.22 Partial Response

Partial response, as used by most authorities means a 50% reduction in the size of the tumor. Scientists differ as to whether partial or complete responses are more important. Drug A may generate a larger number of partial responses but fewer complete ones than drug B. Exactly what should be the appropriate measurement continues to be an area for debate.

2.23 Disease Stabilization

Besides responses, scientists are increasingly examining the concept of disease stabilization. That is, a drug is successful in preventing spread of a tumor even though it does not effect a reduction in tumor size. Some of the newer methods of gene therapy seem to be most successful at disease stabilization.

The opposite of disease stabilization is disease progression, or time to progression which can also be measured. See 11 (arguing that time to disease progression is the most important indicator of a drug's effectiveness).

2.24 Cellular Measurements

While disease response is the most obvious measurement of a drug's effectiveness, there are others. Scientists may wish to measure levels of different proteins and see if a drug is having an effect in that way. For example, if we have a drug which targets the epidermal growth factor associated with lung cancer, we could test levels before and after the drug was used. Sometimes, levels may be reduced, but that does not translate into improved survival. In that event, we try to determine whether the protein tested was really that important, whether reduction in protein levels are only important at certain stages of disease, or whether the reduction did not reach the level to impact survival. The difficulty with lung cancer is that there are many proteins and receptors involved with the disease and it is difficult to assess the relative importance of each. Sometimes we call these measurements endpoints.

2.25 Side Effects

Studies will also identify and classify side effects. Chemotherapy attacks dividing cells, so normal as well as cancerous cells can be affected. Scientists may refer to the number or extent of side effects as "tolerable". While the side effects could be significant, they were not life-threatening nor substantially interfered with body functioning, side effects are generally measured objectively in clinical trials.

Quality of life can be viewed subjectively, comprising various perceptions of pain and discomfort, or objectively. Even though treatments may cause side effects, their impact can be less than the disease itself, with many studies reporting higher quality of life with treatment. Sometimes the purpose of treatment is to improve quality of life. Where treatment is given primarily to relieve pain or improve quality of life, it is called palliative treatment.

2.26 Maximum Tolerated Dose

How do you provide the maximum strength dose of a drug to attack a tumor yet prevent intolerable side effects? Scientists will determine a maximum tolerated dose through clinical trials. That is, what is the maximum amount that can be administered without intolerable side effects.

A similar concept is the maximum effective dose. Most chemotherapy drugs increase in effectiveness with the amount of the dose. In essence, there is no maximum effective dose, the drug's effectiveness increases with dose with only side effects limiting how much can be prescribed. Other drugs may have limits and reach a plateau of effectiveness.

This plateau can be helpful in constructing a cure. Imagine that drug A shows some success in stabilizing disease at a maximum effective dose of 750 milligrams per day with minor side effects. We could combine the drug with another drug and increase our cancer-fighting power without creating substantial side effects.

In clinical trials, the researcher attempts to determine the effectiveness of new drugs and determine their maximum effective doses. The oncologist does something similar, measuring patient response and side effects to provide maximum fighting power without unacceptable side effects.

2.3 MEASUREMENTS OF MORTALITY

2.31 Five Year Survival

Survival is generally measured in years, with five year survival being the most common measurement. For patients with advanced disease, one year survival may be a benchmark, with seriously ill patients sometimes evaluated as to months of post-treatment survival.

2.32 Overall and Disease-Specific Mortality

Scientists keep track of mortality in two ways. First, they determine how many patients were lost from a disease or its consequences. Secondly, they may look at overall mortality, the number of patients who died regardless of cause. At first glance, we might be interested only in disease-specific mortality; after all, the fact that some patients may die of other causes would appear irrelevant.

However, overall mortality can present some tough questions. For example, in a clinical trial, one group receives a new form of chemotherapy, while the other receives the standard treatment. Assume that the group receiving the new treatment has a higher partial response rate, (patients whose tumors are reduced by at least half). However, the treatment group also has a higher overall mortality rate. It may be chance or the new treatment may be impacting other organs in some way. However, the drug would probably not receive FDA approval if its use involved an increased overall mortality.

This illustrates one problem cancer researchers face. The results are not always logical or predictable and may vary based on chance, characteristics of the study group, or unknown factors.

2.4 TYPES OF CANCERS

The most common type of cancer is a carcinoma, a cancer that arises in the cells that form the lining of different parts of the body. Cancers in the lung, breast, prostate, and colon are all carcinomas. Cancers that involve tissue or bone are called sarcomas. Cancers involving blood cells are known as lymphomas or leukemias.

2.41 Treatment

The FDA approves drugs by organ, such as a drug for treatment of lung cancer. While most research is organ specific, studies can cross organ lines. New drugs may be tested on different solid tumors such as breast, colon, and lung, and the drugs may ultimately be used for more than one organ. The results will still be categorized by organ.

2.42 Endpoints for Approval

The FDA issues an approval finding that a drug serves a specific need. In the past, that usually meant the drug provided a higher rate of cure than existing drugs. Today, scientists realize that standard can be too demanding or restrictive, and use a variety of endpoints to evaluate a drug. Thus, if drug B provides fewer side effects than existing treatments, it can be approved. Scientists are struggling to determine whether approvals should be granted if tumor size is diminished or stabilized, or other impact shown, when the effect upon survival is unclear.

2.43 Off-Label Prescriptions

The FDA provides an approval for a specific use, for example, second line chemotherapy for stage 4 patients. Many physicians will restrict the use of the drug to that purpose but, on occasion, a doctor will prescribe a drug, off-label, that is for another use. That is permitted, but if untoward results occur, a doctor could face liability, since some would argue the standard of care is set forth in the FDA approval.

2.5 EPIDEMIOLOGY

Epidemiology comes from the root epidemic, and is the study of patterns of disease. An epidemiologist would investigate what groups contract lung cancer, and make conclusions based upon these patterns. For example, epidemiologists noticed that people who smoked and people who worked with asbestos had substantially higher rates of lung cancer.

2.51 Determining What are Significant Findings

What changes are sufficiently significant that we can attribute causation? Some changes are simply due to chance or differences between groups studied. Assume a study where we study the impact of wives telling their husbands to have a good day on overall health. There are 100 people in each group, one group receiving the greeting and one not and assume that in the group getting the greeting 6 people contract heart disease, while in the group without the greeting 5 do. It would be incorrect to say that the greeting caused heart disease even though there is a slightly increased incidence in the study group.

2.52 The 2-1 Guide in Ascribing Causation or Connection

Some scientists use a 2-1 ratio as a guide to attribute causation. If while investigating a new drug, we find that twice as many people using the drug had complete responses, we can say the drug had an impact. In a trial the group receiving the treatment is called the study group while the group receiving standard treatment is called the control group.

2.53 Determining the Impact of a New Drug

What studies are important and should be given weight? Here are some of the considerations researchers use:

1. **The extent of the difference between the study group and control group.** The greater the difference between the two groups, the more likely the drug is having an impact, and contrariwise, small differences can be attributed to chance.

2. **Whether a dose relationship is identified.** Assume we are testing a new drug. If response rates increase with the amount of the drug given, that indicates the drug is causing the response. However, if response rates do not depend on dose, it may be that other factors are at work. For example, with cigarettes, scientists found that the rate of disease increases with the number of cigarettes smoked, which indicates a causal connection.

3. **Study Group Size** A study with positive findings involving 500 people will be given more weight than one with 20.

4. **Ability to Duplicate Findings in Other Studies.** Drugs generally need to proceed through a number of clinical trials before they are FDA approved. In 1997, a scientist reported that more than half of rats experience a complete elimination of tumors using a new form of treatment. Newspapers reported a new cure. However, when the findings could not be replicated, the weight of the initial report was reduced, and when positive findings were not made in clinical trials, the drug was not FDA approved.

5. **Biological Plausibility** Does the theory make sense and accord with the medical knowledge we have? Note that this can require some detailed medical knowledge. Some complex theories put forth on the Internet may be based on faulty science which would not be apparent to a non-scientist.

6. **Cell Studies and Animal Studies** While no treatment can be FDA approved based simply upon laboratory studies, they can support, undermine, or help explain findings in clinical trials.

2.54 Medline Searches for the Effectiveness of New Drugs.

Assume you read of a new drug and wanted to evaluate its effectiveness. Unfortunately, many news articles are misleading, and may trumpet a new drug though its only effectiveness was shown in a single cell study. With the Internet, many patients and family members are becoming their own researchers.

Using search terms associated with the new drug, you would first go on the Medline database, medscape.com and other portals. You would review cell studies, animal studies, and human clinical trials using the criteria set forth above. Are there human clinical trials showing a substantial impact, mile one? Do cell and animal studies display a significant relationship? You can assemble the published results of studies and, using these criteria, try to make an intelligent determination.

2.55 Applying the Research, How to Measure the Success of New Drugs

With tools like Medline and a basic understanding of cancer research, we can take a first step toward evaluating new drugs. Newspaper and magazine reports can be misleading and company self-reporting can be equally unreliable. The astute patient or family member will want to go to medical journals themselves. Here are some basic standards:

Criteria	Relevant Factors			
Response to the Drug	Percentage of Complete Responses	Percentage of Partial Responses	Mortality Rate and/or Disease Stabilization	Other Endpoints, Growth factor or receptor measurements.
Evaluating the Study	Study Size	Consistency with Other Studies Dose response relationship	Results of Prior Cell and Animal Studies	Biological Plausibility and Studies with Other Tumor types
Side Effects and other Results	Percentage and Type of Side effects	Incidence compared to Placebo or Control Group		

2.6 FORMS OF TREATMENT

The four basic forms of treatment for lung cancer are surgery, chemotherapy, radiation, and gene therapy. Surgery is the ideal treatment with the goal to remove the tumor and surrounding tissue which is or may be cancerous. It is essentially the only treatment that can be completely curative, with survival rates for stage 1 patients in the 65-75% range. Less frequently, surgery is used to remove a significant part, but not all of a tumor.

Radiation is a method of targeting cancer cells in a particular area and using a beam to create a complex process of cell death. In patients with advanced disease, radiation can reduce the tumor and related pain and discomfort, palliative treatment. For advanced cancer patients, radiation is not designed to be a cure. For early stage patients who are ineligible for surgery, radiation is sometimes used with the goal of eradicating smaller tumors.

Chemotherapy is the use of different drugs to fight cancer. The drugs are injected into the blood stream and inhibit the division of cells throughout the body. That is why chemotherapy has side effects, some normal functions are associated with cell division such as hair growth.

Gene therapy is the attempt to identify specific genes which contribute to tumor formation or spread and use specific drugs to target them. A monoclonal antibody, is the use of a specific drug targeted to a single (monoclonal) antibody. The goal of therapies like monoclonal antibodies is to target specific proteins involved in the cell-duplication process, short-circuit the protein, and thereby inhibit the cancer process without affecting normal cells. The difficulty is not only developing an antibody which can successfully come in contact with specific proteins, but determining which proteins are most important in the cancer process.

2.7 THE NATURE OF CANCER EXPERIMENTATION AND TREATMENT

2.71 How Cancer Treatments are Developed

The development of cures or partial cures for cancer involves these steps:

1. Test the new agent in a laboratory on cancer cells, in vitro testing,
2. Evaluate the test on animals,
3. Perform initial tests to see if the new drug is tolerated by humans, define the appropriate dose, (Phase 1 Clinical Trial)
4. Compare the new drug with existing treatment to determine if the new treatment achieves best results, (Phase 3 Clinical Trial)
5. Determine whether the new drug should be combined with other existing forms of treatment to achieve optimum efficiency, evaluate the new drug in different contexts.

2.72 Do Treatments Arise by Design?

Treatments can be developed deliberately or inadvertently. Scientists may notice the positive effect of a particular cell characteristic or interaction, and go about creating a cure based upon its characteristics.

Treatments may be accidental. In the early 60's, some babies were born with birth defects after their mothers took thalidomide, which inhibited the development of new cells and sources of blood supply, necessary for fetal development. To prevent metastasis, the spread of cancer, it is useful to curtail the creation of new sources of blood supply for the tumor. Thus, scientists are investigating the use of thalidomide for patients with advanced cancer.

2.73 In-Vitro Testing

The first step is to test a proposed new cure on cells in a laboratory. "Cell culture is complicated by the tendency of isolated cells to "dedifferentiate" in culture, taking on the qualities of unspecialized cells instead of keeping the characteristics that define them as cells from a specific organ such as the liver." Johns Hopkins Center (1)

Not only may cells behave differently in a laboratory, the endpoints are different. One cannot test a drug to see if it effects a cure, the scientist must use a surrogate measurement such as levels of cell death or division, and postulate that this will translate into positive treatment results in humans. Thus, results from cell culture studies are only a first step, and given only limited weight.

2.74 Animal Studies

After a treatment has shown promise in cell culture studies, it will face evaluation in animal studies. To the extent possible, the scientist will try to create a similar dose and treatment context. Ethical questions arise as we become increasingly aware of animal suffering. As with cell culture, no drug will be approved based simply upon positive results with animals.

2.75 Human Clinical Trials

A new drug will be tested in three phases of clinical trials on humans. In stage 1, the drug will be tested principally to define its optimum dose. Thus patients could be given a new treatment in three doses with the trial attempting to determine which achieves maximum effectiveness without significant side effects. Placebos are rarely given in cancer clinical trials since the testing is objective, what does a CT Scan show about tumor spread, rather than a person's perception. In stage 2, using the optimal dose, scientists will begin taking careful measures of partial and complete response, side effects, and other data to ascertain if the drug is showing sufficient promise to merit FDA approval. In stage 3 after the drug has been determined to be effective, it is tested against the conventional treatment used today.

REFERENCES

1. Zurlo, *Animal and Alternatives in Testing: History, Science and Ethics*, Johns Hopkins Center for Alternatives to Animal Testing.
2. Astra-Zeneca, (manufacturers of Iressa), EGFR-Info.com. *The ErbB Family of Receptors and Their Ligands, Multiple Targets for Therapy*, Signal, Volume 2, Issue 3, 4-11. Signal is a new journal, available online, and focusing on epidermal growth factor treatments and related research.
4. Herbst, *Angiogenesis Inhibitors in Clinical Development for Lung Cancer*, Seminars in Oncology, Vol. 29, No. 1 Supp 4 February 2002: pp. 66-5. Giatromanolaki, *Non-small cell lung cancer: C-erbB-2 Overexpression Correlates with Low Angiogenesis and Poor Prognosis*.
6. M.D.Anderson Medical Center website.
7. Neufeld, *Vascular endothelial growth factor (VEGF) and its receptors*, The FASEB Journal. 1999;13:9-22).
8. Santos, *Enhanced Expression of Vascular Endothelial Growth Factor in Pulmonary Arteries of Smokers and Patients with Moderate Chronic Obstructive Pulmonary Disease*, American Journal of Respiratory and Critical Care Medicine Vol 167. pp. 1250-1256, (2003).
9. Xenia, *Complete Inhibition of Vascular Endothelial Growth Factor (VEGF) Activities with a Bifunctional Diabody Directed against*

Both VEGF Kinase Receptors, fms-like Tyrosine Kinase Receptor and Kinase Insert Domain-containing Receptor, Cancer Research 61, 7002-7008, October 1, 10. 2001.www.targetvegf.com.

11. www.fda.gov/cder/drug/cancer_endpoints/miller/sld033.htm.

12. Holland, Cancer Medicine, (1999), available online at no charge from the National Library of Medicine,http://www.ncbi.nlm.nih.gov.

13. Vasella, *Magic Cancer Bullet, How a Tiny Orange Pill is Rewriting Medical History* (2003).

14. Omitted

15. Heinrich, Cancer Medicine, (2003), available online at www.ncbi.nlm.nih.gov.

16. Robinson, *The Protein Tyrosine Kinase Family of the Human Genome, Oncogene* (2000) 19, 5548-5557.

CHAPTER 3

CHROMOSOMES, GENES, AND CELLS

3.1 CHROMOSOMES AND GENES

Many patients or family members will read about gene therapy and advances in cancer research. New gene therapies target a specific part of the cancer cell or tumor process hoping to have limited impact upon normal cells. A basic knowledge of genes and chromosomes are will help you understand these developments and how they can be important to you.

3.11 DNA and Chromosomes

In the nucleus of our cells is a molecule called DNA (deoxyribonucleic acid). Think of DNA as the brain of these cells. This DNA is arranged in 46 sections called chromosomes, with 23 chromosomes from the father and 23 from the mother.

3.12 Genes

These 46 chromosomes contain approximately 100,000 different genes. Genes determine a person's sex, height, hair color, and virtually every fact about our lives. Genes also manufacture proteins which help us grow and perform other functions. Genes provide signals to other genes to grow, duplicate, die, or signal other genes.

3.121 Two Copies of Most Genes

We have two copies of most genes and a defect in one of the two will generally not cause serious problems. For example, defects in both P-53 tumor suppressor genes are generally associated with cancer. This may be one reason why cancer is a slow process, sometimes dating from 20 years from date of exposure to a carcinogen (cancer-causing agent). At least two mutations are probably needed to alter a single gene, and a number of genes must be altered to create a tumor.

3.13 Chromosome and Gene Location

Think of the chromosome as an X shape. The top part of the X is called p, and the bottom part of the X is called q. Each section of chromosome is also numbered, say from 1-32, going from the centre out, so if you see a gene (or a genetic alteration) as being located at 3p32, that means the top part of chromosome 3 at the very end.

3.14 Types of Chromosome Damage

Cancer involves abnormalities in genes on certain chromosomes. Exposure to toxic substances such as cigarettes can alter our genes and chromosomes. The combination of damage to a number of chromosomes can cause cancer.

Scientists classify the chromosome damage into different types. We have deletions (where some of the chromosome is missing), translocation (where parts of 2 different chromosomes exchange places) and amplifications (where some of the chromosome is amplified). Knowing the specific type of abnormality helps us to identify specifics about a tumor, and to refine our treatment. Here is an illustration of a normal and abnormal adult:

46,XX	Normal female karyotype
46,XY	Normal male karyotype
47,XX,+18	Female karyotype with 47 chromosomes, the additional chromosome being a No. 18
45,XY,–14,– 22, +t(q21.1;21q1 1.1)	A male karyotype with 45 chromosomes with one chromosome comprised of a No.14 translocated (with a breakpoint on the long arm at position q21.1) and fused to a No. 21 (with its breakpoint on the long arm at position q11.1)

3.15 Where Do Damage Causing Lung Tumors Occur?

In the last 15 years, scientists have done much to identify the type and location of gene damage which causes lung cancer.

3.151 Loss of 3P

"Loss of function at 3p has been identified in 75% of non-small cell lung cancer cases. 3p21 in particular is identified. 3p damage appears to be more closely associated with squamous cell cancer." Pass (8) at 509. However, 3p damage occurs in a number of tumors. Pass concludes, "loss of 3p may represent an important generalized tumorrigenic event common to various solid tumors, including NSCLC. Cancers have some common features in terms of development. Scientists have also identified damage at 9p and 17p." Pass (8) at 509.

3.16 Application to Screening

In the future, physicians may perform gene testing to identify early damage to genes, warn smokers of specific damage caused by smoking and detect lung cancer when it is most treatable.

3.2 GENES

3.21 Genes and The Production of Proteins

"Through a number of biochemical steps, each gene tells a cell to make a different protein. Some genes instruct the cell to manufacture structural proteins, which serve as building blocks. Other genes tell the cell to produce hormones, growth factors or cytokins, which exit the cell and communicate with other cells. Still other genes tell the cell to produce regulatory proteins that control the function of other proteins or tell other genes when to turn "on" or "off.""

There is a complex and multi-faceted relationship among genes, with genes signaling and receiving signals, regulating growth, and replicating. Each of these genes is a potential target for cancer research. Clinical trials can help reveal the importance of a particular gene in the cancer process.

3.3 CELL CYCLE

3.31 Why We Need to Understand Cell Cycles

Understanding how and why cells proceed from one stage to another has been a major goal of cell cycle investigation and cancer research overall. If we could stop cancer cells at a specific stage, we could provide a cure or at least a hindrance. Some anti-cancer drugs are directed to specific points in the cell cycle. Understanding cell cycles helps you understand how these drugs work. Some simple cancers have been cured by identifying a specific factor which is influencing the cell's behavior, and creating something, perhaps an antibody, to address it. Unfortunately, lung cancer involves a large group of different factors, and isolating the critical or most potent one has been difficult.

3.32 Phases of the Cell Cycle

The cell cycle process is divided into 4 broad phases: G1 or Gap 1, S or Synthesis, G2 or Gap 2, and M or Mitosis, cell division. The cell progresses to division this way: Gap 1 ± G 2 ± S ± M.

"During progression through the phases of the cell cycle (G_1, S [DNA synthesis], G_2, M [mitosis]), DNA is duplicated and the chromosome sets are distributed evenly over the two daughter cells. To ensure accuracy of the cell-cycle progression, cells need to go through several pauses or "checkpoints". At the checkpoint in late G_1, the cell either exits to G_0 and becomes quiescent or commits to the cell cycle. The G_2 checkpoint allows the cell to repair DNA damage before entering mitosis. Cell-cycle progression is regulated by cyclin-dependent kinases (cdks)."

3.33 Cell Cycle Regulation, Transition and Checkpoints

Growth and replication are carefully regulated:

"The army of protein machines that executes the events of the cell cycle is under the strict control of a regulatory network called the cell-cycle control system. This control system turns the cell-cycle machinery on and off at the appropriate times, and also responds to a variety of intra—and extracellular information to ensure that cell-cycle events are orchestrated perfectly under a variety of conditions. The primary functions of the cell-cycle control system are to trigger cell-cycle events at the appropriate time, in the correct order, and only once per cell cycle." Morgan (16).

"In multicellular organisms, precise control of the cell-cycle during development and growth is critical for determining the size and shape of each tissue. Cell replication is controlled by a complex network of signaling pathways that integrate extracellular signals about the identity and numbers of neighboring cells and intracellular cues about cell size and developmental program." Lodish (14)

If a cell is defective, it may not pass through the cell cycle process. We have checkpoints where defects are monitored and signals sent to stop transition:

"When the cell-cycle control system receives an inhibitory signal such as that generated by an incomplete cell-cycle process, it blocks the cell-cycle at transitions known as checkpoints. There are three major checkpoints. The first is at Start (often called the G1/S checkpoint), where entry into the cell cycle is blocked when cell growth or environmental conditions are inappropriate for continued division. The second major checkpoint is found at the entry into mitosis (G2/M checkpoint), where cell-cycle arrest occurs if DNA replication is incomplete or if the DNA is damaged. The third major checkpoint is the metaphase-to-anaphase transition (mitotic exit or the M/G1 checkpoint), where cell-cycle progression can be arrested if chromosomes are not attached correctly to the mitotic spindle." Morgan (16).

The human body has a number of safeguards to prevent replication of defective cells. We have a system of identifying cellular defects, repairing them, and providing for delayed transition. One hallmark of cancer is a defect in cell repair.

3.34 Apoptosis

"If damage is irreparable, the body then provides signals for cell death, called apoptosis." Cancer Genes (17). Cancer frequently involves defects in the system of cell death. One way this occurs is that anti-apoptotic genes are produced which stop or inhibit the normal process of apoptosis. Cancer represents several areas of damage or failure:

1. Damage to certain genes,
2. Failure of cell repair,
3. Failure to delay transition of damaged cells, and
4. Failure to institute apoptosis.

Cancer is the creation of unnecessary signals to duplicate, and the failure of the body's cell-cycle checkpoints. It's like a bank robbery where we not only need a criminal to do damage, but the failure of our guards and alarm system. It takes a number of gene abnormalities or system signaling failure to create a lung tumor. That is why the disease has a long latency, or time between first exposure and disease diagnosis, typically in the 20 year range. Some chemotherapy drugs induce apoptosis.

3.35 The Role of P-53

P-53 is a gene which monitors malfunctions at various checkpoints and performs critical functions in cell repair and apoptosis. A defect in P-53 is seen in many types of cancers, with about 50-60% of lung cancer patients having P-53 malfunctions.

"The p53 protein functions in the checkpoint control that arrests human cells with damaged DNA in G_1, and it contributes to arrest in G_2. Cells with functional p53 arrest in G_1 or G_2 when exposed to g-irradiation, whereas cells lacking functional p53 do not arrest in G_1. If defects are seen, cellular components can stop division during the cycle. P-53, a tumor suppressor gene detects DNA damage and delays entry into S until the damage is repaired, or causes cell death, called apoptosis." Lodish (14).

Restoring normal P-53 functions is a goal of cancer research.

3.36 Telomers

The body has an inherent protection against excessive duplication. Telomers are essentially counters that allow a certain number of cell replications and count down to zero, terminating cell replication at that point. Each time a cell replicates, it loses a little bit off the end till it can no longer replicate. That is probably one reason why we are not immortal; at some age we lose the ability to replicate cells, with telomers preventing unlimited duplication.

Nonetheless, in the body there are safeguards and means to get around these safeguards. For example, if an individual was severely burned, the body would need to extensively regenerate cells. Something called telomerase allows for additional regeneration of cells, essentially lengthening the ends of cells, so the cell can continue to replicate. Telomerase is seen in embryos and is produced in unusual situations where a number of replications are needed. Unfortunately it is produced in cancer. Some studies have found the existence of teleromerase in the body a sign of a serious carcinogenic process and unfavorable prognosis. Oncologists are looking at ways of inhibiting the production of Telomerase as a way of limiting cell reproduction. Some new drugs address this issue, but none has been FDA approved for lung cancer as of 2003.

3.4 RECEPTORS AND TYROSINE KINASES

Growth and cell duplication are normal bodily functions and as part of that process, cells provide signals to one another. Growth factors prompt other cells to divide and perform other functions:

> "{Highly specific proteins} are essential to the growth and repair of human tissues. Those that directly stimulate cell division are called growth factors . . . . Growth factors bind to receptors on a cell's surface thereby activating proliferation or differentiation. Some growth factors are highly specific in function and cell type while others are more broad spectrum."

3.41 Growth Factors and Receptors

A growth factor binds to a growth factor receptor like a lock and key.

"Growth factors {provide} signals to stimulate the proliferation of target cells. Appropriate target cells must possess a specific receptor in order to respond to a specific type of growth factor. A well-characterized example is platelet-derived growth factor (PDGF) . . . PDGF is released from platelets during the process of blood coagulation. PDGF stimulates the proliferation of fibroblasts, a cell growth process that plays an important role in wound healing. Other well-characterized examples of growth factors include nerve growth factor, epidermal growth factor, and fibroblast growth factor." Cancer Medicine (14)

Receptors are becoming the target of many of the new cancer drugs.

3.42 Structure of the Receptor

Most receptors including EGFR have two parts pertinent to treatment, a ligand binding domain and tyrosine kinase. The ligand binding domain is where the cell receives and processes a signal:

"The cellular response to a particular extracellular signaling molecule depends on its binding to a specific receptor protein located on the surface of a target cell or in its nucleus or cytosol. The signaling molecule (a hormone or growth factor) acts as a ligand which binds to, or "fits", a site on the receptor. Binding of a ligand to its receptor causes a conformational change in the receptor that initiates a sequence of reactions leading to a specific cellular response. The response of a cell is dictated by the receptors it possesses and by the intracellular reactions initiated by binding. Different cell types may have different sets of receptors for the same ligand, each of which induces a different response. Or the same receptor may occur on various cell types, and binding of the same ligand may trigger a different response in each type of cell." Lodish (25).

Once binding occurs, a signal is sent to the tyrosine kinase portion of the cell. There autophosphorylation, alteration of the structure of the protein, occurs. After phosphorylation, the changed residues then interacts with other proteins. It provides signals or interacts with other pathways which regulate cell proliferation, angiogenesis, apoptosis, and differentiation.

"The alteration of cells is critical: Many years ago it was realized that it was a very important process, and there were some clues as to why it was important for transformation. We knew that tyrosine phosphorylation is rare and tightly regulated in quiescent cells, but abundant in rapidly proliferating and transformed cells. We also knew that many transforming viruses encode tyrosine phosphoproteins. Of the over 100 dominant proto-oncogenes known to date, many encode protein tyrosine kinases. These can be hyperactivated by a number of mechanisms, including mutation, overexpression, structural rearrangements, and/or loss of normal regulatory constraints."

3.43 Importance for Treatment

New cancer drugs are directed to the receptor. Some drugs address the tyrosine kinase, trying to prevent phosphorylation while other attempt to prevent binding. For example, IMC 225, is an antibody that binds to the extra-cellular domain of the epidermal growth factor receptor attempting to prevent binding. In contrast, Iressa and Tarceva work at the tyrosine kinase level trying to inhibit phosphorylation.

Additionally patients seem to have different areas of genetic damage. Many patients with bronchoalveolar lung cancer have damage to the tyrosine kinase, and tyrosine kinase inhibitors seem to be particularly effective with them. In contrast, the drugs seem less effective with squamous cell patients most of who do not have damage in the tyrosine kinase. In the near future, we may be testing patients for specific genetic damage, and tailoring treatment to what we find.

3.5 COMPLEXITY OF GROWTH FACTORS AND RECEPTORS

There are many tyrosine kinase receptors in the human body performing various functions. We can identify two receptors associated with cancer, epidermal growth factor receptor (egfr), and vascular endothelial growth factor receptor (vegfr). (See chapter 2). These receptors are important targets for lung cancer research. VEGFR is associated with metastasis or angiogenesis, and how cancerous tissue spreads to other cells and organs.

3.51 Multiple Receptors and Growth Factors

At its simplest level, there would be a single growth factor and an associated receptor, i.e, egf and egfr. The process is more complex and one of the things that distinguishes us from simpler species is the complexity of our signaling network. EGFR is part of the Erb family which includes four receptors in which there are four: egfr or erb 1, erb 2, erb 3, and erb4. It appears receptors at erb1 and erb 2 can interact with the epidermal growth factor. Likewise, there are multiple growth factors that can interact with a receptor.

3.52 Treatment Barriers

The existence of multiple growth factors and multiple receptors shows the complexity of ordinary functioning and the cancer process. This makes developing a cure more difficult. Scientists are working on identifying which growth factors and receptors are most important and the mechanisms by which they are activated.

3.53 Upstream and Downstream Signaling

The basic model of growth factor combining with tumor suppressor (accelerator and brakes) has been supplanted with a model involving participation of many genes. Scientists now look at a gene and talk of upstream, to the gene, and downstream, by the gene. For example, let us look at a simplified model of VEGF: Growth factors ± production of VEGF ± production of blood vessels, other growth factors.

3.6 EPIDERMAL GROWTH FACTOR

There are specific growth factors and related tyrosine kinase receptors involved with lung cancer. One critical one is the epidermal growth factor or (EGF). Epidermal means skin and EGF is associated with the replenishment of skin cells and other cells. EGF is also a part of many cancers with higher levels of EGF shown in tumors. EGF binds to the epidermal growth factor receptor (EGFR).

3.61 Family of ERB Receptors

The epidermal growth factor receptor is called Erb1, and is part of a family of Erb receptors (3). We have Erb 1, 2, 3, and 4. Erb 2 is associated with breast cancer and the drug Herceptin is an Erb2 inhibitor. There is debate over the importance of each member of the Erb family, whether Erb 1 plays the most important role in lung cancer, and the role of Erb2. See Giatromanolaki (5). Signals are also exchanges within the Erb family, cross-talk, and to other growth actors and receptors.

Altering the path of the epidermal growth factor is one type of gene therapy showing significant promise. Scientists are grappling with the question of targeting the specific receptor, Erb1 which Iressa and Tarceva do, another receptor, or the entire Erb family of receptors. The ability of one member of the family, say Erb 1, to provide signals to another member, is called cross-talk. We review epidermal growth factor research in depth in our chapter on Iressa and epidermal growth factors.

3.7 VASCULAR ENDOTHELIAL GROWTH FACTOR

Metastasis is the chief evil of lung cancer, and patients die from distant metastasis rather than consequences in the lung itself. Angiogenesis, the formation of new capillaries, allowing the tumor to expand and infiltrate to nearby structures is essential to cancer growth:

> "By the mid-1980s, considerable experimental evidence had been assembled to support the hypothesis that tumor growth is angiogenesis dependent. The idea could now be stated in its simplest terms: "Once tumor take has occurred, every further increase in tumor cell population must be preceded by an increase in new capillaries which converge upon the tumor. The hypothesis predicted that if angiogenesis could be completely inhibited, tumors would become dormant at a small, possibly microscopic size." Cancer Medicine (12)

In the metastatic process, vascular endothelial growth factor (VEGF) plays a key role.

3.71 VEGF's Role in Developing Tissue

VEGF performs some important functions for normal development. Animals lacking VEGF will die because their cardio-vascular system does not properly develop, and embryos lacking correct VEGF genes have cells that do not properly develop." Neufeld (7) VEGF helps establish new sources of blood supply to damaged tissue. Unfortunately when the process goes awry, VEGF helps connect tumor tissue to adjoining areas and establish new blood vessels for the tumor. There are several types of anti-angiogenic drugs being investigated to inhibit VEGF." Herbst (4).

3.72 VEGF Receptors

Like the epidermal growth factor, VEGF has corresponding receptors.

"Vascular endothelial growth factor (VEGF) binds to and mediates its activity mainly through two tyrosine kinase receptors, VEGF receptor 1 and VEGF receptor 2 . . . The importance of VEGF and its receptors in tumor angiogenesis suggests that blockade of this pathway by antibody therapy would be an effective therapeutic strategy for inhibiting angiogenesis and tumor growth." Xenia (9)

"The VEGF ligand stimulates its functions through binding and activating VEGF-receptor (VEGFR)-1 and VEGFR-2, two membrane receptor tyrosine kinases that are predominantly expressed on endothelial cells within blood vessel walls. Binding of VEGF to these receptors initiates downstream signaling events leading to effects on gene expression, cell survival, proliferation, and migration." Vegf.com (10)

One way to address VEGF would be to prevent VEGF from connecting with one or both of the receptors.

3.73 The Difficulty in Developing a Cure, Multiple Growth Factors and Receptors

If there were a single growth or tumor suppressor gene, our task in developing a cancer cure might only be to identify that gene, and develop a virus or antidote which inhibited the growth factor or prevented it from connecting to its receptor. For example, scientists have isolated a particular gene involved with a particular form of leukemia and developed a therapy to correct that abnormality. See Magic Bullet (12).

With lung cancer our task is unfortunately far more complex. There are a large number of growth factors, receptors, tumor suppressor genes, signaling genes and other cellular products associated with the disease. Indeed, overall, we are beginning to recognize the complexities of cell interaction in the human body:

> "Although our knowledge of these intricate events is increasing at an exponential rate, the complexities appear to be growing even more rapidly. What were once believed to be rather simple and linear pathways have now become multidimensional. Signaling pathways converge, diverge, and cross-talk so frequently that it is becoming difficult to discuss them as individual pathways." Cancer Medicine (14)

In the lung cancer model, outside stimulus causes changes in gene A which prompts changes in growth factor B, which sends a message to receptor C, prompting a reaction in D, ultimately resulting in replication of a cell. We may be working with 10 or more gene components, with the significance of each difficult to ascertain.

Scientists have had some success in developing growth factor inhibitors, with the chances of cures growing as the science improves. The critical questions are essentially these:

1. Will the new drug frustrate the growth factor or growth factor?
2. How important is the growth factor to the cancer process?
3. Can we deliver the drug to the needed area(s) in sufficient amounts to make a large difference in the course of the disease?
4. Can we do (3) without causing substantial side effects? Or put another way,
5. If side effects can be limited, can we combine 1 or more drugs, to increase cancer-fighting ability without significant interference with ordinary bodily functions or side effects?

Chemotherapy drugs can affect different types of cells in the body leading to side effects. Since these growth factor drugs are more narrowly targeted, aiming only at certain growth factors and receptors, they hold the promise of limiting the spread of disease or even preventing its development, without creating significant side effects.

REFERENCES

1. Coleman, *Understanding Cancer* 30 (John Hopkins Press 1998).
2. Chromosome Deletion Outlook, http://members.aol.com/cdousa/intro.htm.
3. Weinberg, *One Renegade Cell* 132 (1998).
4. *The Cell Clock and Cancer*, Scientific American September, 1996, www. Sciam.com.
5. *Cyclin-dependent kinaseinhibitors*, www.cancerprev.org/meetings/2000/abstracts.
6. Coleman (1) at 30.
7. Pass, *Genomic Imbalances In Lung Cancer*, Lung Cancer, (2000).
8. www.inthouchlive.com/cancergenetics.
9. For those interested in a more detailed discussion of cell cycles, we offer the following:
   "A cell will often spend six to eight hours copying its DNA (the S phase) and three to four hours preparing for cell division (the G2 phase). Then begins the complex choreography of cell division, known as mitosis (the M phase), which takes only an hour. After division, the two newly formed daughter cells will take ten to twelve hours to prepare for the next round of DNA copying during the G1 phase. Alternatively, cells in G1 may choose to exist the active growth cycle entirely and enter into a quiescent, non-growing state (the G0 phase) in which they may remain for days, weeks, months, even years . . . . When provided with the proper signals, such sleeping cells will wake up and jump back into the active growth cycle." Weinberg, (3) at 132.

Gap or G1

In G1 or Gap 1, the cell synthesizes proteins which will enable it to grow. G1 represents growth and preparation for replication. P-53 will detect cellular irregularities in G1 and stop division.

G1 Restriction Point

Scientists have identified a specific point in G1 where it is determined whether division will continue called the restriction point or R. More, technically,

"For the cell to pass through R and enter S, a molecular switch must be flipped from off to on. The switch works as follows. As levels of cyclic D and, later cyclic E rise, these proteins combine with and activate enzymes called cyclic dependent kinases. The kinases, acting as part of cyclic-kinase complexes, grab phosphate groups from molecules of ATP and transfer them to a protein called pRB, the master brake of the cell cycle clock. When pRB lacks phosphate, it actively blocks cycling (and keeps the switch in the off position) by sequestering other proteins called transcription factors. But after the cyclic-kinase complexes add enough phosphate to pRB, the brake stops working, it releases the factors, freeing them to act on genes. The liberated factors then spur production of various proteins required for continued progression through the cell cycle." Cell Clock and Cancer (4)

Remember that not all cells will or should replicate. Thus, these brakes such as RB serve an important purpose in restricting cell division, and the failure of these brakes is one reason why cancer or unrestricted cell division occurs.

Iressa and G1

Iressa is a new and promising lung cancer drug which appears to inhibit the cell duplication process at G1. In cell culture studies, "Iressa induced a complete arrest of G1 phase growth after 72 hours of treatment." www.lef.org. While human studies have not demonstrated this type of result nor confirmed that Iressa's primary activity is in the G1 phase, the statement demonstrates why cell cycle research lies at the center of cancer research.

Phase 2, Synthesis

Phase 2 is called S or Synthesis. Here the cell replicates its DNA so it now has 2 complete sets of DNA. S phase genes contain a factor called SPF, S-phase promoting factor, which helps cells go from G1 to S.

Phase 3, G2

During the G2 phase, the cell again undergoes growth and protein syntheses to enable it to divide, creating sufficient protein for two cells.

G2 and Radiation

How does cancer radiation work? One text explains: Many cells exhibit a G2 arrest following exposure to DNA-damaging agents, including ionizing radiation such as drugs such as nitrogen mustard, cisplatinum and adiposity . . . . This arrest may serve a protective function, perhaps allowing cells to repair damage before progressing through the cell cycle.

Interphase Process

The G1, S and G2 phases of the cell cycle are sometimes collectively referred to as interphase.

Mitosis or Cell Division

Mitosis is the final stage where one cell actually becomes two. Mitosis itself may be divided into four stages. Here the DNA is replicated and the chromosomes split and divided into two daughter cells. The process is thus:

prophase— DNA has been replicated, chromosomes become visible and split . . . each chromosome is now a double set of DNA and consists of two chromatids,

metaphase— chromosomes move and line up near the middle of the cell,

anaphase— centromeres split and line up as the daughter sets up separate e chromosomes, telophase— cytoplasm divides, chromosomes distributed to each daughter cell, and the nucleus is reconstituted in each daughter cell. Intouch live (8)

10. Frijhoff, *Second Symposium of Novel Molecular Targets for Cancer Therapy*, The Oncologist, Vol. 7, Suppl 3, 1-3, August 2002.

11. Senderowicz, *Preclinical and Clinical Development of Cyclin-Dependent Kinase Modulators*, Journal of the National Cancer Institute, Vol. 92, No. 5, 376-387, March 1, 2000.

12. Elsayed, *Selected Novel Anticancer Treatments Targeting Cell Signaling Proteins*, The Oncologist, Vol. 6, No. 6, 517-537, December 2001. He explains, "Following mitogenic signals that promote entry into early G_1 phase, progression through the cell cycle is regulated by sequential activation of cell phase-specific cyclins and CDKs. Activation of CDK4 and CDK6 by cyclin D propels the cell through G_1 phase. Activated CDK2 is required for progression through the S phase into G_2 phase where CDK1/cyclin B complex then facilitates its passage into M phase. These steps are negatively regulated by endogenous cyclin-dependent kinase inhibitors."

13. Ryan, *On Receptor Inhibitors and Chemotherapy*, Clinical Cancer Research Vol. 6, 4607-4609, December 2000.

14. Lodish, *Molecular Cell Biology* (2000) (available online at no charge through medline) nlm.nlh.gov.

15. Lee, *Recombinant Adenoviruses Expressing Dominant Negative Insulin-like Growth Factor-I Receptor Demonstrate Antitumor Effects On Lung Cancer*, Cancer Gene Therapy January 2003, Volume 10, Number 1, Pages 57-63.

16. Morgan, *The Cell Cycle: Principles of Control* (New Science Press Ltd 2003).

17. Cancer Genes, www.bimcore.emory.edu/home/Kins/bimcoretutorials/sroper/P53head.htm "{The complex events of the cell cycle} are regulated by a small number of protein kinases. The concentrations of the regulatory subunits of these kinases, called cyclins increase and decrease in phase with the cell cycle. Their catalytic subunits are called cyclin-dependent kinases (Cdks) because they have no kinase activity unless they are associated with a cyclin. Each Cdk catalytic subunit can

associate with different cyclins, and the associated cyclin determines which proteins are phosphorylated by the Cdk-cyclin complex." Lodish (14).

18. Lubec, *Decrease of Heart Protein Kinase C and Cyclin-Dependent Kinase Precedes Death in Perinatal Asphyxia of the Rat*. FASEB J. 11, 482-492 (1997).

19. Carpenter, *Essentials of Signal Transduction*, in Cancer Principles and Practice of Oncology (2001).

20. Chantry, *The Kinase Domain and Membrane Localization Determine Intracellular Interactions between Epidermal Growth Factor Receptors*, JBC Online, Volume 270, Number 7, Issue of February 17, 1995 pp. 3068-3073. Articles in the Journal of BioChemistry are available online at no charge.

21. Miloso in an experiment found that alteration of the chemocial structure of egfr caused it to be produced even in the absence of egf. Miloso, *SHC and GRB-2 Are Constitutively Activated by an Epidermal Growth Factor Receptor with a Point Mutation in the Transmembrane Domain*, JBC online, Volume 270, Number 33, Issue of August 18, pp. 19557-19562, (1995).

22. Cadena, *Receptor Tyrosine Kinases*, The FASEB Journal, Vol 6, 2332-2337, (1992).

23. Wu, *Activator of the EGF Receptor Signaling Pathway in Human Airway Epethelial Cells Exposed to Metal*, Am J Physiol Lung Cell Mol Physiol 277: L924-L931, 1999.

24. Arteaga, *Role of the Receptor Tyrosine Kinase in Neoplastic Transformation* (Focus on HER Axis and VEGF, www.med scape.com.

25. Lodish, Mollecular Cell Biology (available online at medline).

CHAPTER 4

STRUCTURE OF THE LUNG AND LUNG CANCER CLASSIFICATION

4.1 LUNG ANATOMY

Discussion of lung anatomy can help us understand where tumors are located and how they spread.

4.10 The Trachea

The beginning of the airway leading to the lung is called the trachea or windpipe. The trachea is about four and a half inches long and divides into the right and left lungs. Its function is to bring air into the lungs.

4.11 Differences Between The Right and Left Lungs

Air travels from the trachea into the lungs. There are two lungs located in the chest, or in medical parlance, the thoracic cavity. A doctor who specializes in chest surgery is called a thoracic surgeon.

The right lung is more vertical, shorter and wider than the left and as a result, foreign objects that enter can lodge in it. Cancer in the right lung is slightly more common 55% versus 45% than in the left.

The right lung has three sections called lobes. The left lung has two lobes and is smaller because the heart occupies space on the left side. A tumor's location would typically be identified as right upper lobe or left lower lobe. Even more specifically, a place in the lung can be identified as anterior (front) or posterior (back).

4.12 Lung Function

The lung's basic function is breathing, taking in oxygen and eliminating carbon dioxide gas. See Kent (2). Various tests are permitted to assess the level of lung functioning appropriately called pulmonary function tests, or spirometry.

4.121 Pulmonary Reserve and Performance Status

Surgery to remove part of a lung involves removal of healthy tissue near the tumor as well as the tumor itself. Surgeons assess the level of lung functioning before deciding on surgery. If the removal of substantial parts of the lung will significantly impair the patient's breathing ability, surgery may be canceled and other options considered.

One measure of pulmonary function is pulmonary reserve. If a patient has a high pulmonary reserve, that means that some lung tissue can be removed without significantly impairing his breathing ability. The level of functioning of a patient generally, measured by various tests, is called his performance status.

4.122 Why Pulmonary Function May be Impaired

If surgery is considered, usually the tumor is not so advanced as to significantly impair the patient's breathing ability. However, most patients with lung cancer are smokers, and many will have other pulmonary problems. Smokers can have emphysema or bronchitis, both of which impair breathing ability. The two conditions are related and physicians sometimes refer to an overall condition called Chronic Obstructive Pulmonary Disorder, or COPD. If there is serious compromise of pulmonary status, surgery may not be possible.

4.13 The Pleura

The lungs are covered by a thin lining called the pleura. The inner or visceral layer of the pleura is attached to the lungs and the outer, parietal, layer is attached to the chest wall. These two layers are held in place by a film of fluid in a manner similar to two microscope slides that are wet and stuck together. If the pleural cavity fills with air, this is called pneumothorax, and blood in the pleura is called hemothorax. Pleurisy is inflammation of the pleural membrane.

4.131 The Pleura and Mesothelioma

Mesothelioma is a rare form of lung cancer, coming from asbestos entering the pleura and creating tumors in it.

4.14 Mediastinum

The mediastinum is an area between the two lungs. Recall that lymph nodes are part of the lymph system which helps purify the blood and remove byproducts. In the mediastinal area are lymph nodes, and one test of how advanced the cancer is whether the mediastinal nodes are cancerous. A mediastonomy is a procedure where the physician looks at the mediastinal area to detect the presence of cancer in the mediastinal lymph nodes. You will see reference to mediastinal nodes in the description of stage in assessing non-small cell lung cancer.

4.15 The Bronchial Tree

The bronchial system is like a tree with the trunk, the primary bronchus, branches, the bronchioles, and numerous small twigs, the alveoli. Some scientists refer to the bronchi as the larger airways.

4.151 Squamous Cell Cancer and the Bronchi

Some patients have squamous cell carcinoma, which is a tumor involving squamous cells in the bronchus. Since smoke and dust first come in contact with the primary bronchus, it would make sense that many tumors would occur there. Squamous cell cancer in the large bronchi continues to be one of the most common forms of lung cancer.

4.152 Alveoli and Breathing

The bronchi divide to form small bronchi called the secondary or lobal bronchi. Bronchospasm associated with asthma occurs when the muscles of the walls of the bronchioles go into spasm narrowing or closing off the air passageways and causing labored breathing.

Bronchioles subdivide into microscopic branches called respiratory bronchioles, and this in turn divides into microscopic alveoli where air exchange occurs. In the alveoli, carbon dioxide from the outside is converted to oxygen. A descriptive name for alveoli is air sacs. The lungs consist of about 300 million alveoli where this exchange of gas and breathing functions occur.

4.153 Emphysema

During emphysema, the walls of the alveolar are destroyed by smoking:

> "Because emphysema destroys elastic fibers in the membranous walls surrounding individual air sacs these alveoli lose their ability to recoil to their original size during expiration. Then, as an alveolus remains stretched, the rest of the membrane fibers eventually break. The wall is destroyed, meaning the air sac with its neighbor. As the process continues, alveoli become larger and fewer. It is somewhat like tearing down the interior walls in a building of multi-room apartments until each apartment is one large room. The alveoli's membrane walls—which are richly supplied with capillaries, the circulatory system's tiniest vessels—are the actual gas exchange sites." Haas(1)

Foreign substances cause different forms of disease. In emphysema, the area is damaged. The constant duplication of cells to repair damage can cause a growth gene to remain on, and if the duplication and multiplication of cells continues, this is cancer. This is one reason why lung cancer is associated with other lung diseases like emphysema.

4.154 Bronchioalveolar Lung Cancer

One form of lung cancer is bronchio-alveolar, which affects the alveolar regions of the lung. With the advent of filtered cigarettes, smokers inhale more deeply and cancers affecting the deeper airways are occurring more frequently.

4.16 Nodes

One of the chief dangers of cancer is that it may metastasize to other organs through lymph nodes:

> "Because the lungs are so richly supplied with blood vessels, they serve as a convenient route for lung cancer cells to travel to other parts of the body. Most of the cancer cells that enter the bloodstream die, some survive and grow and become metastatic cancer . . . The lungs also have a rich supply of lymph vessels. The system of lymph vessels resembles the system of blood vessels. The purpose of the lymphatic system is to drain the clear fluid called lymph from the body tissues and bring it back into circulation." (Manual 3)

Lymph nodes filter germs and other foreign invaders, such as cancer cells. Trapped cells can create tumorous growth in the lymph nodes causing them to swell, and an enlarged lymph node in the neck region can be an indication of lung cancer. Lung cancer develops in a single spot but when lymph nodes become involved, the tumor spreads to other parts of the body.

4.161 Lymph Node Location

Typically, the lymph nodes in the hilus (hilar lymph nodes) the place where the large airways and blood vessels enter the lung from the mediastinum (towards the center of the chest) are affected first. From there, the cancer may spread to the nodes of the mediastinum and then to the nodes in the neck and /or abdomen. If the tumor cells enter the blood stream, they may migrate (metastasize) to the liver, other sections of the lung, the brain, the bones, and/or the bone marrow." Alcase, Lung Cancer Manual (1998) (at the time of this printing, the lung cancer manual was available at no cost on the Alcase website. Alcase is now called the Lung Cancer Alliance. Lungcanceralliance.org).

4.162 Staging and Measuring Lymph Node Involvement

The extent to which the lymph nodes are involved is an important consideration in determining the stage of disease, and the prognosis. Once there is lymph node involvement, surgery is unlikely to remove all the cancer. Thus, the staging systems below consider as a critical element the presence of cancer in the lymph nodes. A cancer located in the larger bronchi would typically move towards an adjacent hilar lymph node, then a mediastinal lymph node, and then to a node connected with another organ.

4.17 Sources of Pain

A tumor that grows may obstruct a bronchus, causing shortness of breath or chest pain, and these are two indications of cancer. Unfortunately, these problems tend to manifest themselves when the tumor becomes larger and may have already reached a lymph node. Thus, a key to early diagnosis and treatment is not waiting till pain and shortness occur, but developing methods of detecting tumors before they impact bodily functions.

Shortness of breath and chest pain are non-specific symptoms, that is they can indicate a number of different diseases. Heavy smokers may experience heart problems or other pulmonary difficulties which can confuse or delay diagnosis. These facts partly explain why many lung cancers are diagnosed at later stages where treatment is more difficult.

REFERENCES

1. Haas, *The Chronic Bronchitis and Emphysema Handbook* (1990).
2. What is Lung Cancer, www.educ.kent.edu.
3. Alcase, *The Lung Cancer Manual* (2000).

CHAPTER 5

THE CANCER PROCESS IN THE LUNG

5.1 HOW CANCER DEVELOPS

5.11 The Carcinogenic Process in a Smoker

A gradual process of damage to lung tissue creates a tumor. Let us look at the development and spread of squamous cell lung cancer in a smoker:

1. **Columnar Cells Protect the Lung.** Tall columnar cells lining the air passages help keep the lungs clean and secrete sticky mucus which coats the entire respirator tract with a protective barrier. This mucus traps dust particles and cilia sweep the mucus and trapped dirt out of the lungs and throat, through a cough. Cells signal other cells to grow when damage occurs, and the body maintains an orderly system of cellular repair and cellular death.

2. **Irritation to Columnar Cells.** Poisons in cigarette smoke damage the cilia and the sweeping motion slows. Irritation to columnar cells results. In response to this irritation, the lung tissue produces additional mucus. The damage prompts signals for increased production. A wholesale alteration of cell production and signaling is beginning.

3. **Columnar Cells Deteriorate and Metaplasia Develops.** Irritation from smoking continues, and columnar cells deteriorate and change shape. Cilia disappear and columnar cells transform themselves into flat, lacelike cells, a process called metaplasia. Various growth factors are activated, and tumor suppresor genes, the body's monitors are beginning to malfunction. If tissue were analyzed, DNA damage in at least three chromosome locations, 3p14, 9p21, and 17p13, would likely be seen.

4. **The Precancerous Phase Called Dysphasia.** These metaplastic cells become increasing abnormal until they reach a precancerous stage called dysphasia. Considerable changes have now taken place over 10-15 years changing normal tissue to precancerous ones. A number of growth factors signaling tumor replication and related functions have been activated, and the body's system of cell repair and orderly cell death (apoptosis) has been damaged.

   However, these changes will not impact any bodily function, or be apparent on an x-ray, standard blood test, or physical examination. For squamous cell cancer, these changes will be apparent on a sputum cytology test, where the sputum and cells from a deep cough are analyzed. Smoking cessation may allow some of this cellular damage to be repaired and restored, though former smokers will always have an increased risk of lung cancer.

5. **Tumor Development.** A small growth or tumor develops, partly as a result of the body's attempt to repair damaged tissue. Assuming the tumor is non-small cell, the most common, we now have a stage 1 non-small cell lung tumor. If the tumor is surgically removed at this stage, the patient will have an excellent 5 year prognosis. If it is small and less than a centimeter, the tumor can probably be seen only on a chest Ct scan. If it is a little larger, it may be visible on an x-ray. The tumor still will probably not impact normal functions or cause pain or discomfort. In Japan, many lung tumors are detected at this stage through screening. Since no screening program exists in the U.S., most tumors here will be diagnosed later.

6. **Lymph Node Involvement.** Mirroring the process of wound repair, the new cells create sources of blood supply, enabling the tumor cells to migrate to other parts of the body. Cancer cells come into nearby lymph nodes and spread both through lymph nodes and blood vessels. Anti-angiogenic drugs may in the future inhibit this process. Depending upon the location of the affected lymph nodes, the cancer will now be stage 2 or 3. Impacting breathing or causing pain, the tumor may cause some discomfort prompting a medical visit where it can be diagnosed.

7. **Metastasis.** The tumor travels from a lymph node to another organ. Complex proteins manage to break down protective barriers in the basement membrane of other tissue enabling the cancer cells to penetrate. Surgery is not an option given the widespread nature of the cancer. Chemotherapy will be prescribed to inhibit the process of cell reproduction, lengthen life and reduce some symptoms. Since chemotherapy impacts normal cells, the extent must be limited. Newer forms of gene therapy will be prescribed to stop the aberrant cell signaling and inhibit certain growth factors. See Lungcheck (8).

Parts of this process may vary: tumors may take from 15 to 50 years to develop, non-smokers may contract cancer through seemingly different processes, lymph nodes may not always be cancerous, progression of the tumor can vary, and the location of cellular damage will also vary. Scientists have difficulty understanding which cellular changes come first, what is the order of cause and effect, which cellular abnormalities are the most important ones, which cells if repaired would impact cure or frustrate metastasis. Studies show 50 or 60% of cancer patients have a given cell abnormality, and determining which gene malfunctions cause the tumor remains problematic. Here are the major genes associated with lung cancer:

5.2 GENES INVOLVED WITH LUNG CANCER

Name of Gene	Role	Possible Treatment
P-53	Tumor Suppressor Gene P-53 disruptions are identified in many cancers including lung. P-53 helps repair damaged cells and activate processes of cell death when repair is impossible.	While effective in laboratory tests on cells, P-53 treatment has not been proven in clinical trials.
RB Retinoblastoma	Tumor Supressor Gene Associated with small cell lung cancer	None to date
Epidermal Growth Factor	Gene and receptor associated with creation and spread of lung tumors	Iressa has been FDA approved for treatment after chemotherapy. Other drugs like, Tarceva are showing initial success. Trials combining the drugs with chemotherapy have been disappointing.
Erb 2	Part of the EGF family, with some clinical trials showing a role in various cancers.	Herceptin successfully used for breast cancer, significance in lung cancer unclear.
Vascular Endothelial Growth Factor	Associated with angiogenesis	Drugs targeting VEGF and receptors make logical sense, but remain unproven in clinical trials. Avastin and Neovastat, conflicting results. See (17)
Cox 2	Produce in response to various types of inflammation	Celebrex promising in cell studies. Cox-2 inhibitors showing success with various types of cancers and other diseases.
Teleromerase	Cells have limited number of replications. This substance enables tumors to continually replicate	Drugs makes logical sense but remain unproven. Rhodacyanine (MKT077) and FJ5002 address teleromerase but there is little information about these drugs.
Matellomatrixmatellprote inases	Production of MMP's enables basement matrix of organs to be penetrated and cancer cells to enter.	Marimastat trials disappointing
Cyclin D	Cyclin D1 gene is located on chromosome 11q13. This chromosomal region is amplified in a wide variety of human cancers . Associated with RB, production helps cells proceed through cycle.	Flovopirodol (Aventis) decrease of cyclin D1 by repressing the cyclin D1 promoter
BCL-2	Helps prevents apoptosis (cell death).	Scientists are assessing whether levels of BCL-2 can be used as a tumor marker.

5.201 The Reader's Role

Many readers will want as much information as possible about the science behind lung cancer and the drugs that will be prescribed. Others will not and would prefer to simply review the types of drugs customarily prescribed. You may go to later chapters to read about specific drugs, or as I would recommend, try to get a basic understanding of the underlying science.

5.21 Multiple Changes

Multiple genetic changes appear needed to create a lung tumor, though a small number of changes can create other types of cancer. For example, a single change in one gene is associated with a particular type of leukemia. We know that multiple changes are needed in lung cancer.

In one way, that is a blessing. It explains why exposure to a carcinogen such as smoke does not immediately cause a tumor and even multiple changes may not be sufficient. The need for considerable genetic change explains why it takes many years for a smoker to contract cancer and why some may never get it. Once those multiple changes do occur, it is difficult to undo a system of signaling which has undergone considerable disruption. Indeed, the most effective treatment remains removal of the tumor, not attempts to correct the existing disease.

5.22 Gene Repair and Apoptosis

Lung cancer involves damage to various genes and a failure of the body's system of repair. One area of damage concerns apoptosis, the body's mechanism for arranging for the orderly death or elimination of damaged or defective cells. "When nuclear DNA is damaged, normal cells initiate a response that includes cell-cycle arrest, apoptotic cell death, and transcriptional induction of genes involved in DNA repair. Induction of apoptosis is an important response to DNA damage." Bast (16); Wang (10). The system of apoptosis fails to some extent in lung cancer and measurements of apoptotic capacity were associated with survival length. Tumor suppressor genes perform help inducing apoptosis. "P53-specific growth inhibition and apoptosis of tumor cells were observed in both cell lines in vitro."

5.221 Anti-Apoptosis Genes Cox-2

Cox-2 is a protein produced in times of perceived injury to cells. It appears to frustrate the apoptotic process. Cox-2 inhibitors are being examined as a partial treatment for lung cancer, in part to restore the body's apoptotic process.

5.23 Tumor Suppressor Genes

Tumor suppressor genes play a critical role in cancer:

> Although cancer cells use the same cell cycle machinery as normal cells, the cell cycle checkpoints in tumor cells are relaxed. Of the scores of proto-oncogenes and tumor-suppressor genes that have been identified to date, most function in signal transduction pathways that mediate mitogenic stimulation. These signal transduction pathways eventually converge on the cell cycle checkpoint that controls the G0/G1 to S phase transition and activate appropriate CDKs. Influencing the transit of this checkpoint has a major influence on the proliferation of normal and tumor cells by affecting both Tc and growth fraction. Despite the number and variety of these genes involved in signal transduction, relaxation of the G1/G0 to S checkpoint controls in tumor cells is mediated, for the most part, by disruption of two pathways, the Rb and p53 growth control pathways. These two genes, individually, are the most frequently mutated in human cancer cells. Disruption of the Rb or p53 pathways probably occurs in virtually every human cancer." Bast (16)

5.231 P-53

The P-53 gene helps facilitate apoptosis, and acts like a policeman regulating cell development,

> "p53 protein . . . mediates several cellular functions: regulation of the cell division cycle, DNA repair, and programmed cell death. In response to various forms of genomic DNA damage . . . the p53 protein can arrest the cell cycle at the G1 to

S transition point, thus affording time for DNA repair and preventing duplication of a mutant cell, or alternatively, failing DNA repair, p53 protein can implement programmed cell death (apoptosis). Accordingly, p53 has been dubbed the Aguardian of the genome." Etiology of Cancer (7).

5.232 The Retinoblastoma (RB) Gene

The retinoblastoma (RB) gene has a protein that appears to regulate the cell cycle. Most small cell lung cancers have absent or abnormal RB protein. Studies of individuals with abnormalities regarding RB genes showed they develop tumors at 10 times the normal rate. RB abnormalities are also present in NSLC with estimates ranging from 10-60%.

5.24 Growth Factors

In response to perceived cellular damage and other factors, various growth factors are activated in lung cancer.

5.241 Epidermal Growth Factor

The epidermal growth factor is associated with various types of tumors. We developed a chapter to the emerging area of epidermal treatment. A growth factor connects with a corresponding growth factor receptor which begins various cellular processes. Scientists are studying ways of preventing the activation of the growth factor or activation of the corresponding receptor.

Since these treatments target a specific type of cell, their impact upon the overall body will be limited, and the absence of side effects makes these treatments attractive.

5.242 Vascular Endothelial Growth Factor

VEGF is produced and helps the tumor create new blood vessels and connect tissue to facilitate metastasis. Here, too, anti-vegf and vegf receptor drugs are being tested for lung cancer. Vascular endothelial growth factor (VEGF) causes the creation of new blood vessels and the spread of the tumor. One study found that abnormalities of the K-Ras

Gene contributed to VEGF. "Of 14 tumors with mutant K-ras genes, 7 cases (50.0%) had high VEGF expression whereas only 39 of the 167 tumors with wild-type K-ras (23.4%) had high VEGF expression." Konishi, (5). Thus, there is a close relationship among growth factors in the complex mechanism of cell signaling and reproduction.

5.3 WHY ONLY SOME CIGARETTE SMOKERS DEVELOP LUNG CANCER

We know that both growth and tumor suppresor genes are involved with the formation of cancers. This helps explain why some smokers contract cancer while others don't. It may be that cigarette smoke causes some changes but only results in cancer when combined with an existing gene abnormality. That is why people with family histories of certain cancers are more likely to contract the disease. It is somewhat like destruction of buildings in a hurricane. Buildings with defects in the foundation will be damaged while others can withstand the assault.

Additionally, we know that exposure to multiple carcinogens increases the risk of cancer. Thus, people who smoke and were exposed to asbestos are more likely to contract lung cancer than people exposed to only one carcinogen. It would simplify analysis to say that smoking causes a change in a dominant gene while asbestos causes a malfunction in a tumor suppressor gene (or vice versa). However, it appears that each carcinogen can cause changes in both types of genes:

> "Various factors, including cigarette smoking, asbestos, and diet, have been reported to correlate with the development of lung cancer. Of these factors, cigarette smoking is believed as the major carcinogen for lung cancer. Recent studies indicate that cigarette smoke carcinogens cause genetic damages at both oncogenes(K-ras) and tumor suppressor genes(p 53) of lung cancer, and hence initiate and promote the development of lung cancer." Yano, (3).

At this stage in cancer research, we are generally unable to reverse the cell abnormalities though significant progress has been made in identifying them. Clinical trials for patients with advanced cancer are experimenting with various means of correcting or mitigating gene malfunctions.

REFERENCES

1. Devita, *Cancer Principles and Practices of Oncology*.
2. Carney, *Lung Cancer* (Arnold Publishing Co., Great Britain, 1995).
3. Yano, *Causative Agents for Lung Carcinogenesis*, Nippon Rinsho, 2000 May, 58:5, 1017-22.
4. Fleischacker, *Molecular Genetic Characteristics of Lung Cancer* . . . Lung Cancer, Vol. 25 (1) (1999) pp. 7-24.
5. International Journal of Oncology 2000 Mar;16(3):501-11.
6. Fleischacker, *Molecular Genetic Characteristics of Lung Cancer, Useful as Real Tumor Markers*, Lung Cancer, Vol. 25 (1) (1999) pp. 7-24.
7. Etiology of Carcinogensis edcenter.med.cornell.edu./ CUMC_PathNotes/Neoplasia/Neoplasia_04.html.
8. Lungcheck.com (no longer available online). Lungcheck was developed to detect lung cancer or even precancerous changes at an early stage.
9. Here is another description of lung cancer development:

> The current hypothesis is that at least 10-20 genetic mutations are required to produce a lung cancer cell from the normal one. These mutations cause activation of oncogenes (dominant cellular factors, which stimulate or predispose a cell to divide) and deletion of tumor suppressor genes . . . . The development of cancer is due not only to abnormal cell proliferation with loss of growth control, but also to abnormalities in the cells intrinsic cell death programme, (apotheosis). Proto-oncogenes induce cellular proliferation which activate to oncogenes. Activation may occur by point mutation, over expression, or deletion of genetic material. Oncogenes evaluated for prognostic impact in NSCLS(non small cell lung cancer) include the ras oncogeny, c-erb B-2 oncogenies, also called HER-2 and neu oncogeny and Bcl-2 oncogeny (3). These oncogenes have also been evaluated in clinical trials . . . .

All lung cancer cells produce hormones and peptides, which can function as growth factors and generate growth loops. These include epidermal growth factor, transforming growth factor a, platelet derived growth factor, insulin-like growth factor . . . Inactivation of genes that normally regulate cellular growth and thereby have a restraining effect of tumor-genesis (tumor suppressor genes) can lead to uncontrolled cell proliferation. In many cases, inactivation occurs by point mutation of one allele, and, subsequently, loss of an amount of the genetic material of the other. Prevention of cell division may be based on our increased understanding of the effect of growth factors in lung cancer. There are multiple and diverse simulators, meaning that blocking the action of a single growth factor is unlikely to be effective. However, inhibition of intracellular mechanisms that control multiple growth stimulating inputs offers a more realistic potential for intervention.

10. Fas *A6706 Polymorphism, Apoptotic Capacity in Lymphocyte Cultures, and Risk of Lung Cancer*, Lung Cancer (2003) 42, 1-8.
11. Qadr *Selective Cox-2 Inhibition Attenuates Recurrent Tumor Growth*. J Surg Res. 2003 Oct;114(2):269.
11. Jin, *Research on expression and control of p16 and p21 by wild-type p53 gene in two lung adenocarcinoma cell lines*, Zhonghua Yi Xue Yi Chuan Xue Za Zhi. 2003 Oct;20(5):409-12.
12. Shrump, *Inhibition of lung cancer proliferation by antisense cyclin D*, Cancer Gene Ther. 1996 Mar-Apr;3(2):131-5.
13. State of the Science, Lung Cancer www.webtie.org/sots/html/LungAgents.htm
14. Gregorc, *The Clinical Relevance of Bcl-2, RB and P-53 Expression in Advanced Non-Small Cell Lung Cancer*, Lung Cancer (2003) 42, 275-81.
15. Mao, *Clonal Genetic Alterations in the Lungs of Current and Former Smokers*, Journal of NCI, vol. 89, no. 12, (June 18, 1997).
16. Bast, *Cancer Medicine* (2000).
17. "Antibodies that target VEGFR-1 and VEGFR-2 also inhibit the VEGF signaling pathway. Each of these antibodies inhibits VEGF interactions with a specific receptor, leaving VEGF signaling through the other receptor intact. Both of these

antibodies act extracellularly, inhibiting receptors found on the surface of cells . . . . Several small molecules that inhibit the receptor tyrosine kinase activity of VEGFRs are in development. These molecules function intracellularly, inhibiting activity of the cytoplasmically located kinase domains of the VEGFRs and have variable specificity, potentially inhibiting many different kinases. One small molecule inhibitor, currently in phase II clinical development inhibits VEGFR-1, VEGFR-2, PDGF-R, and c-Kit. Another, also in phase II clinical trials, inhibits the kinase activity of VEGFR-2 but not VEGFR-1. This agent additionally inhibits the kinase activity of HER1/EGFR and Flt-3. Similarly another small molecule inhibitor also prevents VEGFR-2 kinase activity but not VEGFR-1 kinase activity. This agent also prevents the kinase activity of the oncogene c-kit, Flt-3 and PDGF, and is currently in phase II clinical trials." www.targetvegf.com.

CHAPTER 6

THE PROCESS OF METASTASIS

6.1 THE CENTRAL ROLE METASTASIS PLAYS IN LUNG CANCER TREATMENT

6.11 The Importance of Understanding Metastasis

The potential for metastasis is a problem for all cancers, and in particular lung cancer. The chief cause of death in lung cancer is not direct damage to the lung but the consequences of metastasis. Most lung tumors are detected in an advanced stage where there has been significant spread of the tumor. Thus, an understanding of how a tumor metastasises, and ways of treating metastatic lung cancer are critical to any discussion of treatment options. Some of the material in this chapter is scientific and some readers may choose to skip or come back to this chapter. Others may find that while the material is weighty, understanding terms like angiogenesis may be helpful in understanding the how and why of new cancer drugs.

6.12 The Steps Involved in Metastasis

Here is a short summary of the metastasis process:

1. **Cancer cells located in an organ such as the lung manage to break down the barrier confining them to that organ.** "Local invasion by tumor cells involves the activation of genetic programs which allow them to pass away from the confines of the primary

tumor mass, through any surrounding tissues and eventually to reach of blood or lymph vessel." Vile, (1). Tumor cells in an organ such as the lung must separate from each other, overcoming the usual restrictions imposed by cell adhesion and cell-contact inhibition.

2. **Tumor cells come to a nearby lymph node or blood vessel** enabling them to use that pathway to ultimately travel to another organ. Tumor cells move to an adjoining lymph node or blood vessel establishing a source of blood supply in that new location.

3. **The tumor encroaches into the protective covering of another organ** breaking down the extracellular matrix. The tumor cells manage to penetrate the protective barrier of another organ, called the basement membrane. Cells move into the new organ, and establish a source of blood supply for future growth. The process by which tumors establish new sources of blood supply is called angiogenesis, and a major source of cancer research is the creation of anti-angiogenesis drugs to frustrate this process.

4. **Tumor cells create a blood supply** (vascularization) by inducing capillary growth into and around the tumor—a process known as angiogenesis. An adequate blood supply is essential so that the rapidly proliferating cells can obtain nutrients and oxygenation, otherwise mass necrosis (cell death) can half the growth of the cells. Tumor cells move to another organ which can sustain its growth.

6.2 HOW CANCER CELLS SEPARATE

Normal cells are connected with one another. For example, cells in a person's arm combine to help perform various tasks. However, in a cancerous tumor, the first step is for cells separate from one another. "Separation of cells from the primary tumor mass must occur before long range spread can be possible. Detachment of single cells or clumps of cells may be directly related to a decreased level of cell adhesiveness in tumor populations." Wile, Id, at 26.

> "The family of cadherin molecules help cells bind to one another, maintaining a sound structure. Cadherin molecules regulate cell adhesion, though we cannot precisely define the role of each type—This study described the expression pattern of

cadherins and catenins in normal bronchial epithelium. The authors' results show that these proteins involved in cell-cell adhesion are abnormally expressed in the majority of non-small cell lung carcinomas . . . . These findings support the hypothesis that alterations in expression, and particularly loss of expression, of cadherins/catenins may play an important role in the development of the malignant phenotype in lung cancer, however, they also point out the complexity of this system and the need for additional study." Cadherin (2).

6.3 HOW TUMORS PENETRATE OTHER ORGANS AND DRUGS TO INHIBIT THAT PROCESS

The boundary that separates one group of normal cells from the next is called the extracellular matrix or basement membrane. Under a microscope, a tumor, a group of cancer cells, can be seen be seen penetrating this basement membrane:

"Cancers can produce substances that attack constituents of the glue that binds cells together (the technical term is extracellular matrix). This matrix contains many different components, such as a substance called collagen, which gives strength to many tissues. Cancers may produce a type of substance called collagenase that attacks and breaks down the substance. Cancer cells can also produce other substances such as hyaluronidase, a group of substances called protease, and probably dozens of others that allow the growing cancer cells to push through normal tissue boundaries. As a result, cancers often have a very ragged, irregular, and indistinct border—a feature that is often important in distinguishing a cancer from a nonmalignant lesion, as nonmalignant areas (such as warts, benign tumors, or cysts) have a border that is clearly visible and quite distinct." Buckman (3).

Certain proteins called metalloproteinases or MMP help enable the tumor to penetrate these barriers.

"Matrix metalloproteinases (MMPs) are a class of structurally related enzymes that function in the degradation of extracellular matrix proteins . . . Increased MMP activity is detected in a wide range of cancers and seems correlated to their invasive and metastatic potential. MMPs thus seem an attractive target for both diagnostic and therapeutic purposes." Dennis (4).

6.31 Drugs to Combat MMP

New drugs are being designed and tested to see if they can frustrate this process of MMP. Many have worked in a laboratory where these drugs succeed in frustrating this process with cancer tissue, and sometimes, animals. However, with humans, there has been difficulty in delivering the particular drug to the tumor area in sufficient quantity to be effective. A later chapter discusses MMP drugs. At present, attention has shifted from preventing MMP, a goal which had been generally unsuccessful in humans to date, to other methods of cancer control.

6.4 ANGIONGENESIS

6.41 Tumors Cannot Grow Beyond a Certain Size Without Creating a Source of Blood Supply

Once the tumor cells have separated, entered a nearby lymph node, and penetrated a distant or nearby organ, the final step is to link to a source of blood supply and nourishment. For clarity we have called this the final step; some scientists would suggest that establishment of a source of blood supply occurs first, or that there are multiple parts of the process.

The creation of a source of blood supply is essential to a tumor's growth, and probably to its ability to sustain itself. Dr. Judah Folkman pioneered the area of angiogenesis research and a book about him explains:

> "No tumor could grow beyond a tiny size until it sent out a chemical message to recruit an ample blood supply. For that chemical signal to be sent out, Folkman believed, an angiogenic switch had to be flipped—a switch that turned on the tumor's production of a growth-producing agent such as B-FGF (basic fibroblast growth factor), or VEGF (vascular endothelial growth factor), which Folkman had long referred to as TAF. It was this

angiogenic switch that made nearby blood vessels sprout and
grow new branches and kick-started the rapid growth of tumors."
Cook, (11).

This process is not unique to cancer, and is part of the body's normal
processes going awry. While writing this book, I accidentally cut my
forehead. Cells signaled other cells to replicate, and sources of blood
supply connected with the damaged area. Angiogenesis is similar to the
process of wound repair. When one smokes, cells may replicate and other
functions are activated to correct the damage. Over time, this process
goes awry and the cell repair function proceeds in an abnormal fashion.

6.42 Anti-Angiogenesis Research

There is continuing research about developing drugs to inhibit
growth factors with so-called anti-angiogenesis drugs. A number of
drugs are attempting to inhibit angiogenesis and there are over 100
clinical trials involving anti-angiogenic drugs. Chemotherapy involves
drugs used to kill cancer cells while anti-angiogenic drugs attempt
to frustrate their spread. Since the two types of drugs work differently,
new research attempts to combine the two types of drugs.

One theme of cancer research in the 21st century is combining
different types of treatment, with each type reaching an optimal level of
toxicity, where it attacks cancer cells but does not do unmanageable
damage to other cells.

6.5 WHERE DOES METASTASIS OCCUR?

6.51 Location and Proximity

"Metastasis is partly explained by geographical proximity: In some
instances, this organ preference of metastasis can be explained simply
in terms of the anatomical relationship of the organ with the site of the
primary tumor growth. Hence, many secondary tumors will develop in
those organs which provide the first capillary bed encountered by
dispersing metastatic cells, since the tumor cells may be carried as
aggregates which pass into a capillary whose lumen is smaller than the
clump diameter. A knowledge of the circulatory anatomical associations
of the primary tumor site with other organs can typically be used to

predict the seeding site of about 60% of the metastasises from that tumor. Metastasises from colon cancer probably occur with high frequency because the liver receives the drainage of the blood supply to the large intestine." Vile (1).

6.52 Chemical and Cellular Attractants

In other instances, there are specific chemical or other attractants which lead cancer cells to particular parts of the body: Usually when tumors are located at a distant site which could not be predicted on the basis of circulatory anatomy, it is because the site expresses specific determinants which actively promote the growth of the metastatic cells.

Structures vary in penetrability, and some areas such as brain, bone, and liver are the subject of frequent metastasis, while others such as feet are virtually never. It may be that those structures where lymph and blood are frequently transmitted have to be receptive to other cells, allowing cancer cells to enter. Using an analogy, a burglar might be able to penetrate some houses whereas others would have sufficient protection.

6.53 Soil and Seed Hypothesis

Eighty years ago, Paget proposed the "seed and soil hypothesis." A seed (the carcinoma) will only give rise to a secondary tumor in organs that sustain its growth (the soil). Cancers can only successfully locate in certain organs; for others, inherent characteristics of the organ prevent or inhibit metastasis. Organs vary in their ability to resist penetration by cancer cells, "The basement membrane of different organs vary in composition and the heterogeneity in binding of tumor cells to components of the extracellular matrix may well be another mediator in the organ preference of metastasis." Vile (1).

6.6 DIFFICULTIES TREATING METASTATIC CANCER

6.61 Staging and Metastatic Cancer

Once a cancer has metastasized, it is more difficult to attack or cure. Indeed, the defining characteristic of stage 4 cancer, or the most advanced, is metastasis to another organ. (Interestingly, within the category of stage 4 tumors, no staging distinctions are made based upon the number of metastasises or their location). Let us look at some of the difficulties metastatic cancer presents.

6.62 Surgery and Metastatic Cancer

Surgery is the first consideration in treating a cancer; simply remove the tumor and an area of surrounding tissue. If the cancer has spread to distant parts of the body, it would be difficult to remove the entire tumor. One might know where the tumor cells are located, and even if we did, operating on many different organs would be risky and time-consuming. Many lung cancer patients are older, with breathing capacity compromised by years of smoking. For such patients, lengthy procedures would create substantial risk. Surgery on the lung is almost never used if the cancer has metastasized to another organ.

Surgery is sometimes used on the particular area of metastasis. Surgery on cranial or bone metastasis is sometimes performed to relieve pain or discomfort.

6.63 Radiation and Metastasis

With metastatic cancer, radiation may be used to target the lung or particular areas of metastasis. Like surgery, this is done to relieve pain or discomfort, not as an effort to eliminate the entire cancer.

6.64 Chemotherapy

Chemotherapy is the use of drugs to kill cancer cells. To date, chemotherapy has been partially effective. It improves quality of life, kills cancer cells, and reduces spread. In many cases, it does not succeed in completely eliminating the tumor, though partial and complete responses are sometimes seen. Here are some reasons for the limitations with metastatic lung cancer.

Chemotherapy generally has only the capacity to kill a certain percentage of cancer cells. Thus, as cancer cells spread and divide, creating a larger number of cells, the ability of chemotherapy to completely combat it decreases. Secondly, as chemotherapy progresses, some cancer cells unfortunately develop the ability to withstand the chemotherapy, called multi-drug resistance. Sometimes, a drug will be used, substantially reduce the size of the tumor, but lose its effectiveness after a period of time. Second-line chemotherapy involves drugs used after the first group has stopped being effective.

REFERENCES

1. Vile, *Cancer Metastasis: From Mechanisms to Therapies*, 10-11 (Wiley 1995).
2. *Cadherin and Catenin Expression in Normal Human Bronchial Epithelium and Non-Small Cell Lung Cancer*, Lung Cancer, Vol. 24 (3) (1999) pp. 157-168.
3. Buckman, *What You Really Need to Know About Cancer* 14 (Johns Hopkins Press 1997).
4. Dennis, *Matrix Metalloproteinases Inhibitors: Present Achievements and Future Prospects*, Invest New Drugs 1997;15(3):175-85.
5. Fu, *Study of Prognostic Predictors for Non-Small Cell Lung Cancer*, Lung Cancer, Vol. 23 (2) (1999) pp. 143-152.
6. Pass, Lung Cancer, Palliative Radiotherapy, (2000).
7. Hanigiri, *Bone Metastasis After a Resection of Stage I and II Primary Lung Cancer*, Lung Cancer, Vol. 27 (3) (2000) pp. 199-204.
8. Quantin, *Concomitant Brain Radiotherapy . . . and Chemotherapy in Brain Metastasis of Lung Cancer*, Lung Cancer 26 (1999) 35-39.
9. Rodriqus, *Brain Metastasises and Non-Small Cell Lung Cancer. Prognostic Factors and Correlation with Survival After Irradiation.* Lung Cancer, Vol. 32 (2) (2001) pp. 129-136.
10. Carney *Lung Cancer* (1995).
11. Cook *Dr. Folkman's War: Angiogenesis and . . . Cancer* (2001).

CHAPTER 7

TYPES OF LUNG CANCER

7.0 THE IMPORTANCE OF CLASSIFICATION

Treatment for lung cancer is dependent upon the stage and type of cancer. To understand your treatment, you must first know the type of cancer your have and its stage.

7.1 NON-SMALL CELL AND SMALL-CELL

Lung cancer is divided into two basic types, non-small cell (NSCLC) and small cell. This classification provides a standardized system useful in estimating prognosis, selecting treatment and reporting data. While both types arise in the lungs, there are mollecular and other differences. "SCLC demonstrate more frequent losses at 4p, 4q, 5q21 . . . 10Q, while losses at 9p21 and 8P21-23 are more frequent in NSCLC's." Miller (10).

About 80% of lung cancers are non-small cell. Non-small cell lung cancer combines three types of lung cancer: squamous cell, adenocarcinoma, and large cell carcinoma. These are classified together because their treatment and prognosis are generally similar:

> "The remaining common histologic varieties of lung cancer-
> adenocarcinoma, squamous cell carcinoma, large cell
> carcinoma—behave as a group in a biologically similar fashion
> and respond similarly to therapeutic intervention. These tumors
> account for approximately 85% of all lung cancers." Aisner, (1).

7.11 Squamous Cell Carcinoma

Squamous cell refers to a type of cell. These line the large bronchi and squamous cell tumors are generally centrally located. Approximately 90% of squamous cell carcinomas arise in subsegmental or larger bronchi and grow centrally toward the main bronchus and infiltrate the underlying bronchial cartilage, lymph nodes, and adjacent lung parenchyma. In time, this progression may lead to the formation of large nodular masses.

Because squamous cell tumors are centrally located, they are sometimes seen on chest x-rays and through other diagnostic tests. Sputum cytology is a device to analyze sputum from a deep cough. Squamous cell tumors can frequently be detected through this test. The cytology can frequently identify early stage cancers and if sputum cytology were used more widely, many lives would be saved.

Epithelial tissue lines body surfaces or tissues, glands, and body cavities, and squamous cell is a type of epithelial tissue. Squamous cells line the pleural cavity and squamous cell cancer can occur outside the bronchi and in other parts of the body. Thus one question is whether a squamous cancer in another part of the body will act similar to a squamous cell tumor in the lung.

7.12 Percentage of Squamous Cell Carcinomas is Decreasing With Smokers Breathing Low Tar Cigarettes More Deeply, Leading to Peripheral Tumors

While squamous cell remains the most prevalent form of lung cancer, its incidence is decreasing. One study found the percentage of squamous tumors in men decreased from 51.8% to 42.7%. Aisner (1) at 251. With filtered cigarettes becoming more prevalent, smokers are inhaling more deeply, leading to the development of more peripheral adenocarcinomas rather than the central squamous cell carcinomas.

7.13 Adenocarcinoma

Adenocarcinoma is the second type of non-small cell lung cancer. It represents about 40% of all cancers and has become the most common lung cancer among women. It generally starts near the outer edges of the lungs, and its increasing incidence is connected with the tendency of smokers to breath the lower-tar cigarettes more deeply.

7.131 Adenocarcinoma, Asbestosis and Silicosis

While smoking remains the largest cause of adenocarcinoma, some scientists see an association with lung scars and occupational exposure to silica, asbestos and other dusts. Where a foreign particle deposits in the lung, and collagen forms to encapsulate the particle, some call this scar formation. For a detailed discussion of silica-related scar formation, See Castranova (2). Asbestosis, silicosis, residuals of tuberculosis along with other scar formations have been linked to adenocarcinoma. Thus, an individual with asbestosis and adenocarcinoma, would likely have a legal claim. See Chapter 22. Some have questioned how closely adenocarcinoma should be associated with the various types of fibrosis or scaring in the lung:

> "For many years, adenocarcinoma was believed to develop on the basis of scar of (a) any kind. Although we do not deny the existence of scar cancer in the lung, . . . We have proposed the concept that central or subpleural scars in most peripheral adenocarcinomas were formed not before, but after, the development of carcinoma, and showed the mode of development of such a scar or a fibrotic focus."

7.132 Bronchioloalveolar Carcinoma

Bronchioloalveolar carcinoma (BAC) is a type of adenocarcinoma which originates in the alveoli. Bronchioalveolar cancer is hard to detect since a clear nodule may not be seen on tests, and it can initially be confused with tuberculosis or other lung disease.

Women are being increasingly diagnosed with this disease. Showing that different subtypes can respond differently to treatment, this type of tumor is particularly responsive to the new drug, Iressa. Indeed, some studies have shown triple or quadruple the number of partial and complete responses to Iressa, particularly among non-smokers. Non-smokers are susceptible to this disease. The different patterns of response indicate that this disease is different from other forms of non-small lung cancer. Since non-smokers contract the disease, one hypothesis is that the disease involves fewer genetic abnormalities than other forms of lung cancer, so that addressing one of the growth factors which prompt cellular reproduction can have a substantial impact.

7.14 Large Cell Cancer

Large cell cancer constitutes about 15% of all cancers and the term large cell refers to large, masses of tissue usually displaying signs of necrosis (cell death). A Undifferentiated large cell carcinoma are defined by the WHO as "a malignant epithelial tumor with large nuclei, prominent nucleoli, abundant cytoplasm and usually well defined cell borders, without the characteristic features of squamous cell, small cell or adenocarcinomas." (9)

Large cell can sometimes be confused with a poorly differentiated adenocarcinoma or squamous cell carcinoma. However, since the treatment for adenocarcinoma, squamous cell, and large cell are generally grouped together, a physician might not be overly concerned with distinguishing cell type within the group. A subtype of large cell carcinoma is giant cell.

7.15 Differences within the Non-small Cell Category

While squamous, adenocarcinoma and large cell have been grouped together for some time, researchers are seeing some important differences. "Studies of large number of lung cancers have shown different patterns of involvement between the two major groups of lung cancer (SCLC and NSCLC) and between the three major histologic types of lung carcinoma" The author goes on to describe different areas of genetic damage, variations in the number of genes impacted, and differences in how the disease arises. Some studies have found differences in survival periods. (1)

These differences mean the broad grouping of three types of cancer with distinct characterstics disease may be analytically incorrect. Instead, in the future, we may develop an approach honed to the specific type of cancer and perhaps analyze areas of genetic damage to create individualized treatment plans. Today, we find that Iressa and anti-epidermal growth factor drugs seem to work particularly well on patients with adenocarcinoma, particularly non-smokers. In conclusion, non-small cell category is still used to denote treatment and prognosis, but the direction of medical research is towards a more focused approach.

7.2 CELL DIFFERENTIATION

Physicians also classify lung cancer by its cell differentiation. Normal tissue is differentiated while cancerous tissue is haphazard, disorganized if you will:

"When a cell grows and develops normally, it becomes more specialized to perform a particular function in life. This process is called differentiation and it results in irreversible changes in the cell's characteristics. Differentiated cells are mature cells that perform a particular function. For example, a lung cell looks and works like other lung cells. As a cell becomes more differentiated, it becomes more restricted in what it can do . . . . As malignant, or cancerous cells grow and divide, they become less and less differentiated. Eventually, they can no longer perform the functions of the tissue where they originated . . . . The term differentiation is also used to describe how the cells of a tumor appear in comparison to normal cells. For example, tumors that are classified as "well differentiated" still contain cells that resemble normal cells of the original tissue." Alcase, (6).

Tumors are classified this way:

1. *Well differentiated*, (a cell at its earliest stage of carcinogenesis).
2. *Moderately differentiated* (more progression in the change to cancer cells).
3. *Poorly differentiated* (a cell seen as clearly cancerous).

Within those categories, there may be subcategories, such as well to-moderately differentiated, or moderately to poor differentiated. Generally, the level of differentiation is a positive factor in survival with the more differentiated the cancer cell, the less chance of metastasis. One study found the DNA content of poorly differentiated adenocarcinoma significantly greater than that of well-differentiated adenocarcinoma. Carney, (7). Thus, one can assume that the loss of differentiation is associated with increasing DNA mutations in the cell. However, stage rather than differentiation remains the primary factor in determining treatment.

7.21 Related Hormonal Syndromes

Small cell carcinoma can cause a number of hormonal syndromes. "The tumor cells may produce ectopic adrenocorticotropic hormone (ACTH), resulting in Cushing's syndrome. Another paraneoplastic hormone syndrome that commonly occurs is the syndrome of inappropriate anti-diuretic hormone (SIADH). This is caused by secretion of ADH from the tumor.

7.3 SMALL CELL STAGING

Small cell cancer is another type of lung cancer. Because it behaves differently than non-small cell, it has its own staging system. Small cell cancer moves quickly, though, initially, it is usually susceptible to chemotherapy, with complete response (no evidence of cancer on x-ray) not unusual. Sadly the tumors frequently return, and preventing that phenomenon is a central goal for research.

Clinical trials generally do not mix small cell and non-small cell patients. Small cell is staged as limited or extensive, unlike non-small cell which has a four part staging system, with subcategories.

Limited stage carcinomas account for 30% of all cases. Limited stage means the small cell cancer is confined to one of the regional lymph nodes. Regional lymph nodes means lymph nodes in the area where the tumor originates. 70% of small cell carcinomas are extensive meaning at the time of diagnosis, the cancer has spread to other organs, or at least beyond the regional lymph nodes. Because extensive disease is common, patients are evaluated with head CT scan, bone scan, liver scan and bone marrow biopsy to see if any metastasis is present.

7.31 Small Cell Location and Appearance

Over 90% of small cell tumors are found in a central location and they typically grow around major bronchi. The tumor typically extends also to lymph nodes and may invade vascular tissue, which explains why many patients have metastasises at the time of diagnosis.

7.32 Role of Surgery in Small Cell Lung Cancer

With non-small lung cancer, surgery is the preferred option and is invariably used for early stage lung cancers, except when the patient has other significant health problems which create risks for surgery. However, a medical article discusses surgery for small cell lung cancer patients:

"In the 1950's, surgical resection was still considered the preferred treatment of SCLC (small cell lung cancer). However, in a study conducted by the British Medical Research Council in the 1960's, patients were randomly assigned to receive surgery alone or radiotherapy alone; in patients with limited disease, the median survival was 199 days for those receiving surgical treatment versus 300 days for those receiving radiotherapy. On the basis of this study and the discovery of systemic chemotherapeutic agents with activity, surgical treatment for SCLC has been abandoned, and chemotherapy has been used for both limited and extensive disease." Midthun, (8).

Some observations:

1. Scientists determine the validity of certain treatment forms through epidemiological studies. The word epidemiological comes from epidemic and epidemiological studies investigate the patterns of disease, sometimes comparing the impact of disease between two groups receiving different types of treatment.

2. Books like this are intended to provide a general overview, and you need to listen to your physician's advice regarding specific types of treatment, since statements in books and articles can be misinterpreted by patients unaware of subtle difference, for example, differences between non-small cell and small cell. Likewise, your physician should be familiar with recent studies and developments.

3. The National Cancer Institute agrees that surgery has limited utility in small cell lung cancer, but would not agree that surgery has been abandoned. See Chapter Four. One has to be careful of making quick conclusions based upon one or two studies, and you need to measure a study's conclusions against your overall medical knowledge in an area. Perhaps a better way of assessing surgery and small cell cancer is to say that many small cell cancers have already had significant spread at the time of diagnosis. Where there has been such spread, that is movement to lymph nodes or other organs, surgical resection cannot accomplish the goal of completely removing the tumor. However, if we can be persuaded that the entire cancer can be removed, surgery might be appropriate.

7.33 Comparison Among the Different Types

The book Lung Cancer categorizes the different forms of cancer

"In lung cancer, we know that the histological type (type of cell) is one of the most important factors, and that SCLC is most malignant of all; squamous cell carcinoma, adenocarcinoma and large cell are intermediate in terms of malignancy; while carcinoid tumor, adenoid cystic carcinoma and mucocpidermoid carcinoma (all relatively rare) are low grade malignancies." Carney, (7).

REFERENCES

1. Aisner, *Comprehensive Textbook of Thoracic Oncology* (Williams & Wilkins 1996).
2. Castranova *Silica and Silica-Related Diseases* (CRC Publications 1997).
3. Dennis, *Matrix Metalloproteinases Inhibitors: Present Achievements and Future Prospect*, Invest New Drugs 1997;15(3):175-85.
4. Brown, *Matrix Metalloproteinases Inhibitors in the Treatment of Cancer*, Med Oncol 1997 Mar;14(1):1-10.
5. Thomas, *Differential Expression of Matrix Metalloproteinases and Their Inhibitors in Non-Small Cell Lung Cancer*, J Pathol, 2000 02, 190: 2, 150-6.
6. Alcase, *The Lung Cancer Manual* 2.4 (1998)
7. Carney, *Lung Cancer* (Little Brown 1995).
8. Midthun, *Chemotherapy for Advanced Lung Cancer*, Postgraduate Medicine, vol. 101, no. 3, March 1997.
9. Virtual Hospital, Lung Cancer, www.vh.org.
10. Miller, *Lung Cancer, Volume 1 Molecular Pathology*, available in part online at no charge through Google. (2003).

CHAPTER 8

LUNG CANCER STAGES

8.1 NON-SMALL CELL LUNG CANCER STAGES

8.11 The Reason for Classification

Non-small cell lung cancer patients are classified by stage:

> "The relationship between prognosis and the extent of disease at diagnosis derived initially from observations that crude survival, or apparent recovery, rates were higher for patients in whom the disease was localized than for those in whom the disease had extended beyond the organ of origin . . . .
>
> Denoix first emphasized the need for a flexible, reliable cancer classification system based on a generally acceptable description of the facts of the case. {They} developed the TNM system for describing characteristics of the primary tumor (the T component), the status of regional lymph nodes (the "AN" component), and the presence or absence of distant metastasis (the "M" component.)." Pass (1), at 590.

The TNM system provides an objective method of classifying non-small cell lung cancer. Patients with similar characteristics will be treated similarly. While we discussed the different types of lung cancer, squamous, adenocarcinoma, it is the TNM system which is given the greatest weight.

8.12 T1 Tumors

The first criterion is the size of the tumor and its relationship to adjoining structures. A T1 tumor is a small tumor confined to a specific area. Not surprisingly, physicians have excellent success in treating T1 tumors by surgically removing the tumor. Here is the T classification scheme:

T1: A tumor that is 3 cm or less in greatest dimension, surrounded by lung or visceral pleura, and without bronchoscopic evidence of invasion.

T2: A tumor which is more than 3 cm in greatest dimension, or invades the visceral pleura and is associated with atelectasis or obstructive pneumonitis that extends to the hilar region but does not involve the entire lung. Pneumonitis is inflamation, and atelectasis is the collapse of one of the air passages in the lung. T2 means there is some observable area of damage in the location of the tumor or the tumor has grown past 3 centimeters.

T3: A tumor of any size that directly invades any of the following: chest wall (including superior sulcus tumors), diaphragm, mediastinal pleura, parietal pericardium. At T3 we are now less concerned with the size of the tumor than its spread within the lung.

T4: A tumor of any size that invades any of the following: mediastinum, heart, great vessels, trachea, esophagus, vertebral body, carina; or separate tumor nodules in the same lobe; or a tumor with a malignant pleural effusion.

A T3 tumor infiltrates the lining of the mediastinum; a T4 tumor has reached the mediastinal structure itself. Metastasis means a tumor has reached another organ, and this tumor grading gives the same indication. Thus, if a tumor has reached the trachea or esophagus, there is a metastasis.

8.13 Nodes

The second criterion is the nature and extent of lymph node involvement. Note that node evaluation is different from the tumor assessment above. We can have tumors where there has been some spread to adjoining areas, but no spread to a lymph node.

N0: No lymph node involvement.

N1: Metastasis to ipsilateral peribronchial and/or ipsilateral hilar lymph nodes, and intrapulmonary nodes including involvement by direct extension of the primary tumor.

N2: Metastasis to ipsilateral mediastinal and/or subcarinal lymph node(s).

N3: Metastasis to contralateral mediastinal, contralateral hilar, ipsilateral or contralateral scalene, or supraclavicular lymph node(s).

8.14 Metastasis

M designates Metastasis or spread of the tumor to other organs. If the cancer has spread to another organ, surgery again is not likely to be a viable option since the cancer cannot be entirely removed. The physician will want to accurately "stage the patient" not only to assess surgery, but to gauge what type of chemotherapy or radiation is preferred. Here, the staging is simple: either M1, metastasis to another organ, or M0, no metastasis.

8.2 THE INTERNATIONAL STAGING SYSTEM FOR LUNG CANCER, STAGE 1, 2, . . .

The international staging system uses the TNM classification and then gives the patients a number, i.e., stage 1, stage 4. This system is used in the United States, with treatment generally based upon patient stage. The importance of stage in clinical decisions led to the creation of substages, 1A and 1B. Here is a summary:

Stage 1. The cancer is located only in the lung, and has not spread to the lymph nodes. This is the least advanced stage. The treatment recommended for Stage I lung cancer is surgical removal of the tumor which is successful for most patients.

Stage 2. The cancer has spread to the nearby lymph nodes found in the chest near the lungs. Lymph nodes are small-bean shaped structures where cells are stored; nodes can trap cancer cells or bacteria traveling through the body. Depending on the size of the nodes as seen on a CT Scan, a physician may recommend a mediastinoscopy to examine the lymph nodes in the chest and perform a biopsy on them to see whether the nodes are cancerous or enlarged because of inflammation associated with the cancer. If the biopsy shows no signs of cancer in the mediastinal lymph nodes, the physician may recommend surgery followed by radiation and chemotherapy directed to the cancerous lymph nodes.

Stage 3. The cancer is found in the lymph nodes in the middle of the chest away from the lungs. Stage III lung cancer has two types. If the cancer is a single tumor, or mass, it is called Stage III-A. Most doctors will recommend beginning treatment for Stage III-A with chemotherapy, or a combination of anti-cancer drugs, and radiation. If the cancer in the chest has spread to more than one area, it is called Stage III-B. Most doctors do not recommend surgery for Stage III-B. A combination of chemotherapy and radiation is usually of the greatest benefit.

Stage 4. This is the most advanced stage of lung cancer. This is when the cancer has spread to a distant part of the body—for example, the liver, bones, brains, or some other organ. For Stage IV, most doctors are in agreement that chemotherapy is the most effective treatment and different types of chemotherapy will be tested. Because the cancer cannot be removed at this stage, surgery will not be performed, and the patients prognosis for long-term survival is not good. Patients in Stage 4 or Stage 3B are clearly candidates for clinical trials. And while the overall statistical probability for long-term survival is not favorable in Stage 5 where there is metastasis, the patient survival time will vary and there are a small number of cases with more favorable outcomes. Excerpted and modified from Cancercare (4).

Using the TNM classification, we get these stages:

Stage IA   T1N0M0

Stage IB   T2N0M0.

Stage IIA   T1N1M0

Stage IIB   T2N1M0. T1, N1, M0 or T2, N1, M0 or T3, N0, M0 or T1N1M0, or T2, N1, M0

Stage IIIA   T1, N2, M0 or T2, N2, M0 or T3, N1, M0 or T3, N2, M0

Stage IIIB   Any T-T4, N3;

Stage IV   Any M or area of metastasis.

8.21 Small Cell Staging

The above classification scheme is for non-small cell carcinoma—squamous cell, adenocarcinoma, and large cell. Unlike nonsmall cell carcinomas, small cell carcinoma is staged only as limited or extensive, depending on whether or not it has spread outside the chest. Limited stage carcinomas account for only 30% of all cases. Limited stage is confined to one hemothorax and regional lymph nodes (including mediastinal, contralateral hilar, and ipsilateral supraclavicular). Given the prevalence of metastasis, small cell patients are usually evaluated with head CT scan, bone scan, liver scan and bone marrow biopsy to see if there has been metastasis. Occasionally books will use the non-small cell terminology for small cell, even though the stages have different meanings for small cell tumors. For example, while surgery would be the usual treatment for stage 1 non-small cell tumors, it would still be unusual for small cell.

8.22 The Importance of Classification

Survival as well as the nature of treatment is related to lung cancer stage as you will see in chapter four. If a tumor is relatively small, confined to a particular location without involvement of lymph nodes, or other organs, surgical removal of the tumor would be the preferred treatment. In contrast, if the tumor had already spread to other organs, surgery would not accomplish the desired goal since parts of the cancer would remain. Let us review what these three items mean before looking at the classification.

8.23 Stage Related to Survival

Finally, tumor size, nodes, and metastasis are directly related to survival. Survival rates of 60-80% have been reported in TXNoMo patients. That is, patients with microscopic tumors with no lymph node involvement or metastasis. In contrast, appreciably lower survival rates apply when the cancer is much larger, lymph nodes are involved, or metastasis to other organs has occurred.

8.3 TREATMENT OVERVIEW

The particular types of treatment are discussed in detail in the succeeding sections. Because the materials can be somewhat technical, you need to understand the terminology which is used in this area.

8.31 Surgical Options

Surgery is the treatment of choice for non-small cell lung cancer. Ideally, a small cancerous tumor is removed with surrounding tissue and that eliminates the cancer. This is done for smaller tumors, ideally without any lymph node involvement.

The lungs are divided into lobes. There are three lobes on the right lung, two on the left. Lobectomy involves removal of the entire section of one lobe.

8.4 SMALL CELL CANCER CLASSIFICATION

8.41 Characteristics and Subclassifications

The other type of cancer group is small cell which has sub-classifications of oat cell and mixed. Small cell, which acts differently than non-small cell, requires different types of treatment, has its own prognosis, and therefore is separately categorized. It usually originates in large central airways and is composed of sheets of small cells. Small cell carcinoma is a tumor of neuroendocrine origin and is very aggressive, metastasizing early and often. Endocrine cells are associated with growth which probably explains why small cell cancers are aggressive. Small cell carcinoma accounts for approximately 15% to 20% of all lung cancers. Small cell is a high-grade tumor meaning it reproduces and metastasises quickly, but is also responsive to chemotherapy.

REFERENCES

1. Pass, *Lung Cancer* (2000).
2. Aisner, *Comprehensive Textbook of Thoracic Oncology* (Williams & Wilkins 1996).
3. Castranova, *Silica and Silica-Related Diseases* (CRC Publications 1997).
4. Cancercareinc Website.
5. www.temple.edu.

CHAPTER 9

DIAGNOSTIC TOOLS

9.0 THE STATE OF LUNG CANCER DIAGNOSIS TODAY

The majority of patients are diagnosed with advanced tumors which are difficult to treat. There have been a number of tests developed or refined during the last ten years which significantly increase our ability to spot even small lung tumors, accurately diagnose existing ones, and identify recurrences of people already diagnosed.

Despite the tremendous gains, no test for early diagnosis is recommended by major organizations like the American Cancer Society or National Cancer Institute, and it appears no test for followup has been adopted either. Outside of some University hospitals, generally we are not utilizing all the tools available. While some HMO's may be happy that expensive tests are not routinely utilized, many patients should be asking why not. Despite its inaccuracy, the chest x-ray continues to be the main-stay of lung cancer diagnosis.

9.1 CHEST X-RAY

The most widely used diagnostic tool is the chest x-ray. It is economical and easy to use; the typical x-ray takes as little as ten minutes and costs less than $100. However, it is not a reliable method of diagnosing lung cancer and many smaller tumors whose early detection could be critical to the patient's survival are missed with the chest x-ray.

9.11 Chest X-Ray Interpretation Problems

Radiologists are called upon to make critical assessments based upon what are frequently almost imperceptible shadows. The chest contains tissues of different consistency, with air next to thick soft tissue and bone. Adequately producing an image which provides clear definition of all structures in the chest requires meticulous technique and attention to detail. The machine (film processor) used to develop the film should be working properly though up to 50% of x-ray film processors may have some deficiency." (1) While this is the most commonly performed examination, it often isdone incorrectly. Studies have shown that from 20B40% of x-rays are incorrectly interpreted. (1) Indeed, there is a discernible difference in skill among radiologists interpreting chest x-ray films. However, even with good equipment and skilled people, the x-ray is still inaccurate.

9.12 Chest X-Ray Misses Over 75% of Treatable
Stage 1 Tumors

An important 1999 study discussed deficiencies in the chest x-ray, contrasting it with the accuracy of the CT or Cat Scan. In this study 1,000 smokers with no symptoms of disease were evaluated with CT Scan and chest x-ray. 27 of the participants were found to have lung tumors which were detected by CT Scan. However, only 7 of the 27 tumors were detected by chest x-ray! Many corporations trumpet less than 1 in 100 defects for various products and the HLA test for detecting paternity is more than 99.7% accurate. The chest x-ray in contrast was shown here to be less than 30% accurate in the patients who would benefit most by early diagnosis. Not surprisingly, but quite sadly, many patients with advanced lung cancer reveal that they had a prior x-ray which failed to detect the tumor.

Stage 1, or beginning stage, cancers are the most treatable. The results of the chest x-ray in this study for small, stage 1 tumors was even worse. With the Ct Scan, 23 of the 27 tumors were detected at stage 1. However, the chest-ray revealed only 4 of the 23 small, stage 1 tumors. Thus "stage 1 tumors were detected six times more frequently on low-dose CT than on radiography." Note, that this study was done in a clinical context at a well-known hospital. The x-ray machines were presumably working correctly and the slides interpreted by capable radiologists. Even in this context, the chest-ray performed poorly.

The study dealt with smokers with at least 10 pack year histories (pack years are computed by multiplying the number of years smoked by the number of packs smoked per day), who had no symptoms of cancer. Most of the persons detected turned out to have highly treatable cancers. Chest x-rays do detect some tumors, but primarily those at advanced stages which are more difficult to treat. It is a test of limited use, better than nothing, but not even 40 or 50% reliable in detecting small tumors.

Given the unreliability of the x-ray, we hope that physicians will begin using CT Scans to test those at high risk. Certainly, where an x-ray is ambiguous or displays some abnormalities, the prudent physician should order an x-ray. Misread chest x-rays are a chief source of medical malpractice claims. The prudent physician will check his equipment and have all slides read by a qualified radiologist. While that can reduce the possibility of error, it cannot eliminate the inherent limitations of the test.

9.2 SPUTUM CYTOLOGY

Sputum cytology is a microscopic analysis of cells from the lung. After the patient takes a deep cough the liquid or sputum is analyzed by a pathologist and a report prepared. Using sputum cytology, a man named Saccamanno in a landmark study was able to detect the progression of lung cancer in a smoker. This test has the following benefits and limitations:

1. **The test is effective at diagnosing central squamous cell carcinomas,** even at microscopic levels, imperceptible on a chest-ray and perhaps a CT Scan. Thus, it has utility in detecting certain tumors at an early stage when the disease can be cured.
2. Non-small cell lung cancer includes squamous cell cancer and adenocarcinoma. **Squamous cell cancer is generally located in the larger central airways, while adenocarcinomas tend towards the smaller, peripheral airways of the lung.** The nature of the test is to retrieve liquid in the lungs, and the patient is more likely to cough up liquid from the larger more central parts of the bronchial tree, than the parts of the smaller airways

that produce adenocarcinoma. Thus, the test is effective at diagnosing squamous cell cancers, but less effective at detecting adenocarcinomas. While squamous cell remains the most common form of cancer, with low tar cigarette smokers inhaling more deeply, the number of adenocarcinomas in the peripheral airways is almost equal.

3. The European Cancer Institutes states, "Sputum cytological analysis is greater for squamous (93%) or small cell (89%) histotypes than for adenocarcinoma (25%) and large cell carcinoma (54%)." (2)

Thus, sputum cytology is a good tool for detecting some lung tumors, but not others. Used with Ct Scan, the two become a reliable method of detecting lung cancer in its early stages. The test is inexpensive, running in the $100.00 range.

9.21 Recent Advances in Detection of Lung Cancer with Sputum Cytology

Sputum cytology is an economical, non-invasive way of detecting lung cancer in its earliest and most treatable stage, with its primary drawback difficulty in detecting adenocarcinomas. However, a recent study indicated progress in refining sputum cytology to improve detection of adenocarcinoma:

> "Lam and colleagues developed a computer-assisted and automated image analysis method that detects aneuploidy and nuclear abnormalities in sputum samples. Between 5000 and 10,000 cells are stained with a Feulgen thionine DNA cellular stain, analyzed with a digital camera, and then screened using computer-assisted algorithms. In a series presented at the presidential symposium, Lam reported results showing that this screening technique was 70% sensitive for stage 0/1 lesions and 80% for adenocarcinomas, with a specificity of 90%." Lynch, 9th World Conference on Lung Cancer, (2000) citing, Lam (3).

Others are testing sputum cytology to detect P-53 mutations. If the test can be developed, we would have an inexpensive and reliable method of detecting lung cancer in its earliest and most curable stages.

9.3 COMPUTERIZED TOMOGRAPHY OR CT SCAN

Computerized tomography or CT uses a beam that rotates around the body to produce a series of pictures taken from different angles. See www.colorado HealthNet.org/cancerlung.symptoms.html. This information is then processed by computer to produce a cross-section of a specific area. CT can reveal the existence of a tumor, and specifics about its location and size. Today, CT is the best non-surgical method of detecting lung cancer and revealing its size and status.

9.31 Accuracy of the CT Scan in Diagnosing Lung Cancer, even Small Nodules

The Early Lung Cancer Detection survey found a high rate of reliability in detecting tumors:

"Compared with chest radiography, low-dose CT greatly increases the likelihood of detection of small non-calcified nodules and, thus, of lung cancer at an earlier and more curable stage. On low-dose CT, non-calcified nodules were detected three times as commonly as on chest radiography, malignant tumours four times as commonly, and stage I tumours six times as commonly. Moreover, the malignant tumours detected on low-dose CT were substantially smaller than those detected on chest radiography, even within stage I (table 3); 15 (56%) of the CT-detected tumours (13 [57%] of those in stage I) were of size 10 mm or less compared with only two of those detected on chest radiography. 26 (96%) of the 27 CT-detected lung cancers were resectable, a striking improvement over the Mayo Lung Project results, in which only 30 (51%) of the 59 tumours detected on baseline chest radiography were resectable. . . . low-dose CT greatly increased the likelihood of detection of malignant disease; ten times as many were detected on CT as on radiography." Hentschke, (4).

9.32 Should X-Rays Continue to Be Used Where We Have a Far More Reliable Test?

The tremendous accuracy of the Ct Scan, combined with the inaccuracy of the x-ray raises serious questions about whether x-rays should continue to be used as a tool for diagnosing lung cancer. Yes, the x-rays are cheaper, but should we continue to use a tool 25% as accurate in diagnosing small tumors simply to save money. Indeed, x-rays can provide a false sense of security.

9.33 CT Scan to Detect the Nature and Extent of Disease

Physicians go beyond using Ct as a device to detect cancer to using it to determine the extent of disease. CT is used to provide a picture of whether a tumor has infiltrated lymph nodes or other organs, and one study found the CT to be 80% effective in determining whether there was cancer in lymph nodes.

9.34 Test Specificity and Accuracy

Let us review these terms which are frequently used with medical tests. A false negative occurs where the patient has a disease or characteristic and the test fails to detect that. Thus, the test is falsely or incorrectly negative; it should have been positive. Another word for false negative is accuracy. That is, what percentage of persons with a given disease are detected. If the CT is 80% accurate in detecting lymph node metastases, its accuracy or false negative rate is 80%.

Specificity is the number of false positives. That is, how many tests are incorrectly read as positive. For example, a person with inflamed nodes could have a CT Scan read as positive for spread of the cancer to the node.

9.4 BRONCHOSCOPY

If Ct Scan is the most reliable non-invasive test, bronchoscopy is the most reliable minimally invasive test. While bronchoscopy should be viewed as a surgical procedure, its risks are generally minimal. The Virtual Hospital is an excellent site which describes bronchoscopy:

> "Bronchoscopy is the examination of the airways under direct visualization. Bronchoscopy began with the use of a candle and a rod with a polished metal disk to visualize the osopharaynx. It has evolved into a wide variety of precision optical instruments capable of visualizing the endobronchial tree to the 5th or 6th generation . . . .

Bronchoscopy is used to obtain peripheral lung samples in the presence of lung parenchymal disease such as peripheral coin lesion(s), hilar adenopathy, or diffuse or focal parenchymal infiltrates. Finally, bronchoscopy is useful in staging lung cancer, evaluating the airways in patients with normal radiographic findings and positive sputum cytology, and evaluating the airways after thoracic trauma, or if there is a suspected airway foreign body." Virtual Hospital, (6).

9.41 How the Patient Feels During a Bronchoscopy?

Here is what the patient will experience:

"The surgeon makes a small incision in the skin on the chest with a scalpel. The biopsy needle is inserted into the lung. You may feel a sharp, temporary pain when the biopsy needle touches the lung. A small amount of lung tissue is removed. Biopsy needle and syringe are removed. Adhesive bandage is applied to the biopsy site. Tissue is sent to the laboratory for analysis." Healthgate (13)

9.42 Reliability of the Bronchoscopy

Reliability seems to depend upon the location of the tumor.

"Tumors may be present in three ways in the lung, as central endoscopically visible lesions, as submucosal or extrinsic lesions, and as peripheral lung lesions. The diagnostic yield and bronchoscospic approach to diagnose these lesions varies among these three presentations. In endobronchial visible lesions, bronchoscopy will correctly diagnose the lesion in 94% of the cases if at least 5 samples of the lesion are obtained . . . ."

By contrast, direct forceps biopsy correctly diagnoses only 27% of patients with extrinsic airway compression or with submucosal oreribronchial disease. The low yield is most likely due to the fact that the forceps biopsy does not sample tissue deep enough. Much better diagnostic results are obtained in this situation by using transbronchial needle aspiration. In this technique, a 1 cm. needle attached to a catheter is placed through the mucosa using the bronchoscopy . . . . The diagnostic yield for peripheral lung lesions varies widely from 30-90% using transbronchial biopsies. In this technique, the forceps are passed through the airways distal to the directly visualized sites using fluoroscopy." Virtual Hospital,(6).

Sadly, some people have gone undiagnosed after a physician failed to detect a tumor during a bronchoscopy. The above highlights the following:

1. Bronchoscopy is not a conclusive test. Where symptoms of lung cancer continue, and a definitive diagnosis of another disease is not made, additional diagnostic tests must be done. Where a patient seems to fit the profile of a lung cancer patient— significant smoking history, loss of weight, fatigue, chest pain, cough, and has other symptoms of the disease, a repeat bronchoscopy, needle biopsy, or even a thoracatomy (surgical biopsy) may be called for with a negative bronchoscopy. Timely diagnosis of lung cancer is critical.

2. Success in detecting the tumor will depend upon the tumor's location and to some extent, the skill of the physician performing the procedure.

3. An adequate sampling is critical. Reports should clearly indicate how many samples have been taken so the extent of reliance on the bronchoscopy can be determined by other physicians.

9.5 PET SCANS

PET or Positron Emission Tomography is a useful tool for diagnosing lung cancer and ascertaining the extent of disease.

9.51 How Does PET Work?

Here is one description of the PET process:

"Glycolysis is increased in tumor tissues. {A glucose analogue is} used in positron emission tomography (PET) to trace glucose metabolism. All 82 patients with lung cancer had increased FDG uptake in the lungs, whereas only 12 of 25 patients with nonmalignant diseases had increased FDG uptake. Sixteen lung cancer patients with mediastinal metastasises had increased FDG uptake in the mediastinum, of whom three had no lymphadenopathy on computed tomography of the chest. Sixteen lung cancer patients without mediastinal nodal involvement had no FDG uptake in the mediastinum. Seven of these patients had lymphadenopathy on computed tomography. FDG-PET imaging is 100% accurate in predicting mediastinal involvement in patients with lung cancer. It is 100% sensitive and 52% specific in predicting the malignant nature of a chest radiographic abnormality." Sazon,(7).

Recent medical literature has trumpeted PET:

"The use of positron emission tomography (PET) with fluorine-18-fluorodeoxyglucose (FDG) has become a valuable tool in the detection of a variety of tumors including lung cancer . . . . FDG-PET had a sensitivity, specificity and accuracy of 98.0%, 78.6% and 93.8%, respectively, in detecting malignant pulmonary nodules. In N staging, sensitivity, specificity and accuracy were 66.7%, 81.3% and 76.0%, respectively. In M staging, the accuracy was 100% . . . . In our observations, whole-body 18FDG-PET images improved diagnostic accuracy in the evaluation of lung lesions and the staging of lung cancer." (8).

Its sensitivity is excellent, and it can detect many small tumors. The difficulty is that some normal areas may show as hotspots causing concerns, and occasionally unneeded surgery. Pet may be useful as an early detection tool for those at risk, such as heavy smokers. The high rate of false positives leads us to question its use as a screening device for the population at large. A new test, combined Pet/Ct, combines the benefits of both sets, creating a diagnostic tool that is both sensitive (detects most tumors) and specific (does not creates false positives).

9.52 Combined PET and Ct Scan

The new device combines a PET Scan with a Ct Scan, providing a reading from both devices for the radiologist and a single seating for the patient. Items which could be misdiagnosed as cancer are eliminated, while the combined tests reduces the possibility that serious lesions are missed:

> "Integrated PET-CT provided additional information in 20 of 49 patients (41 percent), beyond that provided by conventional visual correlation of PET and CT. Integrated PET-CT had better diagnostic accuracy than the other imaging methods. Tumor staging was significantly more accurate with integrated PET-CT than with CT alone (P=0.001), PET alone (P<0.001), or visual correlation of PET and CT."

Some insurers may balk at the increased cost, and the tool may only be available at modern research facilities. However, its greater accuracy means it provides information unavailable in other modalities so insurance should be required to pay the cost.

9.6 OTHER TOOLS FOR MOLECULAR ANALYSIS OF CELLS

9.61 Flow Cytometry

Cancer cells may be analyzed to assess their structure and DNA. Flow cytometry measures how many pairs of chromosomes the cell's DNA contains. See American Cancer Society, (11). If a cell has a normal number of chromosomes, it is diploid. If the cell has severely disrupted DNA, it is said to be aneuploid.

9.62 S-phase Faction, SPF

SPF measures the percentage of diseased cells in the synthesis phase of cell division. If the number is high, a great percentage of cells are in the S-phase and dividing rapidly, indicating the tumor is growing quickly. American Cancer Society, (11). A low SPF indicates a slow-growing tumor. Both flow cytometry and SPF show promise in providing an early indication of disease, though neither are routinely recommended for screening purposes.

9.63 P-53 Analysis

P-53 is an important tumor suppressor gene and we discuss its function in a separate chapter. A few words here. P-53 testing is being investigated as a means to identify early tumors, and changes in tumors already identified.

9.64 EGFR Analysis

The epidermal growth factor receptor binds with the epidermal growth factor and then through its tyrosine kinase initiates a chemical change called phosphylation which can contribute to carcinogenic processes. Patients with a malfunctioning tyrosine kinase may respond to Iressa, a new drug which targets this tyrosine kinase. The Harvard Center for Genetics and Genomics now has a test which measures damage to the tyrosine kinase. (Harvard (14). Patients with such damage may consider Iressa while others without this damage may consider other options. An analysis is performed on exons 18-24, the tyrosine kinase domain of EGFR, but the test does not detect errors in the entire gene.

REFERENCES

1. www.chest.x-ray.com.
2. The European Cancer Institute.
3. Lam et. al, *Lung Cancer Control Strategy in the New Millennium.* Lung Cancer. 2000;29(Suppl 2):145.
4. Hentschke, *Early Lung Cancer Action Project: Baseline Screening,* Lancet, 1999, 354, 99-105.
5. www.chestx-ray.com/StaginglungCa/Lung Cancer.
6. Virtual Hospital, Lung Tumors: A Multidisciplinary Database, Bronchoscopy, www.vh.org/Providers/Textbooks/LungTumors/Diagnosis/Bronchoscopy/bronchosopy.htm.
7. Sazon, *Fluorodeoxyglucose-Positron Emission Tomography in the Detection and Staging of Lung Cancer,* Am J Respir Crit Care Med 1996 Jan;153(1):417-21.
8. *Evaluation of Whole Body Positron Emission Tomography Imaging in the Clinical Diagnosis of Lung Cancer,* Kokyuki Gakkai Zasshi 2000 Sep;38(9):676-81.

9. Dunagan, *Staging by Positron Emission Tomography Predicts Survival in Patients with Non-Small Cell Lung Cancer,*Chest 2001 Feb;119(2):333-9.
10. N. Engl J Med 2000 Jul 27;343(4):254-61.
11. American Cancer Society, *Informed Decisions* 136 (1997).
12. Lardinois, *Staging of Non-Small-Cell Lung Cancer with Integrated Positron-Emission Tomography and Computed Tomography.* N Engl J Med. 2003 Jun 19;348(25):2500-7.
13. www.Healthgate.com.
14. Harvard Medical School, Center for Genetics and Genomics, Cambridge, Massachusetts www.hpcgg.org/LMM/comment/EGFR_info_101404.html.

CHAPTER 10

SURGERY AND DIAGNOSTIC PROCEDURES

10.1 SURGICAL DIAGNOSTIC PROCEDURES

10.11 Types of Biopsies

A biopsy is usually the first surgical procedure a patient will undergo. It involves taking a piece of tissue and having it analyzed by a pathologist to determine its cellular makeup. A biopsy can determine whether the cells taken are cancerous and sometimes determine the level of differentiation in the tissue. The excellent website called Oncolink reviews the different types of biopsies which include aspiration, needle, excisional, and incisional. The approach used depends on the type of tumor suspected, its size, location, and characteristics of growth . . .

Aspiration of cells and tissue fragments through a needle that has been guided to a suspected malignant tissue. Cytological analysis can provide a tentative diagnosis. Since the tumor can be missed, only a positive test is diagnostically significant.

Needle obtaining a core of tissue through a specially designed needle introduced into suspected malignant tissue. Sufficient for the diagnosis of most tumors. Differentiating benign or reparative lesions from malignancies is often difficult with soft tissue and bony sarcomas. Since the tumor can be missed, only a positive test is diagnostically significant.

Incisional Removal of a small wedge of tissue from a larger tumor mass. Preferred method for diagnosing soft tissue and bony sarcomas.

Excisional Removal of the entire suspected tumor tissue. Procedure of choice for small, accessible tumors when they can be done without compromising the ultimate procedure." (1).

10.12 Other Diagnostic Procedures

A mediastinoscopy is a diagnostic procedure to test whether mediastinal lymph nodes are positive. Recall the mediastinum is an area of the chest. If multiple nodes are positive, surgery might not be recommended because it would not eliminate the cancer and open chest surgery could involve significant risk. The procedure involves inserting a crop through a small incision in the neck or chest into the mediastinum where the nodes in that areas are viewed and tested. A thorascopy is a limited surgical procedure that allows the lining of the chest wall and the lungs to be examined for tumor. A thorascopy is inserted through a small incision in the chest wall. These procedures are diagnostic, they do not attempt to cure the cancer, but determine its existence and extent.

10.2 TYPES OF SURGERY

10.21 When is Surgery Performed

Surgery is the preferred form of treatment. In the best of circumstances, surgery involves the removal of the entire tumor and the elimination of disease. That result becomes less possible as the tumor spreads and invades other structures. Thus, surgery is less likely to be an option as the cancer advances.

10.22 Surgery and Stage 1

Surgery is routinely recommended for stage 1 non-small cell patients in good physical condition. For this group, surgery is a complete cure in 55-80% of patients, with results varying upon the precise extent of disease, the physical status of the patients, and differences among study groups.

10.23 Surgery and Stage 2 Patients

Surgery is recommended for most stage 2 patients, that is, patients with limited nodal involvement.

10.24 Surgery and Stage 3 and 4 Patients

Surgery is sometimes performed upon 3A patients. Surgery is generally is not performed upon stage 3B and Stage 4 patients, that is, patients with advanced cancer. The reasoning is that is major surgery, frequently with smokers having other health problems, and the risk associated with surgery are not justified because it will be impossible to remove all the cancer.

Where the patient has other significant health problems, surgery may not be recommended, for example, for an 84 year old man with significant heart problems. Surgery removes the lung tumor and surrounding tissue. If the patient has severe breathing problems, he may lack sufficient pulmonary reserve to permit surgery.

10.25 Lobectomy and Pneumonectomy

There are two basic types of surgery to remove a lung tumor, lobectomy and pneumonectomy. Lobectomy is surgical removal of one of the lobes of the lung. Less intrusive procedures like a wedge resection, removal of part of the lobe have been tried, but cancer reoccurred in greater percentages so they are not generally used. A bilbectomy is the removal of two lung lobes. A pneumonectomy is the removal of the entire lung, and would be used where the cancer may involve substantial portions of the lung. Thoracotomy is the general name for surgery to examine the lung and remove cancerous portions. Yahoo has a good brief explanation:

> "A thoracatomy is a surgical procedure to open the chest and repair or remove lung tissue. While the patient is deep asleep and pain-free (general anesthesia), an incision is made between the ribs to expose the lung. The chest cavity will be examined and diseased lung tissue will be removed. (All or portions of relevant lymph nodes will be removed and undergo pathology testing to see if they are cancerous). A drainage tube is inserted to drain air, fluid

and blood out of the chest cavity and the ribs and skin are closed. Hospital stay is usually 7 to 10 days. Deep breathing is important to help prevent pneumonia, infection and re-expand the lung. The chest tube remains in place until the lung has fully re-expanded. Pain is managed with medications. The patient recovers fully in 1-3 months after the operation." (2).

10.3 VIDEO-ASSISTED THOROSCOPIC SURGERY

10.31 Benefits of Laparoscopic Surgery

In recent years, surgeons have utilized modern technology in surgery, particularly the television camera. Laparoscopic surgery, use of a laparoscopy together with a television camera has now been used for a number of years in many gall bladder removals and certain gynecological procedures. Recently, some have begun using this type of television aided surgery in lung procedures. The advantages of the camera-aided procedures are as follows: by using and moving a camera during surgery, much smaller incisions can be used. For example, with laparascopic gall bladder removal, four small incisions are used instead of the large one with traditional surgery. Thus, there is an appreciably smaller scar and shorter recovery period. With this video-assisted lung surgeries, it may not be necessary to break a rib to enter the area where the lung is located, as is done with standard surgery. Thus, we have a less intrusive surgery, reduced pain, smaller scar, and quicker recovery time.

10.32 Potential Problems with Laparoscopic Surgery

Using our knowledge of laparoscopic procedures, we can suggest the following drawbacks with video-assisted thorascopic surgery. In nine out of ten procedures, the result is a quicker, less intrusive surgery, with a smaller scar and quicker recovery. However, using these new procedures requires significant skill and there is a high learning curve. There is less, or at least different, visibility with a video-assisted procedure; the surgeon now relies on a television camera. Thus if there are anatomical anomalies or other problems, the surgeon could be hindered by his lack of direct visibility. If a serious problem arises, the procedure will have to be converted to an open or traditional procedure, creating a small amount of added risk.

We can identify two potential problems. First, a surgeon inexperienced with this type of procedure will present greater risks. With such a procedure, you want a surgeon highly experienced with this procedure, at a hospital which it is also routinely done. Secondly, given the reduced or at least different visibility and the need to convert the procedure if problems arise, use may be limited for patients with other significant health problems.

RELEVANT FACTORS	IDEAL PROFILE	PROBLEM PROFILE
DR.'S EXPERTISE	Extensive experience, over 100 surgeries of this exact type performed.	Limited experience (note that this will not be quickly revealed)
HOSPITAL	Excellent hospital with years of experience performing this particular type	New to hospital, nurses and others learning how it works
GENERAL HEALTH	Excellent health other than the cancer	Existing health problems such as COPD Chronic Obstructive Pulmonary Disorder or heart problems, present additional risks
STATUS OF THE TUMOR	Small stage 1 tumor	Stage 2, or 3, more complicated surgery.

10.4 HOSPITAL STAYS

U.S. News and World Report provides an excellent rating system for cancer centers. With experience and specialization, we can expect that care at these top hospitals will be better.

10.41 Specialization

A recent study found lower rates of mortality when patients were operated upon by thoracic surgeons, rather than general surgeons. Silvestri, (3). Likewise, hospitals which perform a large number of particular procedures report better results. Begg,(4) ("Hospitals that treat a relatively high volume of patients for selected surgical oncology procedures report lower surgical in-hospital mortality rates than hospitals with a low volume of the procedures.").

> "The volume of procedures at the hospital was positively associated with the survival of patients (P<0.001). Five years after surgery, 44 percent of patients who underwent operations at the hospitals with the highest volume were alive, as compared with 33 percent of those who underwent operations at the hospitals with the lowest volume. Patients at the highest-volume hospitals also had lower rates of postoperative complications (20 percent vs. 44 percent) and lower 30-day mortality (3 percent vs. 6 percent) than those at the lowest-volume hospitals."

Thus, as in many other areas, experience in doing the same task is the best predictor of success. The more delicate, unusual, or risky the procedure, the more likely you want it performed by a surgeon experienced with the surgery. In some cases, this may prompt to consult a specialized university hospital.

10.5 REDUCING THE RISKS OF SURGERY

10.51 Problems at Night

Care in ICU (intensive care units) following surgery is usually excellent. One nurse may monitor 3 or 4 patients, constantly checking for small changes in heart rate and other vital functions, and ready to notify physicians of potential problems. Outside of ICU, even the best hospitals are facing increasing financial pressures, with HMO's constantly looking to reduce costs and limit reimbursement.

HMO's typically negotiate fixed reimbursements to participating hospitals. A large HMO will approach a hospital offering to list the hospital on its participation list, in exchange for the hospital's agreement to accept reduced sums for care. Those hospitals which refuse such arrangements may find the number of patients reduced. Hospitals in the last 10 years have accepted lower reimbursement rates, placing increasing pressure on the hospitals to cut costs, which may include limiting the number of nurses per shift.

Care during days at most hospitals may be sufficient, with problems occurring at night. Few nurses and staff wish to work at night, and with limited budgets, there are frequent staffing problems at many hospitals which will not be apparent to the average patient or his family. Hospitals limit visiting hours and family members may not think to visit at 2:00 or 3:00 A.M. In some city hospitals, a single nurse may be responsible for monitoring many patients in serious condition, and the care can be substandard but unnoticed.

10.511 Private Duty Nurses and Family Monitoring

Consider hiring a nurse or health care aid to assist in monitoring the patient during the night when problems are least likely to be detected. Unfortunately, insurance is unlikely to cover this type of expense. A private duty nurse may cost from $250-500 for an 8 hour shift, with a health care worker costing somewhat less. Such costs can strain the budgets of many families.

Alternatively, consider having a family member sleep over or remain in the room through the night to help the patient and alert nurses to any problems. If a private room is available, the sleeping accommodations are easy. Alternatively, a family member might have to remain in a chair or sleep during the day. It is important because we do not have the luxury of 24 hour closely monitored care in most hospitals. It is appropriate that all family members help after surgery and one will note that the Sixth Commandment is not limited to women.

Legally, injuries arising from a lack of staff are not always malpractice, and in any case, may be difficult to detect. One is not entitled to the best care, but simply care which meets average standards. Thus, following major surgery with most hospitals having limited staff, many family members will want to play the important role in checking the patient and notifying hospital staff of problems.

10.6 DEALING WITH YOUR DOCTOR

As medical testing has become more sophisticated and expensive, personal contact has decreased. The number of calm and compassionate physicians who can spend an hour with a patient dealing with not only medical questions but the entire patient is decreasing. Some doctors may see 35-40 patients per day and spend some of the scarce remaining time arguing with insurance carriers over reimbursement issues. What does this mean?

As a patient, you need to prepare for your examination. If you are experiencing pain or discomfort, try to identify the nature and type.

REFERENCES

1. http://oncolink.upenn.edu.
2. http://health.yahoo.com.
3. Silvestri, *Specialists Achieve Better Outcomes than Generalists for Lung Cancer Surgery*, Chest, Vol 114, 675-680.
4. Begg, *Impact of Hospital Volume on Operative Mortality for Major Cancer Surgery*, JAMA 1998 Nov 25;280(20):1747.
5. Bach, *The Influence of Hospital Volume on Survival after Resection for Lung Cancer*, Vol. 345: 181-88 New England Journal of Medicine, July 19, 2002.

CHAPTER 11

CHEMOTHERAPY

11.0 OVERVIEW

11.01 Chemotherapy's Role in Lung Cancer

Most patients are diagnosed with later stages of this disease, and chemotherapy is the primary form of therapy for later-stage disseminated forms of lung cancer. Chemotherapy has the capacity to limit the tumor's growth, improve quality of life, and reduce pain and discomfort.

For some cancers, chemotherapy serves as a cure. That is, unfortunately, not the case with lung cancer and chemotherapy's purpose is instead, to relieve symptoms and prolong life. Patients survive longer with chemotherapy, though the benefits are not enormous. "Several meta-analyses were required in the 1990s to convince many clinicians that chemotherapy does have a small, but statistically significant, impact on survival when compared with best supportive care."

Since the ordinary course of lung cancer is metastasis, chemotherapy holds out the best possibility of cure or extension of life. Without any treatment, the patient is not likely to survive an extended period and chemotherapy remains the standard treatment for metastatic disease, though gene therapies are being developed and studied. Clinical trials measure partial response, and with most chemotherapy drugs partial responses are in the 20-25% range. That is, 50% of tumor volume has been reduced as seen on x-ray or Ct Scan, though it may later return.

11.02 Cure

The number of complete responses or overall cures is limited, though they do exist. Willis wrote the Cancer Patient's Workbook three years after her diagnosis of stage 4 lung cancer, surprising her doctors with excellent results from chemotherapy. Participants in online newsgroups report survival 2, 3, and even 5 years from diagnosis, encouraging others to have a positive attitude. Long-term or 5 year survivals are also seen in clinical trials. With both complete and partial responses, tumors can reoccur through a complex process called multi-drug resistance (MDR) where the cancer cells become resistant to chemotherapy. Cures are rare though not unknown.

11.03 Statistical Problems

Statistics vary, so defining chemotherapy's benefit is difficult for several reasons. First, the majority of statistics are maintained through clinical trials. Many patients enter clinical trials with very advanced disease, lessening the possibility of cure. Thus, these statistics are likely to understate the possibility of cure. In addition to an increase in survival time, many studies show an improvement in quality of life. This is because the chemotherapy can reduce the symptoms associated with lung cancer. While the drugs may cause side effects, many scientists believe that chemotherapy related side effects are less than the effects of the disease without effective treatment.

11.04 Platinum-Based Therapy as the Principal Regimen

The American Society of Clinical Oncology treatment guidelines in 1997 for unresectable disease concluded: "In stage IV disease, chemotherapy prolongs survival and is most appropriate for individuals with good performance status. Chemotherapy given to NSCLC patients should be a platinum-based regimen." Schiller (17)

11.05 No Optimal Drug Combination Has been Determined

Specific drugs and combinations continue to be studied and debated. There are at least six drugs with roughly equal effectiveness; that is the percentage of partial responses in scientific studies are within 5% of one another. The percentage of partial responses remains in the 25% area, with some variation from study to study, or drug to drug. The advantages of one drug or drug combination over another remain small and two physicians could legitimately prescribe different drugs for the same patient.

Clinical trials continue to investigate the success of different combinations, with trials yielding varying and sometimes contradictory results. Trials generally divide patients by stage and category and it is possible that the particular type of tumor, squamous, adeno or large cell, might play a role in a drug's effectiveness, or other factors as well.

Cisplatin (and its analogue Carboplatin), Taxol, Gemcitabine and Etopiside are the major drugs; but 5 or 6 other drugs have shown results in clinical trials.

Scientists are improving ways of relieving chemotherapy-related discomfort. The nausea and vomiting associated with some chemotherapy has been significantly reduced. A book entitled Living Well with Cancer states,

> "We would like to stress the fact that cancer treatment has changed dramatically in the past decade. Almost all of the nausea and vomiting that people experienced in the past is now controlled or even prevented by excellent and readily available antinausea medication." Moore (15)

Drugs have been altered and improved, and medicine to minimize nausea is sometimes prescribed with the therapy. For some patients however, the effects of chemotherapy must be constantly reevaluated and those who find the treatment particularly difficult, and who are in poor health from the disease, may choose to end chemotherapy. The decisions can be difficult for the family and patient. Second-line chemotherapy refers to the second drug used, and while many will try chemotherapy, at some point many with advanced stage 4 disease will stop. Chemotherapy for patients with advanced disease can release the symptoms of the disease and prolong life but usually cannot provide a cure.

11.06 "Chemo" or Chemical Therapy

The term "Chemo" means chemical and chemotherapy can be broadly defined as the use of drugs to treat cancer. In that vein the term anti-cancer drug is simpler.

Chemotherapy generally mean drugs which target dividing cells. By preventing or inhibiting cell division, chemotherapy drugs frustrate the cancer process, though they can also impact normal cells. Chemotherapy drugs may affect the immune system since white blood cells reproduce and divide quickly and thus may also be affected by chemotherapy.

In contrast, some forms of gene therapy like Iressa, are narrowly crafted to attach only to certain growth factor receptors. While reducing the impact on normal cells and tailoring a drug to attach specific areas are laudable goals, the question remains whether that type of limited approach will be as successful as chemotherapy. In any case, we should try to distinguish traditional chemotherapy drugs which impact numerous types of dividing cells, from the newer gene therapies which attempt to deal with the cancer process by attacking receptors or specific targets. There have been few studies comparing traditional chemotherapy with gene therapy. Laboratory studies indicate that since the two approach cancer in different ways, ultimately they will be used together. Semantically, I will use the term chemotherapy to denote those therapies which target the cell division process, though I must acknowledge there is no completely clear dividing line.

11.07 The Advantages of Multi-Modal Chemotherapy

The mechanisms by which chemotherapy drugs attempt to attack cancer are varied. Since the drugs perform different functions, if side effects could be managed, it would make sense to use a number of different drugs simultaneously to attack cancer and that is what is being done today. For patients who are in otherwise good health and not of advanced age, drug combinations are prescribed, sometimes with radiation.

Generally, chemotherapy targets any area where cancer cells are located, in comparison to surgery and radiation which target defined areas. Chemotherapy may be used to reduce tumors, or in some cases, prevent the development of cancer in particular areas. These drugs generally destroy cancer cells by stopping them from growing or multiplying at one or more points in their life cycle. Most oncologists will recommend multi-modal chemotherapy (more than one drug), though the best mix of drugs is not known with clinical trials yielding varying results. The task is to provide a large enough dose to successfully attack the cancer while not unduly affecting the normal cells.

11.1 THE FDA APPROVAL PROCESS

The Food and Drug Administration (FDA) regulates prescription drugs. Prescription drugs must be given with a doctor's supervision and have FDA approval for use in the United States. FDA approval comes after review of clinical trials and other data to determine the safety and effectiveness of a particular drug. For example, the FDA refused to approve Thalidomide in the early 1960's believing that adequate information about its safety had not been provided, notwithstanding the drug's use in Europe. Subsequently, it was found that the drug caused serious birth defects.

11.11 FDA Approval is Organ and Treatment Specific

Cancer or chemotherapy drugs are not approved for all purposes. Instead the FDA generally recommends their use to certain organs and sometimes in certain doses. For example, look at this FDA approval:

> "FDA today approved Taxotere for treating non-small cell lung cancer that does not respond to cisplatin-based chemotherapy . . . Taxotere was approved for treatment of patients with locally advanced or metastatic non-small cell lung cancer after failure of prior cisplatin-based chemotherapy. Most patients with non-small cell lung cancer are found to have metastatic disease (cancer which has spread to other organs) when diagnosed, and curative treatment is not possible. Two randomized controlled clinical trials demonstrated that patients treated with Taxotere had increased survival compared to patients receiving supportive care or cancer therapy consisting of either vinorelbine or ifosfamide." FDA. (18).

The approval denotes the type of cancer covered, the status of the patient, and the circumstances of use.

11.12 Off-Label Use

While the approval is for a specific use, a doctor may decide to utilize the drug for other purposes, so-called off-label use. Such use varies since a physician may worry that an unusual use of a drug may lead to liability if a patient's condition worsens. Some insurers do not cover off-label use.

11.13 Regular and Accelerated Approval Programs

Most drugs are approved under the FDA's regular approval program. However, where there is no existing cure for a disease at a particular stage, the FDA may utilize an accelerated approval program:

> "Regular approval is based on end points that demonstrate that the drug provides a longer life, a better life, or a favorable effect on an established surrogate for a longer life or a better life. Accelerated approval (AA) is based on a surrogate end point that is less well established but that is reasonably likely to predict a longer or a better life . . . . End points other than survival were the approval basis for 68% (39 of 57) of oncology drug marketing applications granted regular approval and for all 14 applications granted accelerated approval." Johnson (16)

11.2 HOW DOES CHEMOTHERAPY WORK

11.21 Chemotherapy Generally Targets Rapidly Growing Cells

Chemotherapy attacks all body cells to some extent, but targets rapidly dividing cells such as cancer cells. Its effect on other rapidly dividing cells such as hair follicles, cells lining the stomach, and red blood cells, accounts for many of its side effects. Almost all of the drugs used in chemotherapy suppress cancer by somehow altering the cells' DNA and thus their ability to reproduce. See Bruning, (1) (an excellent book written by a woman with breast cancer).

11.22 What Does Cell-Cycle Specific Chemotherapy Mean?

Almost all the drugs used in chemotherapy suppress cancer by altering the cells' DNA and thus their ability to replicate or reproduce. Since DNA is most vulnerable to drug interference during the reproductive phases of the life cycle, cancer cells are more likely to be affected than are the bulk of the body's normal cells, which reproduce at a much more relaxed pace. Thus, the very characteristic that makes cancer so dangerous has in some cases helped to contribute to its undoing. Indeed, some rapidly growing cancers such as small cell cancer are particularly susceptible to chemotherapy.

11.23 Adjuvant Therapy, Combining Chemotherapy with Other Therapy

Sometimes chemotherapy is the only therapy a patient receives. One advantage of primary chemotherapy is that because the cancer cells have not yet been exposed to anticancer drugs, they may be more vulnerable. A case of primary chemotherapy could be a patient with a severe heart problem who could not tolerate surgery and chemotherapy would be the exclusive form of treatment. The disadvantage of such chemotherapy is that the drugs must destroy a larger target, since none of the cells were removed by surgery or diminished by radiation.

Chemotherapy used in addition to surgery or radiation is called adjuvant therapy (adjuvant or in addition to). Chemotherapy is sometimes used after surgery and/or radiation therapy to help destroy any cancer cells that may remain.

11.24 Considerations Before Treatment Begins

Because chemotherapy can be harmful to certain organs, preliminary tests are conducted. For example, cells in the bone marrow frequently divide and therefore like other rapidly dividing cells are susceptible to the effects of chemotherapy. Thus, a blood test would be conducted to determine that the patient has a healthy number of red and white blood cells and platelets. Liver, kidney, and heart would normally also be checked.

11.3 CHEMOTHERAPY TERMINOLOGY

11.31 Activity

The first question that must be asked is whether the drug has some favorable impact upon a particular type of cancer. If it does, the drug is "active". That a drug is active does not mean it will always or usually be used. Its level of activity may be less than other drugs, or its side effects could be significant.

11.32 Partial and Complete Response

There are some objective ways of categorizing activity. Most scientists call a partial response, a 50% decrease in the size of the tumor. Thus, if we have an 8 centimeter tumor, and with a particular drug, the tumor is reduced to 4 centimeters, the drug is active and the patient had a partial response.

If the tumor is completely eliminated, for example, it cannot be seen on an x-ray, that is called a complete response. A complete response must unfortunately be distinguished from a cure. Chemotherapy might temporarily eliminate a tumor, only to have it later return, or it might leave microscopic traces indiscernible by x-ray or perhaps even Ct Scan.

11.4 RESERVED

11.5 PARTICULAR DRUGS

11.51 Platinum Drugs

11.511 Cisplatin

Cisplatin is one of the first and still most widely used drugs for lung and other types of cancer. Most studies show at least 25% of patients treated with Cisplatin receive at least a partial response, elimination of 50% of tumor volume. Nonetheless, the response is usually not permanent and chemo-resistant cells generally develop.

Lung cancer patients treated with chemotherapy generally have a longer life expectancy, but whether that is a matter of months or more is difficult to determine. Some clinical trials dealing with particularly ill patients show only modest gains from Cisplatin versus best supportive care. In other cases, the number of patients with partial response and the occasional complete response show the drug is working, and a few patients with 2,3, and 5 five year survival rates show the drug's effectiveness is not always limited to a brief extension of life.

11.5111 Side Effects

Cisplatin is associated with some side effects. Nausea and vomiting have been particularly troublesome which has lead to the development of platinum drugs like Carboplatin which are designed to match Cisplatin's effectiveness with fewer side effects. Patients using Cisplatin will want to consider using other drugs to minimize stomach disorders. Less common side effects include hearing abnormalities and neuropathy or leg weakness or discomfort. (BC Cancer Agency 12). Chemotherapy side effects are reviewed in the next chapter. Even though these side effects exist, most studies still find higher quality of life with chemotherapy than without.

11.5112 Chemistry and brand Name

Cisplatin is formed by an atom of platinum surrounded by chlorine and ammonia atoms. "The prefix "cis-" in cis-diamminedichloroplatinum refers to the arrangement of the atoms of this molecule around the central platinum atom." (13). Platinol is the commercial name of Cisplatin. Cisplatin is generally given by injection.

11.512 Carboplatin

Carboplatin produces less nausea, and other side effects with approximately the same effectiveness. It is a clear liquid also given intravenously and Paraplatin is its commercial name. Carboplatin reduces nausea but can affect white blood cells:

> "[Carboplatin can cause a] Temporary reduction in bone marrow function. This can result in anaemia, risk of bruising or bleeding and infection. This effect can begin about 7 days after the treatment has been given and usually reaches its lowest point at 10-14 days after the chemotherapy. Your blood count will then increase steadily and will have usually returned to normal within 21-28 days." (British Cancer Agency 13)

The manufacturer's insert states, "Bone marrow suppression (leukpenia, neutropenia, and thrombocytenia) is dose dependent, and is also the dose-limiting toxicity." (Paraplatin 14). Thus the amount of

Carboplatin that will be prescribed is limited to avoid these side effects. Patients have their blood tested regularly with the dosage reduced or the drug eliminated if a problem presents itself.

11.52 Taxol

Taxol is one of the newer drugs which have shown effectiveness and less nausea than Cisplatin. In addition to lung cancer, it is used to treat ovarian, testicular, breast, head, neck and melanoma. Taxol is an extract from the bark and needles of the yew tree, Taxus brevi folia. The history of Taxol is supplied on a webpage entitled The Taxol Molecule:

> "Taxol was discovered at Research Triangle Institute in 1967 when Dr. Monroe E. Wall and Mansukh C. Wani isolated the compound from the Pacific Yew Tree, taxus brevi folia and noted its antitumor activity in a broad range of rodent tumors. Interest in Taxol waned for nearly a decade. . . . In 1980, scientists at Albert Einstein Medical College reported that Taxol has a unique mechanism of action, making it the prototype for a new class of chemotherapeutic drugs. Taxol binds tubulin, thereby inhibiting cell division . . ." RTI.org. (Research Triangle Institute)

Taxol is a white powder which is liquified and given intravenously. It is commonly used in combination with other chemotherapy drugs such as Carboplatin, and Cisplatin. Dosages may vary but it is frequently generally given once every three weeks. Generally Taxol's side effects are tolerable, less than drugs like Cisplatin. One well-known side effect is numbness or tingling in toes and fingers. This may be because Taxol affects bone marrow. Taxol is metabolized in the liver and dosage may be reduced for patients with liver dysfunction or liver metastasis.

11.523 Taxotere

Just as Carboplatin was designed to provide similar efficacy with fewer side effects than Cisplatin, Taxotere is designed to be better than Taxol.

11.53 Vinorelbine

This drug is active or effective with non-small cell lung cancer and has been successfully combined with cisplatin. Vinorelbine has been investigated in 4 randomized trials and found to improve survival. The combination of vinorelbine to cisplatin has been compared in two randomized trials to vinorelbine alone with significant response rate improvement with survival increase in one (5) and not in the other (6). In the first one, the comparison was also performed with a third arm treatment made of cisplatin and vindesine, with a marginal effect on survival. It should be noted that both trials have obtained high quality scores in our review (89 and 79,8%).

11.54 Gemcitabine

Gemcitabine is a newer drug whose strength is that it provides the same, or almost the same effectiveness as the platinum drugs, but with fewer side effects. Known by its trade name, Gemzar, it is a clear liquid usually given intravenously. It is a frequent choice for elderly patients or those in poorer health because of its mild side effects. It has been shown in randomized trials to be better tolerated than the Cisplatin combinations.

Unlike Cisplatin, side effects do not usually include nausea or vomiting. Instead drop in bone morrow or fatigue may occur. Anecdotally, my father-in-law felt better after taking the drug.

11.541 Gemcitabine and Platinum Combinations

Scientists continue to investigate combining Gemcitabine with other anti-cancer drugs. One study found the two drug combination more effective than Gemcitabine alone (Hitt 11). Hitt suggests that "the higher response rate, prolonged time to progression, and improved survival in the GCB arm appears to support the use of combined platinum-based therapy for patients with advanced NSCLC." Hitt (11). Hitt did note that thrombocytonopenia was more pronounced in the combination group. Thus, for persons in otherwise good health, Gemcitabine combinations for advanced lung cancer patients are becoming more prevalent. For persons in poorer health, Gemcitabine may be used alone to reduce side effects.

11.6 THE ERA OF MULTI-MODAL OR COMBINATION CHEMOTHERAPY

From a search for the magic bullet or cure, has come a recognition that success is most likely to come from a combination of drugs, each of which has an incremental impact. While combining four drugs with 20% response rate will unfortunately not lead to an 80% response, it will yield success beyond that of any one drug:

> "Four principles underlie the design of chemotherapy combinations. First, each agent in a regimen should be independently active against the tumor. Unless there is unexpected synergy, adding an agent with the same mechanism of action or inhibiting the same enzyme is unlikely to enhance the response with an additive effect, but will add to the toxicity. Secondly, each drug in the regimen should have an independent mechanism of action, preferably with each drug in the combination targeting different steps along a biochemical pathway. Third, there should be no cross resistance among the drugs in the regimen, so that if one drug selects a resistant tumor subpopulation, it is unlikely to be cross-resistant to another drug in the combination that kills through a different mechanism. Fourth, each of the drugs should have a different dose-limiting toxicity. Two drugs with the same toxicity profile given at maximum tolerated dose can produce unacceptable toxicity." Chemotherapy pitt.edu (10)

Here is a comment from the 1998 Cuneo Lung Cancer conference:

> "During the two decades from 1970 to 1990, the results of chemotherapy for stage IV disease have been unimpressive. Cisplatin was demonstrated to have modest activity, and appeared to be synergistic with etopiside and vinca alkaloids. Numerous phase III studies compared different cisplatin combination chemotherapy regimens and failed to identify a "standard" program (2,3). Furthermore, phase III studies comparing chemotherapy to supportive care had mixed results, with others failing to demonstrate an advantage for chemotherapy in stage IV disease. Only from a recent meta-analysis a small advantage for the combinations containing cisplatin could be demonstrated (4)."

During the past 5 years, several new agents have been evaluated in NSCLC (Non small cell lung cancer) and demonstrated improved results compared to older regimens. The taxons (paclitaxel and docetaxel) have also demonstrated activity, with a 20-30% single agent response. In the U.S., paclitaxel achieved a 40% 1 year survival in studies by Eastern Co-operative Oncology Group (ECOG) and M.D. Anderson, ECOG subsequently performed a phase III study in 571 valuable patients, randomizing patients to cisplatin (75 mg/m) + etopiside, versus cisplatin (75 mg/m) + paclitaxel, given as a 24 hour infusion at a dosage of 135 mg/m or 250 mg/m with G-CSF. Response rates were 12%, 27% and 32% and there was improved survival with the two paclitaxel arms (7).

Gemcitabine is one of the most extensively evaluated single agents in NSCLC, with response rates of 20-30% world-wide (8).

11.61 Side Effects and Multi-Modal Therapy

While the addition of another drug may improve survival, it will also increase potential side effects. For the young person with early disease, an aggressive regimen may be recommended, while others with impaired health may wish to limit side effects, by perhaps using only type of drug.

11.7 MULTI-DRUG RESISTANCE

Chemotherapy works best when there are (1) small numbers of cancer cells that are (2) actively dividing. Chemotherapy is highly effective with small cell lung cancers promptly diagnosed, since this type of cancer rapidly divides. The effectiveness of chemotherapy with non-small cell lung cancer is less clear. One writer states,

"Whereas radical surgery or radiotherapy are potentially curative treatments for disease which is localized, chemotherapy is the only major modality with the potential to eradicate disease which has disseminated. In some less common malignancies, chemotherapy is indeed curative in a large proportion of patients. Examples of such diseases are acute leukemias, lymphomas and testicular teratoma. For the more common solid tumors, however, long-term disease eradication by chemotherapy is rarely seen.

The main reason for this is the relative lack of selectivity displayed by current anticancer drugs. Their differential toxicity towards malignant cells within the body is such that they cannot be administered at dose level which may eliminate the malignant population without killing the patient. Some progress has resulted from the development of combination regimens which combine several drugs with different modes of action and nonoverlapping toxicities." Twentyman, (7).

In "cell kinetics" experiments it has been shown that drugs destroy a constant fraction or percentage of cells, not a constant number. So if there are 10 trillion cancer cells and 99 percent are killed, 100 billion are still left after the first treatment. After the second treatment, 1 billion cells are left, and after the third 10 million remain. The proportion of cells killed is the same, but each time a smaller number of cells is killed. The cells that are resting rather than actively reproducing escape the drugs' killing effects.

In between treatments, when it is safe, the resting cells resume production and replace the ones that have been killed. Chemotherapy under the best of conditions is a matter of taking two steps forward and one step back, and it is very difficult to make enough progress to kill off every single cell. Kinetic studies have also shown that as the cancer increases in size-the more cells it contains-the number of actively reproducing cells (the "growth fraction") decreases. The higher the number you start with, the harder and longer you have to work at getting the cell population down, because not only are there more cells to kill, there are more cells that are not vulnerable.

11.71 The Development of MDR, Multi-Drug Resistance

Unfortunately cancer cells develop resistance to certain drugs. While initially successful, chemotherapy becomes ineffective. PGP (P-glycoprotein) is produced which inhibits the ability of the drug to reach cancer cells, thus reducing "intracellular drug concentrations and hence reduced cytotoxicity." Twentyman, (7):

"At least three different MDR (multi-drug resistance) phenotypes exist, two of which are relatively well defined. The best known is the so-called 'classical' or P-glycoprotein-related

MDR phenotypes, in which resistance is due to reduction of the intracellular drug accumulation via a 170 kDa protein pump (P-glycoprotein)." Jensen, (8)

11.72 Why Dosage and Scheduling Can Be Critical

Dosage scheduling can be important and is the subject of clinical trials.

"Rapidly growing tumors tend to be most sensitive to chemotherapy. Also, damage to normal tissues at short intervals after chemotherapy or wide-field radiation is most often observed in organs such as the bone marrow or the intestine, which are renewal tissue known to contain rapidly proliferating cells. These observations suggest that rapidly proliferating cells may be more susceptible to therapy and have led to several studies of the relationship between cytotoxicity and proliferative rate . . . ."

"Several investigators have proposed that drug treatment might be scheduled at intervals that allow the surviving tumor cells to progress to a drug sensitive phase of the cell cycle, or, conversely, such that cells in critical normal tissues are again in a drug-resistant phase. In practice, the wide heterogeneity of cell cycle parameters makes this difficult to achieve. It has been demonstrated that therapeutic outcome is markedly dependent on scheduling interval for drug treatment of experimental tumors, but it has been difficult to predict the optimum scheduling interval from knowledge of cell kinetics." National Cancer Institute. For updated information visit its website(s) at www.nci.org.

Chemotherapy administrations should not be missed without a reason. If an administration is missed, the doctor should be promptly informed.

11.8 HOW DRUGS ARE SELECTED

The oncologist's choice of drug depends on the type of cancer, its impact on bodily functions, the patient's general health, and his assessment of various clinical trials or studies. For dual agent chemotherapy, most U.S oncologists choose Taxol and Carboplatin. In Europe, Cisplatin is more widely used. Gemcitabine is used as second agent chemotherapy, as are the tyrosine kinase inhibitors like Iressa and anti-angiogenic agents like Thalidomide.

11.9 CHEMOTHERAPY ADMINISTRATION

11.91 Where is Chemotherapy Administered?

Chemotherapy for lung cancer is generally administered in a physician's office, a clinic or hospital's oncology department. When the patient first begins chemotherapy, a hospital stay might be needed to assess the medicine's effects.

11.92 How Often Will Chemotherapy be administered?

How often the therapy is administered will vary. Chemotherapy is sometimes given in on-and-off cycles that include rest periods so that the body has a chance to re-build new cells and the patient regain its strength. The time and amount are generally based upon results from clinical trials.

11.93 Goals of Chemotherapy

Chemotherapy helps patients live more comfortably by eliminating cancer cells which cause pain, discomfort or other problems. This is called palliative care, where the goal is to help the patient better function, not cure. Currently, chemotherapy is generally not an overall cure for advanced lung cancer, the type of cancer for which it is prescribed. Chemotherapy is not given for stage 1 cancer as standard treatment though clinical trials are investigating whether it would be beneficial.

11.94 Methods of Administration

One common way for the drug to be given is by mouth. This is more convenient and less costly than other methods. The disadvantage is that there may be many instructions given with the drug, and the patients should follow these instructions explicitly and maintain careful records of when the drugs are taken.

Drugs may also be injected into a vein where the cancer cells appear to be circulating. Two kinds of pumps—external and internal—may be used to control the rate of delivery of chemotherapy. External pumps remain outside the body. Some are portable and allow a person to move around while the pump is in use. Other external pumps are not portable and may restrict activity. Internal pumps are placed surgically inside the body, usually right under the skin. They contain a small reservoir (storage area) that delivers the drugs into the catheter. Internal pumps allow people to go about most of their daily activities.

Generally the goal with chemotherapy is to attack cancerous cells circulating throughout the body. Occasionally, chemotherapy may be given in a manner to directly attack cancer cells in a particular area.

11.95 Does Chemotherapy Hurt

Getting chemotherapy by mouth, on the skin, or by injection generally feels the same as taking other medications by these methods. Having an IV started usually feels like drawing blood for a blood test. Some people feel a coolness or other unusual sensation in the area of the injection when the IV is started. Report such feelings to your doctor or nurse. Be sure that you also report any pain, burning, or discomfort that occurs during or after an IV treatment.

Many people have little or no trouble having the IV needle in their hand or lower arm. However, if a person has a hard time for any reason, or if it becomes difficult to insert the needle into a vein for each treatment, it may be possible to use a central venous catheter or port. This avoids repeated insertion of the needle into the vein. Central venous catheters and ports cause no pain or discomfort if they are properly placed and cared for, although a person usually is aware that they are there. It is important to report any pain or discomfort with a catheter or port to your doctor or nurse.

11.96 Use of Other Medication During Chemotherapy

Some medicines may interfere with the effects of your chemotherapy. That is why you should take a list of all your medications to your doctor before you start chemotherapy. Your list should include the name of each drug, how often you take it, the reason you take it, and the dosage. Remember to include over-the-counter drugs such as laxatives, cold pills, pain relievers, and vitamins. Your doctor will tell you if you should stop taking any of these medications before you start chemotherapy. After your treatments begin, be sure to check with your doctor before taking any new medicines or stopping the ones you already are taking. A patient's ability to work will depend upon his stage and performance status. The disease more than the therapy is likely to be the cause of a termination of employment.

REFERENCES

1. Bruning, *Coping with Chemotherapy* (Ballantine Books 1993).
2. Devita, et. al. *Principles and Practice of Oncology* (1999).
3. Pritchard, *Other Chemotherapeutic Agents: Do We Need Them.*
4. Cuneo-Lung Cancer Study Group, M. Tonato, *From Nitrogen-Mustards to Cis-Platinum and Beyond,* www.culcase.org.
5. Le Chevalier, J Clin Oncol 12: 360; 1994.
6. Depierre, Ann Oncol 5: 37; 1994.
7. Twentyman, *Mechanism of Drug Resistance in Lung Cancer Cells,* excerpted in Carney, Lung Cancer (Arnold Publ. Co. Great Britain 1995).
8. Jensen, et. al., *New Directions in Drug Therapy of Small Cell Carcinoma Based on In Vitro Studies,* 234, in Carney, Lung Cancer (1995).
9. *About Com Pharmaceutical Guide* Quoting December 23, 1999 Press Release by Events Co.
10. *Chemotherapy.*www.pitt.edu/~super1/lecture/lec0701/124.htm.
11. Hitt, *Gemcitabine for NSCLC,* (presentation before the American Society of Clinical Oncolology Asco, excerpted on medscape.com).
12. Online summary from the British Columbia Cancer Agency www.bccancer.bc.ca/HPI/DrugDatabase/DrugIndexALPro/Cisplatin.htm.
13. *Cisplatin: The Platinum Standard,* www.chemheritage.org/EducationalServices/pharm/chemo/readings/cisplat.htm
14. http://www.cancerbacup.or.uk/info/carboplatin.htm.

15. Moore, *Living Well with Cancer* (2001).
16. Johnson, *End Points and United States Food and Drug Administration Approval of Oncology Drugs*, J Clin Oncol. 2003 Apr 1;21(7):1404-11.
17. Schiller, *Platin or No Platin? That Is the Question, Journal of Clinical Oncology*, Vol 21, Issue 16 (August), 2003: 3009-3010.
18. www.FDA.gov

CHAPTER 12

CHEMOTHERAPY SIDE EFFECTS

12.0 OVERVIEW

12.01 Limits of this Book

It is important to discuss, but not overemphasize, the significance of side effects from chemotherapy. With the emergence of new drugs, medication to reduce side effects, and refinements in dose, some of the traditional side effects have been reduced. And while side effects are important, many studies show that quality of life is better with chemotherapy than without. I discuss side effects generally, but only your oncologist can give you a case-specific analysis based upon the nature of your disease and the type of chemotherapy provided.

Let me add a personal note to this. It is much easier for me as author, to characterize nausea or other side effects as minor, than if I were experiencing this myself. If I have not taken the time to empathize with the patient or family member, it is because I felt that a clear, if unemotional analysis was the best way for me to communicate information. A book cannot provide the support a family member or close friend can provide.

12.02 Support Groups

Support groups play an important role in dealing with side effects.

A clinical trial can only categorize side effects, it cannot give a description of what a person experiences and how to deal with that. Physicians can be busy, and the best way to discuss the pain or discomfort associated with chemotherapy can be a support group.

Association of Online cancer resources, Acor.org currently provides 3 online support groups. These are categorized by disease, for example, non-small cell lung cancer, and can provide an excellent resource. Alcase.org is a leading lung cancer advocacy group which also provides support group information. Lungcanceronline.com provides support group information as well as material about side effects. The American Cancer Society and many hospitals also provide support.

To note side effects associated with chemotherapy paints an incomplete picture. The disease itself creates many serious consequences, some of which are relieved by chemotherapy. Thus, many studies report higher quality of life with chemotherapy, along with extended survival.

12.03 Medical Reasons for Side Effects

An American Cancer Society Guide discusses the reason for side effects:

> "All the tissues and organs of the body are subject to an anticancer drug's action, which is to destroy rapidly dividing cells or prevent them from reproducing. Cancer cells, which continuously and quickly replace themselves, are obviously targets. But some healthy cells that also divide rapidly, such as those in the hair follicles and lining the intestinal tract, are vulnerable to the drugs as well. Consequently, temporary hair loss and nausea are common side effects. The challenge, then, for the oncologist is to balance the cancer-destroying benefits of a particular drug or combination of drugs against their toxic effects. It is sometimes quite a delicate balance, but with good emotional and physical care and support the side effects can be managed in most cases and, if not fully controlled, at least made tolerable." The American Cancer Society *(1)*.

12.1 CHEMOTHERAPY CAN IMPROVE QUALITY OF LIFE BY REDUCING THE SYMPTOMS OF DISEASE

Chemotherapy causes side effects in some patients. However, it is incorrect to therefore conclude that the decision to use chemotherapy represents a tradeoff between length and quality of life. For example, one study analyzes quality of life with the chemotherapy drug Vinorelbine. (2).

First, the study found that Vinorelbine extended life among stage 3b and 4 lung cancer patients. Survival rates at 6 months and 12 months were 55% and 32% in the chemotherapy treated group versus 41% and 14% in the group receiving best available care without chemotherapy. Indeed, the trial had to be stopped because physicians were increasingly reluctant to assign patients to the control group whose mortality rate was demonstrably higher. There is increasingly little debate that chemotherapy extends life even among advanced lung cancer patients, at 3b and 4. In the Vinorelbine chemotherapy group, there was one patient with a complete remission and 14 partial responses of 50% or more reduction in tumor volume (of approximately 76 in the group). There should be little question that chemotherapy has proven to be effective even with patients whose cancer has metastasized to lymph nodes or other organs. Chemotherapy will extend life in many cases, and in a few it had the capacity to serve as a cure. Based upon this study and some others, the only realistic question is what type of chemotherapy should be prescribed.

Equally important to cancer patients were the findings of quality of life. Quality of life or (Qol) can be statistically measured using a questionnaire given to patients in the clinical trial, and comparing results in the group receiving chemotherapy and the one given best supportive care. Vinorelbine-treated patients scored better on quality of life, and the study found a reduction in cancer-related symptoms such as pain and dyspnea, loss of breath. This would presumably correlate with the reduction in the size of the tumor in many cases. The study did find an increase in certain chemo-related side effects. Constipation was observed in three patients, heart arrhythmias in two, loss of hair—alopecia in three, and other side effects in approximately five. Thus there is a sad tradeoff between chemo-related side effects and those of the disease itself, but most would prefer the chemotherapy and the prospect of extending life with the drug. The study concludes, "we obtained a survival advantage that was not at the expense of a worse Qol (quality of life)."

12.2 NAUSEA AND ANTI-EMETIC DRUGS

Some anticancer drugs cause nausea and vomiting because they irritate the stomach lining and regurgitation can be a natural response to irritation. The severity of these symptoms depends on several factors, including the chemotherapeutic agent(s) used, and the patient's reaction. Some patients will experience only limited side effects with a drug while others will have greater ones. In most clinical trials, only a minority experience a particular side effect, and the side effects will vary from patient to patient. Diet may play a role with the patient who eats oily foods probably more likely to experience nausea when a foreign drug comes in contact with his body.

Management of nausea and vomiting occasioned by chemotherapy is an important part of care for cancer patients when it does occur. Note that our ability to combat nausea has improved, and do not assume that side effects encountered by a patients 10 years ago will occur with the same severity today.

12.21 Compazine

The Chemotherapy and Radiation Therapy Guide says:

> "[Compazine] has been the mainstay of antinausea treatment for over thirty years. It acts in the CTZ (chemotherapy trigger zone) by blocking Dopamine receptors. Dopamine is released by the body in response to some chemotherapy drugs and can cause nausea. Compazine can be used alone for preventing nausea when you are getting mildly nauseating chemotherapy or radiation treatments. It is available in many forms." (6) at 70.

12.22 Atavan

Atavan is also frequently prescribed for nausea:

> "This drug is a tranquilizer in the same family as valium. It doesn't't block dopamine at the CTZ or speed up the digestive tract, but works by making you relaxed, forgetful, and sleepy. It is sometimes used alone, but often in combination with other antinausea drugs." Chemotherapy and Radiation Therapy Guide (6) at 70.

Not surprisingly, side effects are sedation and forgetfulness, and the drug should not be used before driving.

12.23 Kytril

Kytril "works by preventing seratonin from getting through to the CTZ and causing nausea." (6), at 71.

12.24 Tropisetron

This newer drug was found as effective as Kytril in a recent Chinese clinical trial (7). Another recent article reports, "These results indicate that continuous administration of tropisetron could contribute to preventing patient QOL influenced by cisplatin treatment."

12.25 Substitution of Carboplatin for Cisplatin

While effective, in treating lung cancer, Cisplatin has been associated with nausea. Some suggest that substituting Carboplatin, another Platinum drug, maintains the same level of effectiveness with fewer side effects.

12.26 Marijuana and Nausea

There has been some interest in the use of marijuana to treat a number of medical problems, including chemotherapy-induced nausea and vomiting in cancer patients. Delta-9-tetrahydrocannabinol (THC), is available by prescription for use as an antiemetic. The U.S. Food and Drug Administration has approved its use for treatment of nausea and vomiting associated with cancer chemotherapy in patients who have not responded to the standard antiemetic drugs.

THC may be useful for some cancer patients who have chemotherapy-induced nausea and vomiting that cannot be controlled by other antiemetic agents. The expected side effects of this compound must be weighed against the possible benefits. Dronabinol can causes a "high" (loss of control or sensation of unreality), which is associated with its effectiveness; however, this sensation may be unpleasant for some individuals."

12.27 Diet

Many believe that diet plays an important role. Eating light, non-oily foods, may reduce the nausea associated with some forms of chemotherapy. One guide suggests the following:

15. Eat bland foods, toast, sherbert, crackers,
16. Be wary of foods with strong aromas,
17. "Sometimes sweet juices are hard to tolerate after treatment",
18. "Fresh air and mild physical activity help prevent nausea."

These things vary from patients to patient. Change mealtimes when needed. My father-in-law tended to eat better at breakfast and sometimes ate better at his daughter's home. Note the patient's eating habits and adjust schedules accordingly.

12.3 CHEMOTHERAPY AND BLOOD CELLS

Chemotherapy can increase the risk of infection. White blood cells fight infection and are constantly reproducing and may therefore be affected by chemotherapy.

12.31 Neutropenia

Drugs which inhibit the cell reproduction process can cause a reduction in white blood cells called neutropenia making the body more susceptible to infection:

"Chemotherapy and extensive radiotherapy often interfere with the formation and maturation of blood cells (hematopoeises) . . . According to a Gallup poll of chemotherapy patients, nearly half had their treatment postponed at least once because their white counts were alarmingly low. White cells safeguard us against infection, particularly the neutrophils, which make up 60 percent of all white cells. Their job is to intercept and destroy bacteria. A person is said to be mildly neutropenic when her absolute neutrophil count (ANC) is between 2,000 and

1,000. The ANC is determined by multiplying the percentage of neutrophils by the total white-blood-cell count. Oncologists will generally continue chemotherapy so long as the number says in the 500-1000 range, which is considered moderate netrupenia . . . ."

"Most chemo regimens suppress your immune system for perhaps a week to ten days, after which time the neutrophil count starts climbing back. The other key players in fighting off disease are the lymphocytes which track down viruses. Although chemotherapy depletes the number of lymphocytes, says Dr. Rajagopal, the ones that remain are functional. During this period of impaired immunity, the major concern is to immediately treat any bacterial infections that develop. The GI tract, along with the skin and the respiratory tract, is a haven for bacteria." Teeley(3)

12.311 Colony Stimulating Factor

Some doctors may recommend colony stimulating factors. "In 1991, small cell lung cancer (SCLC) was reported as the first tumour type where colony stimulating factor (CSF) support was clinically effective." Feinglass (7) Valley (8). Your doctor may prescribe Neupogen, a medication that stimulates your body to produce more white blood cells. (Neupogen website 6)

12.32 Thrombocytopenia

A low level of platelets is called thrombocytopenia. One method of treatment is platelet transfusion. Transfused platelets act as mature "stand-ins" for your developing cells until your body becomes able to produce enough platelets on its own.

12.33 Anemia and Procrit

Anemia is having less than the normal number of red blood cells or hemoglobin. "The hemoglobin (Hb) in red blood cells carries oxygen to all parts of the body, providing the strength you need. When you are anemic, less oxygen is able to reach your muscles and organs. This can leave you fatigued and unable to do the things you love to do every day."

Procrit (9) "Hemoglobin is measured in grams (g) per deciliter (dL). The average hemoglobin value for men is 16 g/dL and for women is 14 g/dL." Procrit (9).

One popular drug to address anemia is Procrit, also called Epogen or epoetin alfa. The drug can increase the number of red blood cells, restore strength, and allow chemotherapy to continue. Erythropoietin is a protein produced in the kidney that stimulates red blood cell production. Procrit mimics Erythropoietin prompting increased red blood cell production. The drug is taken intravenously and generally takes 2-6 week to show results. Procrit (9). The manufacturer suggests that Procrit is generally well-tolerated, though possible side effects include elevated blood pressure, headache and diarrhea.

Another less widely used drug for anemia is Aranesp. It also mimics the body's own Erythpoientin and its manufacturer suggests that fewer injections are needed. See Aranesp.com (11). Research and experience with this drug are more limited. Similar side effects are noted.

12.34 Testing Procedures

A common and easy test is CBC or complete blood count. On almost all laboratory tests, there is a standard or benchmark and the patient's reading is compared to that. CBC will generally measure white blood cells, red blood cells, hemoglobin. platelets and others.

12.35 Precautions and Reducing Infections

Chemotherapy presents enhanced risk of infection and danger from infection. Most physicians recommend that the patient immediately consult a doctor if they have a temperature above 101. The chemotherapy patient needs to be carefully monitored with precautions taken to prevent infection. Some general precautions against infection:

- Wash your hands frequently. Be sure to clean under your nails and between your fingers. Take a warm bath or shower each day and wash between folds of skin. Germs may locate inside the groin, between a woman's breasts—anywhere than skin touches skin and is not exposed to air.
- Stay away from anyone with a cold or disease. Do not share

drinking glasses, washclothes or other items which may carry germs.
- When you are done preparing food—particularly meat, poultry, and eggs, disinfect countertops and cutting boards.
- Avoid small groceries and check food expiration dates. Avoid food leftover for more than a day. Check that your refrigerator and freezer are working properly.
- Cook fresh vegetables. Avoid raw foods like shellfish or sushi.

12.4 CHEMOTHERAPY AND LIFESTYLE CHANGES

Any observer must express tremendous admiration for the typical patient. Chemotherapy can bring major changes to a person's life. It can affect overall health, threaten a sense of well-being, disrupt day-to-day schedules, and put a strain on personal relationships. No wonder, then, that many people feel tearful, anxious, angry, or depressed at some point during their chemotherapy. These emotions are perfectly normal and understandable, but they also can be disturbing. Fortunately, there are ways to cope with these emotional "side effects," just as there are ways to cope with the physical side effects of chemotherapy. (Some time after this was written, a close member of my family contracted a form of cancer, not of the lung. However, I realized that it is far easier to talk about calmness and relaxation as an onlooker, than as a patient or family member).

12.5 SOURCES OF SUPPORT

There are different sources of support for the patient:

Counseling professionals. Counselors can help you express, understand, and cope with the emotions cancer can cause. Psychiatrists, psychologists, or social workers, or someone with specialized experience with cancer patients, can discuss difficult questions.

Doctors and nurses. Some doctors may be easy to speak with about side effects, while others may be distant and clinical. Try to find a knowledgeable and sympathetic person at your hospital or physician's office to discuss side effects and other issues. Be prepared to clearly and concisely tell the doctor about particular side effects, and listen carefully about remedies.

Support Groups. Alcase provides support for lung cancer patients on a national level. Your hospital's social work department, the American Cancer Society, and the National Cancer Institute's Cancer Information Service may have information. Ideally, you want a lung cancer support group, with people experiencing the same illness and treatment as you.

Online Groups. Acor.org has online support groups for non-small cell lung cancer, small cell, and mesothelioma. You can give your name or speak anonymously, and see how others deal with similar problems.

Religious Groups. Your priest, minister, or rabbi is qualified to talk about the difficult questions you may experience during treatment. It is perfectly appropriate to reach out to your clergyman even if you have not attended services.

Close Friends and family members. Talking with friends or family members is useful though friends and patients respond in different ways. Some may be able to provide comfort and reassurance that no one else can.

Friends and Neighbors. Some people do not understand cancer, and may withdraw from you because they're afraid of your illness. Others may worry that they will upset you by saying "the wrong thing." You can help relieve these fears by being open in talking with others about your illness, your treatment, your needs, and your feelings. Let people know that there's no single "right" thing to say, so long as their caring comes through loud and clear. Once people know they can talk with you honestly, they may be more willing and able to open up and lend their support.

Here are some tips from the National Cancer Institute:

- Try to keep your treatment goals in mind. This will help you keep a positive attitude on days when the going gets rough. Remember that eating well is very important. Your body needs food to rebuild tissues and regain strength.
- Set realistic goals and don't be too hard on yourself. You may not have as much energy as usual, so try to get as much rest as you can, let the "small stuff" slide, and only do the things that are most important to you.
- Ask your doctor or nurse about a safe and practical exercise program. Using your body can help you feel better about yourself, help you get rid of tension or anger, and build your appetite.

12.51 Dealing with Your Doctor

Addressing chemotherapy side effects is one of the most important tasks for the oncologist, but one done with varying skill and empathy. Some doctors can be cold and clinical and others empathetic.

Note that we are in a managed care health system where doctors see substantial numbers of patients each week. Thus, you will want to clearly and concisely explain the nature of your discomfort and side effects. Consider writing down what is occuring, noting frequency, stimuli, and particular sensations.

12.6 RELIEVING STRESS

Some believe muscle relaxation techniques are useful:

Muscle tension and release. Lie down in a quiet room. Take a slow, deep breath. As you breathe in, tense a particular muscle or group of muscles. For example, you can squeeze your eyes shut, frown, clench your teeth, make a fist, or stiffen your arms or legs. Hold your breath and keep your muscles tense for a second or two. Then breathe out, release the tension, and let your body relax completely. Repeat the process with another muscle or muscle group.

Rhythmic breathing. Get into a comfortable position and relax all your muscles. If you keep your eyes open, focus on a distant object. If you close your eyes, imagine a peaceful scene or simply clear your mind and focus on your breathing. Breathe in and out slowly and comfortably through your nose. If you like, you can keep the rhythm steady by saying to yourself, "In, one two; Out, one two." Feel yourself relax and go limp each time you breathe out. You can do this technique for just a few seconds or for up to 10 minutes. End your rhythmic breathing by counting slowly and silently to three.

Visualization. Visualization is a method that is similar to imagery. With visualization, you create an inner picture that represents your fight against cancer. Some people getting chemotherapy use images of rockets blasting away their cancer cells or of knights in armor battling their cancer cells. Others create an image of their white blood cells or their drugs attacking the cancer cells. Visualization and imagery may help relieve stress and increase your sense of self-control. But it is very important to remember that they cannot take the place of the medical care your doctor prescribes to treat your cancer.

Hypnosis. Hypnosis puts you in a trance-like state that can help reduce discomfort and anxiety. You can be hypnotized by a qualified person, or you can learn how to hypnotize yourself. If you are interested in learning more, ask your doctor or nurse to refer you to someone trained in the technique.

12.7 LOSS OF WEIGHT, ANOREXIA AND CACHEXIA

Anorexia, the loss of appetite or desire to eat, is a common symptom in cancer patients that may occur early in the disease or later as the cancer grows and spreads. *Cachexia* is a wasting condition in which the patient has weakness and progressive loss of body weight, fat, and muscle.

Anorexia and cachexia can occur together, but cachexia is present in patients who are eating an adequate diet but have malabsorption of nutrients. "Tumor cells deprive normal cells of nutrients. Meanwhile the body is expending extra energy as it heals from the effects of cancer surgery, radiotherapy, or chemotherapy. In order to sustain vital functions, the body retrieves nutrients stored in fatty tissue. Once all available fat has been broken down for fuel, it sets to work on muscle. Of all nutrients, protein is the one most essential for building muscle, bone, skin, and blood cells. If the body's cells consume more protein than you take in, muscle mass rapidly wastes away, causing the emaciated look often associated with cancer." (3). Maintenance of body weight and adequate nutritional status can help patients feel and look better, and maintain or improve their performance status. Teely recommends the following:

COMPLETE PROTEINS: canned humas, skinless turkey, steak, whitemeat chicken, whole milk, hard-boiled eggs, nuts, wheat germ.

NUTRIONAL SUPPLEMENTS with your oncologist's approval.

LIGHT EXERCISE to stimulate your appetite.

The author of that book, a cancer patient himself, recommends foods dense in high-quality protein such as meat, chicken, fish, eggs, and dairy products. Some patients may not easily tolerate these foods, and you will need to structure a diet which provides the necessary nutrients without creating nausea.

12.8 LOSS OF HAIR

Loss of hair can be a disturbing side effect of chemotherapy. We associate hair with virility and beauty and its rapid loss can cause significant pain. Today many sports stars like Michael Jordan are bald voluntarily with many others choosing to shave their head. Insurance policies should cover hair replacement since hair loss is a consequence of disease. One should obtain a prescription or note.

12.9 PREPARING FOR CHEMOTHERAPY

12.91 Family Assistance and Personal Information

Chemotherapy can be fatiguing. Have a family or friend accompany you if possible. Prepare an information sheet so a doctor or nurse can quickly get the necessary information about a patient's history and status.

Personal Information. John Smith, age 63, height, 5-9, weight 165 41 Stone Street, Boston, Massachusetts, Home telephone (948)512-0121, work telephone 943-343-5512.

Current Diagnosis. Non-small cell lung cancer, adenocarcinoma, date of diagnosis 1/7/03, stage 4 metastasis to two areas of bone.

Treatment history. Radiation to lung 10 treatments, currently taking Taxol and Carboplatin.

Physician. Dr. Gordon Johnson, New York Presbyterian Hospital, Office No. 212-565-4300, Beeper 212-656-3222. *Emergency Contact.* Wife, Evelyn Smith, home 914-963-5114, office, 914-565-4300.

Allergies. None.

The hospital may already have this information, but checking that things are done correctly, done in a pleasant way, is important.

REFERENCES

1. The American Cancer Society Guide, *Informed Consent,* 172 (1997).
2. *Effects of Vinorelbine on Quality of Life and Survival of Elderly Patients with Advanced Non Small-Cell Lung Cancer,* 91, No. 1 66-72 (Jan. 6, 1999).
3. McKay, *The Chemotherapy & Radiation Survival Guide* (New Harbinger Pub. Co. 1998).
4. Teeley & Bashe, *The Complete Cancer Survival Guide* 707-08 (Doubleday 2000).
5. Wang, *The Clinical Effect of Tropisetron in the Prevention of Nausea and Vomiting Induced by Anti-Cancer Drugs,* Zhonghua Zhong Liu Za Zhi 2001 May;23(3):251-3.
6. www.neupogen.com.
7. Feinglass, *G-CSF as Prophylaxis of Febrile Neutropenia in SCLC,*Expert Opinion on Pharmacotherapy 2002, vol. 3, no. 9, pp. 1273-1281.
8. Valley, *New Treatment Options for Managing Chemotherapy-Induced Neutropenia,* J Health Syst Pharm 2002 Aug 1;59(15 Suppl 4):S11-7 Am.
9. www.Procrit.com.
10. *www.Nci.org* (Section on treatment of non-small cell lung cancer).
11. www.Aranesp.com.

CHAPTER 13

RADIATION

13.0 PURPOSE OF RADIATION

Radiation is designed to kill cancer cells in a specified area. Radiation is frequently given in the area of the lung tumor, and sometimes in areas of metastases such as bone. It is designed to improve quality of life by reducing pain and discomfort emanating from a specified area. Radiation does not eliminate metastasis because it does little to alter the overall carcinogenic process.

13.01 Radiation and Stage 1

For early stage tumors where surgery is not an option (for example the patient has a severe heart condition), radiation may be used with the goal of eliminating a small tumor.

13.02 Radiation and Advanced Cancers

More commonly, the goal of radiation is palliative, that is to relieve pain and discomfort. Thus, in a stage 4 patient with metastases, radiation would be used to reduce the tumor in the lung or at the location of the metastasis. Physicians refer to radiation as palliative or local control. The radiation may reduce the size of the tumor and its direct impact, but it generally does not provide an overall cure for advanced cancer patients.

13.021 Radiation as Part of an Overall Treatment Plan

Thus radiation will commonly be used with chemotherapy or gene therapy as part of an overall treatment plan. Scientists continue to debate whether radiation before, after, or concurrent with chemotherapy is most effective.

13.1 HOW DOES RADIATION THERAPY WORK

Radiation in high doses can kill cells or prevent them from dividing:

"Radiation therapy (RT) is the use of focused high energy electromagnetic waves (photons) or electrons to treat cancerY. These beams strike and transfer varying amounts of energy to carbon, nitrogen, and hydrogen atoms in or near the DNA chains in the nucleus of cells thereby producing breaks, deletions, or cross linkages in the DNA chains, some of which are lethal to the cell. A few cells may die within minutes after being hit, but after sustaining lethal damage most cells survive until they attempt to go through mitosis and cell division. Cells are most sensitive to RT when they are in mitosis or shortly after cell division. Tissues in which a high proportion of cells are actively multiplying tend to be more sensitive to high energy photons than are tissues where most cells divide relatively infrequently."

"By giving daily doses of RT large enough to kill a high proportion of the rapidly dividing cancer cells while killing only a small proportion of the more slowly dividing normal tissue cells in the area, a malignant tumor can be eradicated. The factors which determine whether or not a cancer can be eradicated by radiation therapy include the sensitivity of the tumor to RT, the volume of tumor cells to be eradicated and the tolerance of the most radiation sensitive vital tissues in the area. This latter factor is influenced by how effectively these structures can be shielded from the irradiation received by the tumor and whether the vital tissues can be sacrificed without mortality. Thus, RT is most effective when the volume of tumor cells to be treated is small, i.e. microscopic deposits of tumor cells left behind after the visible part of a tumor has been surgically excised, or when the tumor can be given a high dose of high energy photons or electrons without destroying the function of the vital structures in the area."

13.2 TYPES OF RADIATION

The primary type of radiation used for lung cancer is external beam radiation which directs radiation from a machine to the area of the tumor. A type of radiation frequently used with other cancers is brachytherapy, in which a radioactive source is placed inside the body in the area of the tumor.

13.21 Hyperfractionated Radiotherapy

The standard dose of radiation is once daily. In hyperfractionated radiation, the daily dose is divided into smaller doses that are given more than once a day. One study showed beneficial results but increased side effects:

"Patients were randomly allocated in a 3:2 ratio to CHART (Continuous hyperfractionated accelerated radiotherapy) or conventional radiotherapy Y. {In the Chart group} there was a 24% reduction in the relative risk of death, which is equivalent to an absolute improvement in 2-year survival of 9% from 20% to 29% (p = 0.004, 95% CI 0.63-0.92). Subgroup analyses (predefined) suggest that the largest benefit occurred in patients with squamous cell carcinomas (82% of the cases), in whom there was a 34% reduction in the relative risk of death (an absolute improvement at 2 years of 14% from 19% to 33%). During the first 3 months, severe dysphagia occurred more often in the CHART group than in the group on conventional radiotherapy (19 vs 3%). Otherwise, there were no important differences in short-term or long-term morbidity . . . CHART compared with conventional radiotherapy gave a significant improvement in survival of patients with NSCLC." Saunders, (2)

13.211 Cost Issues with Hyperfractioned Radiotherapy

Some HMO's may balk at the cost of this type of radiation even if there is some research showing its effectiveness. See Coyle(3). However, hyperfractionated radiation is not an unusual or strange therapy, it has been used with other forms of cancer, and there are clinical findings indicating its effectiveness with lung cancer. Thus, it should be a decision of the physician and patient as to its use. I suspect that confronted with a vigorous well-documented presentation, most HMO's would provide reimbursement for this treatment, even if they initially rejected its use, and did not approve its use for lung cancer on a routine basis.

13.22 Stereotactic Radiosurgery or Gamma Knife

Another newer form of radiation is stereotactic radiosurgery. Currently this is being used to treat cranial metastases. Gamma waves are narrowly directed to specific areas.

13.3 HOW RADIATION IS PERFORMED

13.31 Personnel Involved

There are different medical professionals involved with radiation as follows:

Radiation Oncologist. A physician specializing in treating cancer with radiation. He makes many of the decisions as to the type and frequency of radiation.

Radiation Physicist. An expert in medical physics trained in planning radiation treatment. He helps determine the treatment plan and the specifics of the radiation.

Dosimetrist. A technician who also plans and calculates the dosage of radiation and how it will be administered, sometimes with a computer program.

Radiation Technologist. A specially trained technician who operates the radiation equipment. A nurse trained in radiation

therapy may help patients deal with any side effects. See American
Cancer Society, *(5)*.

13.4 SIDE EFFECTS

Generally there are not significant or long-lasting side effects with
radiation. Radiation therapy does not hurt, though some people
experience a sensation of warmth or tingling. While chemotherapy kills
some normal cells as well as tumor cells, the goal of radiation is to kill
only cancerous cells. The goal of radiation is to attack the tumor without
damaging normal tissue. While injecting a drug into the bloodstream
one cannot control its effect, however, when directing radiation one
can, and there are fewer side effects associated with radiation than
chemotherapy.

13.41 Tiredness

Tiredness and fatigue are associated with radiation, though the
precise causes are not known. According to the American Cancer Society
Guide, "fatigue is likely to begin early and increase using the course of
treatment, peaking between the third and fifth weeks . . . . Why the
body reacts to radiation in this way isn't exactly understood, though
there are a number of plausible explanations. It may be that the healing
process drains the body's energy. Another reason may be the buildup of
toxic wastes resulting from cell destruction. An increase in the body's
metabolism may play a role, too. Furthermore, daily trips to a radiation
center disrupt the normal activities of life." (5).

Are there different types of fatigue, one writer suggests so :

> "There are three types of fatigue: neuromuscular, attentional,
> or subjective fatigue. Neuromuscular fatigue involves the inability
> to move or use the physical body in the usual capacity. Attentional
> fatigue is the inability to concentrate and direct attention for a
> period of time. Subjective fatigue describes any sense of unusual,
> abnormal or excessive whole body tiredness unrelated to any
> level of activity or exertion. All three types may be experienced at
> the same time. The key is to assess the level of fatigue and its
> symptoms. Pinpoint the factors, such as when it begins, when it
> peaks, or if it is constant. Develop a plan to contain your level of

fatigue and incorporate it into your life rather than letting it control you. Tiredness is usually relieved with rest, good nutrition, stress management, and/or exercise."

13.411 Measurements of Fatigue

Some use the Piper Fatigue Scale as an objective way of measuring fatigue. A general measure of quality of life is The Lung Cancer Symptom Scale.

13.42 Poor Appetite

Related to fatigue, loss of appetite can result. Changes in some cells affect hunger signals or the stress of illness reduces appetite. However, since cachexia, (loss and body weight and muscle from tumor) can arise, maintaining good appetite and eating habits is important. One study found that while fatigue and loss of appetite were common symptoms, there was no clear correlation between the two. "Fatigue and nutrition are major problems for patients with lung cancer, but nutritional changes do not correlate with fatigue." Beach (8)

13.43 Skin Problems

Skin in the radiation area may undergo temporary changes such as redness, dryness, or itchiness.

13.44 Addressing Side Effects

With any side effects, the physician and nurse should be informed. Doctors vary, with radiation we can have skilled physicians with limited empathy for the patient. Consider cancer support groups and speak with groups like the American Cancer Society. You should consult with your oncologist before making any changes since that could affect treatment in some way.

13.45 Measuring the Positive Consequences of Radiation

The primary purpose of radiation is generally to relieve pain or symptoms associated with the disease. For a small group of stage 1 patients ineligible for surgery, radiation's purpose is curative. In the majority of patients, radiation is designed to kill tumor cells in a specific area and relieve symptoms caused by the tumor. That process may extend life but since a metastatic tumor cannot be completed eradicated by radiation, it generally is not intended to provide an overall cure.

As a tool in relieving pain and discomfort, radiation is frequently successful. "(R)esults suggest symptomatic benefit from radiotherapy even in those NSCLC patients with advanced disease." Lutz (12) "The rate of palliation of local symptoms is high, being 60-80% for chest pain and hemoptysis, while breathlessness and cough are controlled at a somewhat lower rate (50-70%)." Numico (9) "Radical radiotherapy offers palliation of respiratory symptoms and improved QoL (quality of life) in a substantial proportion of patients with NSCLC who have relatively good prognostic features." Langendijk (10).

13.5 CURRENT DEBATES WITH RADIATION

13.51 Radiation and Small Cell Cancer

Should radiation be used for small cell cancer? While local control is helpful, its utility is debatable since metastasis is the primary danger of small cell lung cancer. A 1997 article argues for its use,

"Although chest irradiation has been used to treat SCLC for over four decades, its standard role in the management of limited-stage disease was established only during the last decade. Multiple prospective randomized trials have shown that the addition of thoracic radiation therapy to chemotherapy usually halves local failure rates, from >60% with chemotherapy alone to about 30% with chemoradiation therapy." Kumar (1). Ali (11)

If distant metastases occur, the significance of local control is limited. Many would argue that radiation's use would be palliative, not curative.

REFERENCES

1. Kumar, *The role of thoracic radiotherapy in the management of limited-stage small cell lung cancer: past, present, and future*, Chest 1997 Oct;112(4 Suppl):259S-265S.

2. Saunders, *Continuous hyperfractionated accelerated radiotherapy (CHART) versus conventional radiotherapy in non-small-cell lung cancer: a randomized multicentre trial. CHART Steering Committee* Lancet 1997 Jul 19;350(9072):161-5.

3. Coyle, *Costs of conventional radical radiotherapy versus continuous hyperfractionated accelerated radiotherapy* (CHART) Clin Oncol 7 Coll Radiol) 1997;9(5):313-21.

4. McGuire, *73.6 Gy and Beyond: Hyperfractionated, Accelerated Radiotherapy for Non-Small-Cell Lung Cancer.* J Clin Oncol 2001 Feb 1;19(3):705-711.

5. American Cancer Society, *Informed Decisions* 1997.

6. West Virginia University Oncology Page http://www.hsc.wvu.edu/ radrx/patfatig.htm.

7. Beach *Relationship between Fatigue and Nutritional status in Patients receiving Radiation Therapy to treat Lung Cancer,* Oncol Nurs Forum 2001 Jul;28(6):1027-31.

8. Lutz, *Symptom frequency and severity in patients with metastatic or locally recurrent lung cancer: a prospective study using the Lung Cancer Symptom Scale in a community hospital.* J Palliat Med 2001 Summer;4(2):157-65.

9. Numico, *Best supportive care in Non-small cell Lung Cancer: is there a role for Radiotherapy and Chemotherapy,* Lung Cancer 2001 Jun;32(3):213-26.

10. Langendijk, *Prospective study on quality of life before and after radical radiotherapy in non-small-cell lung cancer,* J. Clin Oncol 2001 Apr 15;19(8):2123-33.

11. Ali, *Phase II study of Hyperfractionated Radiotherapy and Concurrent weekly alternating Chemotherapy in limited-stage small cell Lung Cancer.* Lung Cancer 1998 Oct;22(1):39-44.

12. Lutz, *A retrospective Quality of Life analysis using the Lung Cancer Symptom Scale in patients treated with palliative radiotherapy for advanced nonsmall cell Lung Cancer.* Int J Radiat Oncol Biol Phys 1997 Jan 1;37(1):117-22.

CHAPTER 14

DEALING WITH THE CONSEQUENCES OF CANCER: PAIN, WEIGHT LOSS, FATIGUE

14.1 FATIGUE

Fatigue may be the most frequently reported symptom of cancer and cancer treatment. It is defined as a sustained sense of exhaustion and decreased capacity for physical and mental work that is not relieved by rest or sleep. (1) (2). Another chapter discussed fatigue in relation to radiation though it occurs in many contexts. Generally fatigue, as well as the other symptoms, is associated with the severity of the disease. The causes may be physiological, psychological, disease-related, treatment related, or a combination.

14.11 Disease-related Causes

The tumor's theft of nutrients, a state related to tumor growth, infection, and disruption of cellular processes can account for fatigue. (2) (3)

14.12 Treatment-Related Causes

Radiation is sometimes reported to cause fatigue. One possible cause may be the increased energy needed to repair damaged tissue. Fatigue is likewise associated with chemotherapy. Where anemia results from chemotherapy, fatigue may occur as a result.

14.13 Remedies for Fatigue

Your oncologist should be consulted about fatigue and may identify a specific factor associated with the disease or treatment. Depending on the severity, treatment may be changed, or dosage reduced to manage fatigue. "A study of breast cancer patients demonstrated a reduction in fatigue in women who participated in a low intensity-walking program." (1) An exercise advocate writes:

> "Regular exercise has been shown to benefit most cancer patients, as discussed in a recent article in the *Annals of Behavioral Medicine*.[1] According to the 24 studies reviewed in this article, exercise contributes to improvement in quality of life, physical strength, and endurance; reduces fatigue and depression; and increases the number of immune cells which may have implications in actual cancer control." (3)

Any program should be approved by a physician and is dependent upon the patient's physical status. Fatigue may be associated with depression. Providing support through family, friends, in-person and on-line support groups can help. Acor.org runs specific programs for lung cancer.

14.2 THE SIGNIFICANCE OF WEIGHT LOSS

"About half of all cancer patients experience a wasting syndrome called cachexia in which the tumor induces metabolic changes in the host leading to loss of adipose tissue and skeletal muscle mass." (Tisdale 7). "When the problem is tumor-induced weight loss, increasing food intake isn't the answer, as the metabolic alterations that occur in these patients would appear to prevent the effective use of additional calories, resulting in ongoing wasting." Rogers (2) Substantial weight loss is a negative sign in a patient's prognosis. "Tumor-induced weight loss (TIWL) is a common cause of morbidity and mortality in patients with advanced cancer. It differs from simple starvation in that it cannot be reversed by the provision of apparently adequate nutrition." Barber (5), Rogers, (6).

14.21 Distinguishing Cachexia from anorexia.

Anorexia is eating significantly less than normal requirements and should be distinguished from cachexia:

> "Unlike simple starvation, where body fat is lost preferentially, cancer cachexia is associated with depletion of both fat and skeletal muscle mass. Although anorexia is frequently associated with cachexia, a reduction of nutrient intake alone could not explain the progressive wasting. Instead, the process appears to be mediated by circulatory tumor-produced catabolic factors acting either alone or in concert with certain cytokines. Various phenomenon are associated with cachexia." Tisdale (7).

14.22 Increased Consumption of Protein

"Whole body protein turnover has been found to be increased in the majority of advanced cancer patients compared with starved normal individuals and weight-losing noncancer patients and appears to increase further with progression of disease." Barber (1) "Cachectic cancer patients exhibit relative glucose intolerance and insulin resistance with an increased rate of glucose production and recycling via lactate (the Cori cycle). These changes may become more pronounced with progression of the disease." Barber (1)

The precise mechanisms are unclear. While weight loss is associated with poor prognosis and is frequently seen in advanced cancer patients, cachexia can occur early in the course of cancer. A clear correlation between, for example, cancer size and the extent of cachexia is not seen.

14.221 Influence of Cytokines

One theory is that cytokines such as tumor necrosis factor "mobilize fatty acids and amino acids from adipose tissue and skeletal muscle respectively."

14.23 Nutritional Programs

Increasing calorie intake can help mitigate the effects of cachexia.

Helping the cancer patient to eat may mean some modifications. "If the patient indicates that they eat best in the morning, the largest meal should be served in the morning and small snacks eaten throughout the remainder of the day. Dietary restrictions should be eliminated since adherence to restrictions may decrease the caloric intake that is essential to the individual with cancer." Rogers (6).

One study found that "a nutritional supplement enriched with fish oil will reverse weight loss in patients with pancreatic cancer cachexia." Barber (5). "In animals bearing a murine colon adenocarcinoma, EPA— one of the most important fish oil w-3 fatty acids—has been shown to inhibit cancer cachexia . . . Diets in which 50% of total energy was provided as fish oil also reversed tumor-associated weight loss in rats with an experimental prostate tumor." (Burns 11).

The problem is not easily solved. In one study, a program of Total Perenteral Nutrition or (TPN) failed to produce significant improvement in small cell lung cancer patients. Some patients benefit from appetite stimulants like Megace. Disease combined with chemotherapy diminish many patient's desire to eat. "The appetite stimulant megestrol acetate (Megace) has been reported to induce a weight gain of greater than 5% in 15% of the patients treated, although significant changes in lean body mass were not generally observed." (Tisdale 9).

14.3 DEPRESSION

14.31 Incidence

Approximately 40% of lung cancer patients encounter depression with the incidence related to the severity of the disease and its symptoms. Aldridge (13). Various people and people can provide support during this difficult time including: family and friends, nurses and counseling professionals, psychologists and social workers, clergman, cancer organizations like the American Cancer Society and Alcase devoted to lung cancer, and online cancer support groups like Acor.

REFERENCES

1. *Fatigue in Cancer Patients*, Cancerbacup www.cancerbacup. org.uk/reports/fatigue-mac.htm.

2. Winningham, *Fatigue in Cancer* (Jones & Bartlett 1999).
3. *Exercises for People With Lung Cancer: A Suggested Exercise Program for Improving Quality of Life After Diagnosis*, Vol. 20, No 10 (November/December 2000).
4. Hoseman, *Fatigue: The Multidimensional Side Effect*, M. D. ANDERSON ONCOLOG Volume 44, Number 1 (January 1999).
5. Barber, *Advances in the Management of Tumor-Induced Weight Loss*, Medscape.com (2002, Continuing education program).
6. Rogers, General Weight Loss in Cancer Patients: An Approach to Assessment and Care, Medscape.com (2002, Continuing education program).
7. Barber, *Effect of a fish oil-enriched nutritional supplement on metabolic mediators in patients with pancreatic cancer cachexia*, Nutr Cancer 2001;40(2):118-24.
8. *Evans, Limited impact of total parenteral nutrition on nutritional status during treatment for small cell lung cancer*, Cancer Research, Vol 45, Issue 7 3347-3353.
9. Tisdale, *Wasting in Cancer*, Journal of Nutrition Vol. 129 No. 1 January 1999, pp. 243S-246S.
10. Tisdale, *Clinical Trials for the Treatment of Secondary Wasting and Cachexia*, Presentation at the 1999 American Society for Nutritional Sciences Meeting.
11. Burns, *Phase I Clinical Study of Fish Oil Fatty Acid Capsules for Patients with Cancer Cachexia: Cancer and Leukemia Group B Study 9473*, Clinical Cancer Research Vol. 5, 3942-3947, December 1999.
12. Klein S, Simes J, Blackburn G. *Total parenteral nutrition and cancer clinical trials*. Cancer. 1986;58:1378-1386.

CHAPTER 15

IRESSA AND EPIDERMAL GROWTH FACTOR INHIBITORS

15.0 THE EPIDERMAL GROWTH FACTOR PATHWAY_

15.01 Normal Cell Signaling_

Duplication of genes is a normal process in the human body. Proteins called growth factors provide signals for cell replication, but malfunctions in these growth factors are a critical part of cancer. A basic model of cancer suggests it is a product of a growth factor prompting unnecesary duplication of cells and the failure of a tumor suppresor gene to regulate them.

A more sophisticated model suggests cancer presents a complex system with many growth factors, multiple tumor suppresor genes, and damage to other cellular regulators. As we enter the 21st century we are learning that both models may be correct for different types of cancers—there are simple ones with only a few components of growth and more complex ones with numerous contributing factors. In the 60's and 70's, we learned that cancers acted differently depending upon their site; today we are seeing that lung cancer represents a heterogenous group of cancers, some of which respond very differently to treatment than others. We now look to one important growth factor, (EGF) and its treatment.

15.02 Epidermal Growth Factor

The epidermal growth factor EGF and its associated receptor (EGFR) plays a role in normal human development with functions which include repair of damaged tissue and development of_new tissue in fetuses. Klein (49). Its role in healthy non-developing adults is unclear, and scientists are not sure whether functioning EGF is needed for normal processes. EGF is a critical factor in various cancers.

"The epidermal growth factor receptor (EGFR) autocrine pathway contributes to a number of processes important to cancer development and progression, including cell proliferation, apoptosis, angiogenesis, and metastatic spread. The critical role the EGFR plays in cancer has led to an extensive search for selective inhibitors of the EGFR signaling pathway. The results of a large body of preclinical studies and the early clinical trials thus far conducted suggest that targeting the EGFR could represent a significant contribution to cancer therapy. A variety of different approaches are currently being used to target the EGFR. The most promising strategies in clinical development include monoclonal antibodies to prevent ligand binding and small molecule inhibitors of the tyrosine kinase enzymatic activity to inhibit autophosphorylation and downstream intracellular signaling." Tartora, (2), See also FDA (1). See also Baselga (24).

15.03 EGFR's Inhibition of Normal Apoptotic Processes

The body has mechanisms to deal with chromosome damage, one of which is apoptosis, the elimination of damaged cells. When activated EGF appears to frustrate that process, and has an anti-apoptotic effect protecting mutated cells from orderly elimination. EGFR activation seems to promote tumor growth by sending signals for growth downstream, to other cellular regulators and growth factors.

15.04 EGF and EGFR

To initiate cell reproduction, a growth factor links with an associated receptor, like a lock and key. EGF links with EGFR, the epidermal growth factor receptor. "Growth factor receptors are found on the surface of cells and normally play a role in the regulation of cellular growth and differentiation processes. The discovery that these receptors are present in unusually high_numbers in many tumours then suggested that they play a role in carcinogenesis. Various attempts were therefore made to selectively inhibit {EGFR} signaling pathways. In one approach, antibodies that block the extracellular part of these receptors were developed, while another approach resulted in the development of low-molecular-weight substances known as cell signaling inhibitors that block the intracellular part of the receptors." In recent years, the receptor rather than the growth factor itself has become the target of new drugs.

15.1 THE STRUCTURE OF EGFR

15.11 Receptor Structure

The receptor has two basic parts. The first part is called the extracellular ligand-binding domain. There the receptor receives a signal from a growth factor and a process called ligand binding occurs. Once binding occurs, a signal is sent to the second part of the receptor called the tyrosine kinase domain, and a process called autophosphorylation occurs. A chemical change occurs and signals are sent to other cells:__"In each receptor a molecule of adenosine triphosphate (ATP) becomes attached and an energy-rich phosphate group is transferred to the amino acid tyrosine. Activation of tyrosine kinase and phosphorylation of tyrosine residues leads to activation of intracellular signaling pathways." Roche (61).

15.12 The Tyrosine Kinase Portion of the Receptor_

What does the tyrosine kinase do?

"Tyrosine kinases are proteins that can attach a phosphate group to the amino acid tyrosine. This action serves at least two basic roles: It allows two proteins to bind to one another, and it can serve as a switch that turns a function on or off. Thus, tyrosine kinases act like small keys that can regulate a cascade of events, including cellular division. Tyrosine kinase can be a freestanding enzyme within a process or it can be associated with a receptor that is a trigger for a cascade of processes—aptly named a tyrosine kinase receptor. A receptor is simply a docking point for an outside chemical, much like a docking port for the space shuttle on the space station." Tyrosine Kinase (66).

In cancer, the signals generated by this chemical process are abnormal, and other cells are told to duplicate or perform other aberrant functions. Tyrosine kinases are becoming a primary target for cancer research:

> "Cancer is characterized by successive changes in cell behavior caused by accumulated genetic alterations. Two kinds of cellular changes are particularly important in cancer pathology. First, the cell division cycle becomes deregulated, causing overproliferation and tumor growth. Second, these transformed cells may gain mobility: they lose contacts with their neighbors and the extracellular matrix (ECM), become mobile, crawl into the circulatory system, and crawl out at a new location distant from the original tumor."
>
> "This mechanism accounts for metastasis, the systemic spread of cancer. Both of these pathological behaviors are controlled by cell signaling pathways that employ tyrosine phosphorylation as a molecular on/off switch (Hunter, 1998). Numerous oncogenes encode overactive mutant forms of protein tyrosine kinases (PTKs), whose normal counterparts regulate cell division and differentiation in response to extracellular signals. PTKs also contribute to regulation of the cytoskeleton and cell adhesion systems that determine whether a cell will remain in place or migrate." Cancer pathology & tyrosine phosphorylation (65).

Cancer drugs can work in two basic ways, they can try to prevent binding, or autophosphorylation. The fact that there are two separate functions means that drugs may later be combined, and anti-EGFR drugs are likely to have different degrees of effectiveness depending upon the specific area of cell damage in the epidermal growth factor receptor.

15.13 The EGF Family_of Receptors

EGFR is part of the Erb family of receptors, and is also called Erb1. There are four receptors in the Erb receptor family, Erb1, 2, 3, and 4. It would be simple if there were a single growth factor and single receptor. Unfortunately the human body is far more complex. Multiple growth factors can contact EGFR to initiate signaling. The primary one we address here is the epidermal growth factor. In a simple model, EGF contacts EGFR. In a more complex but accurate model, other growth factors may contact EGFR, and when binding occurs, EGFR will send signals to other members of the Erb family, "cross-talk."

15.2 CLINICAL TRIAL RESULTS

15.21 Initial Results and Grouping

Initial studies with Iressa found that about 12% of patients achieved a partial response, that is, reduction of 50% of the tumor. More patients found their diseases stabilized. FDA Trial 16 found about 35% of patients experienced disease stabilization._FDA (1). In addition to extending life, the drug improved quality of life, with one third of patients reported relief of at least one pulmonary related symptom. FDA Advisory Committee (1). Funokuora reported symptom improvement rates of 40.3% and 37.0% in his study. (45). Nonetheless, Iressa did not significantly extend life for most patients, though disease stabilization and symptom relief were clearly important.

Based upon these studies, the FDA approved Iressa for third line treatment of non-small lung cancer. That is, Iressa would be recommended after two types of chemotherapy were no longer effective. Chemotherapy has response rates of about 20%. Because these response rates were higher than Iressa's 12%, the new drug could not be recommended for routine treatment. Nonetheless, Iressa was reported to improve symptoms and stabilize disease in some patients along with providing responses in some. Therefore, Iressa was approved as third line therapy, to be used after platinum based chemotherapy (Cisplatin or Carboplatin) and Taxol. While the FDA's recommendation is important, physicians can prescribe the drug off label, in other ways. Further studies reported in 2003 and 2004 have provided important information about who is likely to benefit from Iressa.

15.22 Who Responds to Iressa

The category non-small cell lung cancer includes adenocarcinoma, squamous cell carcinoma, large cell cancer, and a host of subgroups within these categories. In the past 40 years, many similarities among these types were found, particularly their responsiveness to radiation, chemotherapy, and surgery. Non-small cell lung tumors share the common characteristic of behaving differently than small cell cancers. Within the non-small category, treatment has been essentially the same for all three types for the last half century. This may change with Iressa.

Recent studies found that patients with bronchioloalveolar lung cancer (BAC), a subtype of adenocarcinoma, particularly seemed to respond to Iressa. Additionally, non-smokers with lung cancer also benefited:

1. The first study was published in the prestigious New England Journal of Medicine (56, full-text available online at no charge). Nine patients were found to respond to Iressa. Four had BAC, a subtype of adenocarcinoma while five had adenocarcinoma itself. None of those who responded had squamous cell or large cell lung cancer. None of the responders were smokers, six had never smoked, while 3 were former smokers. Lynch (55). For the 9 who responded, mutations were observed in eight clustered within the tyrosine kinase domain of EGFR. Iressa inhibits autophosphylation from the tyrosine kinase which helps explain why the drug would be effective with patients having tyrosine kinase cellular malfunctions.

2. A second study also found that response to Iressa could be predicted by the existence of abnormalities in the tyrosine kinase region of the EGFR: "While sequencing of the kinase domain (exons 18 through 24) revealed no mutations in tumors from the four patients who progressed on gefitinib, all five tumors from gefitinib (Iressa)-responsive patients harbored EGFR kinase domain mutations." Paez (56).

The authors then tested tissue from lung cancer patients and found the type of damage to the tyrosine kinase to be relatively rare. Only one of sixty one randomly selected patients had it. However, almost all who responded to Iressa had it.__Cell analysis confirmed the efficiency of Iressa. When cells from patients with the defect were tested, Iressa was effective at 100 milligrams. However, 100 times the dosage was required to duplicate that response with other cell lines. Paez (56). Genetic testing of patients to determine whether they are likely to respond to

Iressa makes sense. The how, why, and cost of such testing remains to be determined.

Other studies have shown similar results. In one study, non-smokers had a response rate of 29.4% (10/34) compared with 4.6% (5/108) for smokers. FDA (1) (43). In Wong's study, "6 out of 7 responders were non-smokers." FDA Center (48, at 7). In Shah's study, "bronchioalveolar carcinoma and having never smoked were the only predictors of response." FDA Center (48, at 7).

Study Name	Characteristics	Characteristics of Non-responders	Importance of the Study
Lynch, Specific Activating Mutations in the Epidermal Growth Factor Receptor Underlying Responsiveness of Non-Small-Cell Lung Cancer to Gefitinib. The New England Journal of Medicine (online April 29, 2004).	9 patients benefit, 4 with BAC, 5 with adenocarcinoma. responders had detectible mutations in the kinase region of EGFR	0 patients with squamous or large cell had responses.	Initial study finds that BAC and adenocarcinoma patients benefit from Iressa and have specific defects in tyrosine kinase domain.
Sloan Kettering Study_Pao, EGF receptor gene mutations are common in lung cancers from Never smokers'and are associated with sensitivity of tumors to gefitinib and erlotinib, PNAS ISeptember 7, 2004 vol. 101 no. 36 13306-13311	Nine of 12 (75%) mutation-positive tumors in this study had adenocarcinoma histology and were derived from never smokers.Mutations in the TK domain of EGFR are common in surgically resected NSCLCs derived from never smokers but infrequent in former or current smokers.	None of eight Iressa-resistant tumors contained mutations within exons 18-24 of EGFR."	Found non-smokers_and very light former smokers had tyrosine kinase mutation, few found in smokers. Identified specific genetic area where response is likely to occur.

15.23 Implications for BAC and Adenocarcinoma Patients

A clear pattern is arising. Iressa is very effective with patients with tyrosine kinase defects. Nonsmokers, patients with BAC, and some adenocarcinoma patients appear to have that genetic damage, it plays a prominent role in their cancers, and Iressa is effective for a substantial percentage. The response rates for BAC patients and non-smokers far exceed those with chemotherapy or radiation.

Nonsmokers are unlikely to have the extensive genetic abnormalities affecting growth factors, receptors, and tumor suppressor genes that smokers have. Instead their tumors appear to be largely EGFR driven, and for some, Iressa the silver bullet that attacks the specific abnormality. For non-smokers and brief former smokers, a single or small number of gene abnormalities is causing or prompting their cancers. Thus, if that area of damage can be identified and addressed, the prognosis may be good.

15.231 Should Iressa be First-Line Treatment for BAC Nonsmokers and Adenocarcinoma Patients?

Physicians will need to investigate whether Iressa should be first-line treatment for patients in this group. Currently Iressa is recommended as third-line treatment after two forms of chemotherapy. See FDA (1). However, Iressa's 35-40% response rates with certain groups dwarfs the 20% response rates found in chemotherapy. Additionally, since Iressa targets only a specific kinase, it generates far fewer side effects than chemotherapies which impact a large number of dividing cells.

Whether oncologists will accept these results and prescribe Iressa first-line for BAC and adenocarcinoma patents, particularly nonsmokers, remains to be seen. Some will follow the current FDA recommendations which recommend Iressa as third-line treatment, and wait for a pronouncement from a major organization before adopting a different approach. Major research institutions may be more agressive and innovative in treatment strategies. Patients will have some tough decisions and may switch oncologists to obtain what they see as the most beneficial treatment.

15.232 Insurance Questions

Insurance issues will arise. The studies indicate cell testing can predict who is likely to respond to Iressa. Will insurance pay for such testing? Since that test is not publicly available, the cost is uncertain.

15.24 Iressa and Squamous Cell and Large Cell Patients

Results are discouraging for squamous cell and large-cell patients. Few responses came in these two groups and the pattern of genetic damage in the tyrosine kinase region does not appear to be generally present in squamous cell or large cell patients.

The FDA recommendation and findings would seem accurate for these groups. That is, Iressa is third line treatment to be used after two forms of chemotherapy are no longer effective. The overall response rate for Iressa was about 11%, we now know that the rates are appreciably higher for certain forms of cancer, and correspondingly lower for squamous cell and large cell. For the squamous cell and large cell groups, Iressa may stabilize disease and relieve symptoms. This is presumably because EGF plays some role in cancer spread, but not a critical or dispositive one for these patients.

An ASCO presentation (American Society of Clinical Oncology) suggested there are three groups involved with Iressa response. First are adenocarcinoma and BAC patients, non and former light smokers with tyrosine kinase damage, who will substantially benefit from Iressa, secondly, squamous cell and other patients may secure a modest benefit from Iressa, and thirdly, those with properly functioning EGFR but other abnormalities who will receive no benefit from Iressa.

15.241 Other Forms of Treatment

Some of these patients may look to other forms of treatments. If the patients do not have the defect in the tyrosine kinase region, a tyrosine kinase treatment seems misdirected. For EGFR treatment, they might consider Tarceva which attacks the binding process or other drugs. Perhaps their cancers are not primarily EGFR driven in which case other types of treatment like cox-2 inhibitors and anti-angiogenic drugs are preferable. More research is needed. In the upcoming months, cell tests may be developed, and drugs could be tested in a laboratory rather than on the patient.

15.25 Duration of Response

For patients of all types, when can a response be expected? Trial 39 reported, "the majority of patients (72%, 16/22) who achieved a response did so by the third (4 patients) or fourth week (12 patients); 3 patients achieved a response by week 7, 1 by week 12, and 2 by week 16. FDA (46). The final FDA report likewise concluded that those who benefit do so relatively quickly: "Many patients had a prospectively defined improvement in disease-related symptoms: the symptom improvement rates were 40% in IDEAL 1 and 43% in IDEAL 2. Symptom relief was rapid: the median time to improvement was 8 days in IDEAL 1 and 10 days in IDEAL 2 (the times of the first post-baseline assessment for each study).

There was a significant improvement in disease-related symptoms in most patients with a partial/complete response or stable disease in the FDA Ideal studies. Natale (8). Response is correlated with the development of a rash.

15.26 Dosage

Optimal dosage remains unclear. Some studies reported no significant increase in efficacy from 250mg to 500mg. The FDA evaluated both 250 mg (milligrams) per day and 500 mg dosages, but reached no clear conclusion. In their studies, the efficacy was similar between two dosages with some fewer side effects at the lower dose. FDA (46), at 51. The FDA also noted a higher response rate for women than men. More women experienced tumor responses at either the 250-mg/day and 500/mg day doses." (FDA 47). In trial 39, the response rate (diminution of 50% tumor volume) for women was 17.5% but 5% for men." FDA statistical review, 48 at 4. Janne found all those who had responses were women. FDA statistical review. _FDA Approval Package at 62.

15.3 IRESSA AND CHEMOTHERAPY AND RADIATION

15.31 Complimentary Impact Seen in Cell and Animal Studies

The use of different drugs in combination has become standard in treating lung cancer. Logically one could believe that Iressa would compliment chemotherapy and there are cell studies supporting that hypothesis:

"The cooperative growth inhibitory effect of cytotoxic drugs and ZD 1839 was shown to involve the induction of apoptosis (cell death). In fact, treatment with ZD 1839 potentiated cytotoxic drug induced apoptosis by approximately 2 to 3.5 fold . . . Studies have also used ZD 1839 and cytotoxic drugs (paclitaxel, topotecan or raltitexed) in vivo in murine models of human tumors. A cooperative antitumor effect was observed with each combination; there was a significant suppression of tumor growth and prolonged survival. This effect was most pronounced with the ZD 1839 plus paclitaxel cogitation." Ciardiello (13). Studies showed Iressa reduced or eliminated at a considerable percentage of solid tumors on laboratory mice, and also reduced other factors associated with cancer. Fortunate (12).

While commentators suggested that Iressa would improve chemotherapy's effect, a positive result was not demonstrated in a recent clinical trial.

15.32 Clinical Trials Using Iressa and Chemotherapy Failed to Demonstrate a Benefit from the Combination

Two large scale clinical trials found Iressa did not improve the effects of chemotherapy. (50). The well-publicized clinical trial compared patients who took chemotherapy and Iressa with those who took chemotherapy alone. The group taking the combination did no better than the group using chemotherapy alone. Rates of survival, partial response, and complete response were similar between the two experimental groups using 250mg and 500 mg Iressa + chemotherapy, versus the control group taking chemotherapy alone with placebo.

15.33 Explanations and Conclusions

The lack of benefit may be a product of a plateau effect known in other areas where the addition of new drugs does not significantly improve results. For example, adding a third chemotherapy drug to a patient's treatment does not significantly improve response rates or survival. The patients were in a group with very advanced cancer, so either chemotherapy alone or with Iressa could provide only limited help. The study was limited to patients with advanced lung cancer. It remains to be seen whether earlier intervention with a combination of chemotherapy and Iressa would be beneficial to patients with less advanced disease.

15.4 SIDE EFFECTS

Because Iressa targets a specific part of the cell, its side effects are limited. In comparison, most chemotherapy drugs affect large numbers of dividing cells.

15.41 Rash

The most prevalent side effect is a localized rash. Patients have reported it but it appears to be localized and is not usually serious. Additionally, some studies have found the existence of a rash indicates Iressa is working with patients with rashes having longer survival rates, though other studies found no impact. (53)

15.411 Treatment of the Rash

Some suggest a moisturizing product is helpful in addressing the rash. At a non-small cell lung cancer newsgroup, patients and care-givers discuss dealing with drug side effects and offer suggestions. See *www.acor.org.*

15.42 Diarrhea

Diarrhea though not particularly severe has also been reported.

15.43 Pneumonitis

One serious side effect has been an unusual form of pneumonia. Pneumonia is associated with lung cancer and chemotherapy generally. However, there have been a series of pneumonitis deaths linked to Iressa initially reported in Japan:

> "We assessed four patients who had non-small cell lung cancer causing severe acute interstitial pneumonia in association with gefitinib. Although two patients recovered after treatment with steroids, the other two died from progressive respiratory dysfunction. On the basis of autopsies and bilateral distribution of diffuse ground-glass opacities in chest CTs, we diagnosed diffuse alveolar damage, which was consistent with acute interstitial pneumonia. Patients with interstitial pneumonia also had other

pulmonary disorders such as previous thoracic irradiation and poor performance status. Physicians should be aware of the alveolar damage induced by gefitinib, especially for patients with these characteristic features." Inoue (22).

15.431 Presentation of Pneumonitis

FDA describes the onset this way, "patients often present with the acute onset of dyspnea (difficulty breathing), sometimes associated with cough or low-grade fever, often becoming severe within a short time and requiring hospitalization." FDA (1).

15.432 Monitoring

Careful monitoring for this side effect has been recommended. Patients on Iressa should monitor temperature rises, fevers, and immediately report problems to their oncologist. FDA suggests that "persons with concurrent pulmonary fibrosis have a higher mortality rate." This would presumably include people with silicosis, asbestosis and similar fibrotic disease.

15.5 OTHER EPIDERMAL GROWTH FACTOR THERAPIES

15.51 Tarceva

Tarceva (also called OSI-774 or Orlotinib) is a less publicized epidermal growth factor inhibitor. Like Iressa, it is directed to the tyrosine kinase portion of the epidermal growth factor receptor. A phase 1 clinical trial reported, "OSI-774 was well tolerated, and several patients with epidermoid malignancies demonstrated either antitumor activity or relatively long periods of stable disease." (17). One study found a 12% response rate with symptom improvement, findings similar to Iressa. Perez-Soler (59). Like Iressa, the occurence of a rash correlated with response to the drug. An important study compared Tarceva with a placebo and found it improved survival. Asco (63).

15.511 Who is Likely to Benefit?

Initial results are similar to Iressa, with a response rate of 9%, a small bit lower than Iressa but within the range of chance. As with Iressa, non-smokers seem to benefit most with Iressa. 25% of non-smokers responded compared with 4% of smokers. Asco (63). For smokers, the survival rate was almost the same with or without the drug. See Asco (63) citing Tribute trial.

15.512 Asco Report of Tribute Trial

The percentage of adenocarcinoma responders was 14% compared with 4% for other. Women had a 14% response rate compared with 6% for men. Interestingly, performance status, a measure of how sick the patient is as indicated by mobility and like factors was not a significant factor. As with Iressa, there appears to be a narrow group of non-smokers with adenocarcinoma who benefit greatly from Tarceva. At the other end, smokers with squamous cell cancer and normal functioning EGFR seem to benefit little, if at all. In the middle, there seems to be a group who have a modest benefit in disease stabilization, and a mild increase in survival, with that group perhaps having small abnormalities in EGFR, or multiple growth factors.

15.513 Side Effects

An important blind trial assessed side effects, with patients not knowing whether they were being given placebo or Tarceva. Many side effects were reported including anemia, vomiting and fatigue. However, the results for most side effects were essentially the same for placebo and drug.__Two were significant. Again, patients reported a rash at substantially higher rates. Diarhrea was higher with the drug. Patients participating in the Acor online newsgroup reported though, that it could be controlled.

15.514 Chemotherapy + Tarceva

One study showed no substantial benefit from adding Tarceva to chemotherapy, mirroring results with Iressa. Asco (63).__However, favorable results were reported with a combination of Bevacizubak and Tarceva. (Asco (63). The 51% one year survival rate was higher than the 34% one year rate reported in the Tarceva trial alone.

An application has been submitted to the FDA, with a presentation similar to Iressa focusing on disease stablization and symptom relief.

Since its mode of action is similar to Iressa, it is unclear what Tarceva does that Iressa does not.

15.52 Erbitux

Erbitux (IMC-C225 or Cetuximab) is a monoclonal antibody (Maps) directed against ligand binding in the extracellular domain of EGFR. While it is an epidermal growth factor inhibitor like Iressa, it has a different mode of action, since it prevents ligand binding rather than autophosphylation. Erbitux has been used with colon cancer. (58)

15.521 Erbitux and Chemotherapy

Adding Iressa to chemotherapy provided no additional efficacy. However, the combination of Erbitux and chemotherapy did create higher response rates in a clinical trial. Molecular mechanisms predicting response to cetuximab therapy are currently not well understood and studies are ongoing to assess the single-agent activity of cetuximab in metastatic NSCLC. Mattar (56).

15.522 Erbitux and Chemotherapy for Squamous and Large Cell Patients

As we saw above, squamous cell and large cell patients generally had few responses from Iressa. These patients generally did not have the tyrosine kinase damage that is the hallmark of the non-smoker BAC lung cancers that responded to Iressa. For squamous cell and large cell patients, Erbitux should be considered since its mode of action may conceivably be more effective against these cancers. More research is needed and how much weight a single clinical trial should be given is difficult to say.

15.53 Herceptin

Herceptin (Trastuzumab) has been FDA approved for metastatic breast cancer. The drug targets Erb2 which is a "molecular marker of ductal breast cancer although it is overexpressed in other adenocarcinomas as well (e.g. endometrial, colorectal and lung cancers)." While drug effectiveness is organ specific, lung, colon, and breast are categorized as solid tumors and have some common characteristics. For example, the chemotherapy drug Taxol is used for both breast and lung cancer.

15.531 Basis for FDA Approval of Breast Cancer

"The safety and effectiveness of Herceptin were studied in two trials with women whose metastatic breast cancers produced excess amounts of HER-2. In one clinical trial, women received either Herceptin and chemotherapy or chemotherapy alone. The women who received Herceptin and chemotherapy had slower tumor growth, greater reduction in tumor size, and longer survival than the women who received chemotherapy alone. In another trial, women received Herceptin by itself. In 14 percent of these women, the tumor got smaller or disappeared. Scientists continue to study the safety and effectiveness of Herceptin in clinical trials."

The FDA has not approved Herceptin for lung cancer. Since it is an FDA approved drug, a few physicians might consider it for lung cancer. The role of Erb2 in lung cancer is unclear. A 2002 report found that patients who overexpressed erb2 had poorer survival. Predictive Role of Her-2 (30).

15.532 Side Effects of Herceptin

The National Cancer Institute provides this list of side effects for breast cancer patients taking Herceptin.

"Side effects that most commonly occur during the first treatment with Herceptin include fever and/or chills. Other possible side effects include pain, weakness, nausea, vomiting, diarrhea, headaches, difficulty breathing, and rashes. These side effects generally become less severe after the first treatment with Herceptin." (NCI) (31).

There were also a small number of reports of heart problems.

15.54 CI-1033

Iressa is designed to inhibit one specific epidermal growth factor receptor at erb1. A new drug developed by Pfizer, CI-1033 was created to inhibit the entire family of receptors at erb-1, and erb-2-4.

"The erbB receptor family is part of the receptor tyrosine kinase superfamily and consists of four members, erbB-1, erbB-2, erbB-3, and erbB-4. A majority of solid tumors express one or more members of this receptor family, and coexpression of multiple erbB receptors leads to an enhanced transforming potential and worsened prognosis. The erbB receptor family has been shown to play an important role in both the development of the normal breast and in the pathogenesis and progression of breast cancer. Receptor overexpression has also been shown to be a negative prognostic indicator and to correlate with both tumor invasiveness and a lack of responsiveness to standard treatment. Clinically, blockade of the erbB-2 receptor has recently been shown to provide benefit in a subset of chemotherapy-resistant breast cancer patients. CI-1033 is an orally available pan-erbB receptor tyrosine kinase inhibitor that, unlike the majority of receptor inhibitors, effectively blocks signal transduction through all four members of the erbB family. In addition, it blocks the highly tumorigenic, constitutively activated variant of erbB-1, EGFRvIII, and inhibits downstream signaling through both the Ras/MAP kinase, and PI-3 kinase/AKT pathways. CI-1033 is also unique in that it is an irreversible inhibitor, thereby providing prolonged suppression of erbB receptor-mediated signaling."

15.541 Side effects

If targeting one receptor has caused only limited side effects, targeting the family of receptors seems to have increased adverse effects. A study reported about a one forth of patients experiencing nausea, vomiting or diarrhea. (Asco 33).

15.542 Irreversibility

It appears the impact upon epidermal growth factors is irreversible. (34). That fact may indicate it is more powerful, but should be used only on patients with advanced cancer.

15.55 Relationship Between EGFR and Erb2

Some preliminary studies have found that two or more of the epidermal growth inhibitor drugs can be used together with increased effectiveness. Normanno (26). EGFR or Erb1, the target for Iressa, and Erb2, the target for Herceptin, are part of the Erb family. Some suggest that activation of Erb1 may prompt or coincide with activation of Erb2. "Co-expression of EGFR and its ligands has also been found in primary breast carcinomas, suggesting that an autocrine loop may be operating in these tumors." Given that the two receptors are related, using two drugs to target the combination makes logical sense.

15.6 COMBINING DRUG THERAPIES_

15.61 Iressa and Chemotherapy_

Surprising and disappointing many, Iressa and related therapies have not improved the efficacy of chemotherapy according to two clinical trials.

15.62 Combining Two Types of Epidermal Growth Factor Treatments

Combining two types of drugs makes sense particulary among those patients without a clearly identifiable tyrosine kinase defect. Some have found success with dual treatment in cell studies.

"The combined treatment with gefitinib and cetuximab resulted in a synergistic effect on cell proliferation and in superior inhibition of EGFR-dependent signaling and induction of apoptosis. In a series of in vivo experiments, single-agent gefitinib or cetuximab resulted in transient complete tumor remission only at the highest doses. In contrast, suboptimal doses of gefitinib and cetuximab given together resulted in a complete and permanent regression of large tumors. In the combination-treated tumors, there was a superior inhibition of EGFR, mitogen-activated protein kinase, and Akt phosphorylation, as well as greater inhibition of cell proliferation and vascularization and enhanced apoptosis. Using cDNA arrays, we found 59 genes that were coregulated and 45 genes differentially regulated, including genes related to cell proliferation and differentiation, transcription, DNA synthesis and repair, angiogenesis, signaling molecules, cytoskeleton organization, and tumor invasion and metastasis. Conclusions: Our findings suggest both shared and complementary mechanisms of action with gefitinib and cetuximab and support combined EGFR targeting as a clinically exploitable strategy." Mattar (57).

Given the limited response to Iressa among squamous cell and large cell patients and tolerability of EGFR drugs, a combination makes sense for these groups. For these groups, Iressa is unlikely to provide significant relief, while a drug combination holds forth that possibility.

15.63 Iressa and Cox-2 Inhibitors

Celebrex is a Cox-2 inhibitor. Since Cox-2 plays an important role in lung cancer, scientists have looked at combining the two treatments.

"In this study, we have evaluated the possibility of obtaining a control of tumor growth without using cytotoxic drugs, by the combined blockade of EGFR, PKAI, and Cox-2 three molecules that interact in nodal points of distinct yet related signaling pathways. To translate this hypothesis in an experimental setting, we have used three novel agents with specific properties, including oral activity: the selective EGFR tyrosine kinase inhibitor ZD1839; a hybrid DNA/RNA MBO AS-PKAI; and thee Cox-2 inhibitor SC-236. All these agents have demonstrated antiproliferative and antiangiogenic properties in different tumor models, alone and in combination with cytotoxic drugs. We have demonstrated, in human colon and breast cancer cell types, that these agents in combination have a cooperative growth inhibitory effect, achieving maximal activity when the three agents are used together, even at very low doses. The antitumor effect is accompanied by down-regulation of the expression of Cox-2 as well as of VEGF and bFGF angiogenic proteins. Moreover, secretion of VEGF (a growth factor connected with metastasis) in the CM was inhibited by combined treatments."

15.7 CELL TESTING

15.71 The Harvard EGFR Test

The Harvard Gene laboratory is now offering a test to detect EGFR mutations. Their press release states:

"The Harvard Medical School—Partners HealthCare Center for Genetics and Genomics (HPCGG) has begun to offer a test that gives doctors a valuable new tool to guide the treatment of certain lung cancers. The test B known as EGFR Kinase Domain Sequencing B was developed in cooperation with the pathology laboratories of Brigham and Women's Hospital and Massachusetts General Hospital, and detects mutations in a critical part of the gene called epidermal growth factor receptor (EGFR). The gene mutation is present in a subset of non-small cell lung cancers, most commonly adenocarcinomas and bronchoalveolar carcinomas arising in nonsmokers. When the mutation is present, it is associated with a response to the anti-cancer drug Iressa (gefitinib). Iressa works by blocking the function of the mutant EGFR protein that these cancer cells need to survive and proliferate. Last April, two teams of investigators B one led by Thomas Lynch, MD, and Daniel Haber, MD, PhD, at Massachusetts General Hospital, and one by Bruce Johnson, MD, William Sellers, MD, and Matthew Meyerson, MD, PhD, at the Dana-Farber Cancer Institute B discovered the molecular marker that identifies lung cancer patients whose tumors will respond to Iressa. Until then, doctors had been unable to understand why Iressa caused tumors to shrink significantly in only 13.6 percent of patients, even though some of those responses were rapid and dramatic. The discovery of the EGFR mutation provided the answer.

Now, less than six months after the gene mutation discovery, the HPCGG Laboratory has prepared a molecular test to screen lung cancer tumors for the mutation. The test, which takes approximately two weeks to complete, involves extracting DNA from a tumor tissue sample. The test is significant because it gives doctors the information they need to decide which patients may benefit from Iressa at the earliest possible time, within weeks of diagnosis.

The MGH and DFCI investigators have applied for a patent for the test and are in the process of licensing the EGFR test to a commercial diagnostic partner so that it can be performed throughout the country and eventually the world. In the meantime, HPCGG will continue to offer the test through its Cambridge lab."

It appears the test will cost $895.00. What type of sample is needed is unclear, though samples from a standard bronchosopy may be sufficient. One can presume cost will decrease, health care insurers will arrange for volume discounts, and other laboratories will develop similar tests. At this time, doctors and patients will want to consider tests to identify the treatment most likely to benefit them. Basically, adenocarcinoma and BAC patients, particularly non-smokers and light former smokers will want to consider Iressa and have the test to confirm tyrosine kinase mutations. Smokers with squamous cell cancer may want to use the test to exclude Iressa, or use it in conjunction with other drugs.

Name of Drug	Mechanism of Action	Area of Success	NonResponders	Questions
Iressa_	Inhibits tyrosine kinase portion of EGFR	Adeno-carcinoma, BAC, nonsmokers, patients with defined damage to tyrosine kinase binding area of EGFR	Smokers, squamous cell cancers, patients without damage to tyrosine kinase.	1. Will patients without tyrosine kinase damage benefit from the drug?
Tarceva	Similar to Iressa, Inhibits tyrosine kinase portion of EGFR	Less data than Iresa but appears to have similar findings, helping adeno-carcinoma, BAC, nonsmokers with tyrosine kinase damage.	Similar to Iressa.	1. Are there any significant differences from Iressa?
Erbitux-IMC-C225 or Cetuximab	Prevents ligand binding of the EGFR	A study found that Erbitux combined with chemotherapy had better survival than chemotherapy alone. This is contrasted with studies finding Iressa added to chemotherapy did not improve survival....	Limited data with lung cancer. . . . The reasons for the difference remains unclear. Erbitux has been FDA approved for colon cancer, and can be prescribed off-label for lung.	1. Should this drug be used in areas where Iressa is not successful? 2. Will a drug combination make sense?

REFERENCES

1. FDA. *Advisory Meeting Document for the Use of Iressa*, FDA. Gov.

2. Tartora, *A novel approach in the treatment of cancer: targeting the Epidermal Growth Factor Receptor*, Clin Cancer Res 2001 Oct;7(10):2958-70.

3. Pass, Lung Cancer, 186 Lippincott, 2000) citing Tateshi, *Immunohistochemical evidence of autocrine growth factors in adenocarcinoma of the human lung*, Cancer Res 1990; 50: 7077.

4. Cox, *Matrix metalloproteinases 9 and the epidermal growth factor signal pathway in operable non-small cell lung cancer*, Clin Cancer Res 2000 Jun;6(6):2349-55.

5. Ohsaki, *Epidermal growth factor receptor expression correlates with poor prognosis in non-small cell lung cancer patients with p53 overexpression*, Oncol Rep 2000 May-Jun;7(3):603-7.

6. Kostyleva, *EFR-like peptides and their receptors as prognostic factors for the survival of patients with non-small cell lung cancer*, Vopr Onkol 1999;45(6):617-22.

7. Ferraro, *New Ammunition in Cancer War, New York Post 5/20/01*, p. 28.

8. Natale, *ZD1839 (Iressa): What's in it for the Patient*, The Oncologist, Vol. 7, Suppl 4, 25-30, August 15, 2002.

9. Oncology 1997 Mar-Apr;54(2):134-40.

10. Ferry, *Intermittent Oral ZD1839 (Iressa), a Novel Epidermal Growth Factor Receptor Tyrosine Kinase Inhibitor (EGFR-TKI), Shows Evidence of Good Tolerability and Activity: Final Results from a Phase I Study.*" www. asco.org. 2.

11. Uejima, *A phase I intermittent dose escalation trial of ZD1839 (IressaJJ) in Japanese patients with solid tumors*. Annals of Oncology, Vol 11, Suppl.4 October 2000, page 110.

12. Fortunate, *Inhibition of Growth Factor Production and Angiogenesis in Human Cancer Cells by ZD1839 (Iressa), a Selective Epidermal Growth Factor Receptor Tyrosine Kinase Inhibitor*, Clin Cancer Res 2001 May;7(5):1459_1465.

13. See Ciardiello, *EGFR-Targeted Agents Potentiate the Antitumor Activity of Chemotherapy and Radiotherapy*, Signal, Volume 2, number 2, (2001) 4.6.

14. Ciardiello, *EGFR-Targeted Agents Potentiate the Antitumor*

Activity of Chemotherapy and Radiotherapy, Signal, Volume 2, number 2, (2001).

15. Hainsworth, NSCLC: An Overview of Current and Upcoming Trials, 2nd Int. Lung Cancer Congress, July 18, 4.

16. Sololer, *Phase II Trial of the Epidermal Growth Factor Receptor (EGFR) Tyrosine Kinase Inhibitor OSI-774, Following Platinum-Based Chemotherapy, in Patients (pts) with Advanced, EGFR-Expressing, Non-Small Cell Lung Cancer (NSCLC).*2001, www.Medscape.com.

17. Hidalso, *Phase I and pharmacological study of OSI-774, an epidermal growth factor receptor tyrosine kinase.*18. Lung Cancer, Oncologist 2001; 6 (5): 407-14.

19. www.astrazeneca-us.com/news/article.asp?file.

20. Zhonghua, *The Growth Inhibition of anti-EGF receptor monoclonal antibody to human lung adenocarcinoma cells,* Jie He He Hu Xi Za Zhi 1998 Apr; 21(4):233-5.

22. Inoue, *Severe Acute Interstitial Pneumonia and Gefitinib (Iressa),* Lancet 2003 Jan 11;361(9352):137-9.

23. Janne, *Inhibition of epidermal growth factor receptor signaling in malignant pleural mesothelioma,* Cancer Res 2002 Sep 15;62(18):5242-7.

24. Baselga, *Why the Epidermal Growth Factor Receptor? The Rationale for Cancer Therapy,* The Oncologist, Vol. 7, Suppl 4, 2-8, August 15, 2002 (currently available online at no cost).

25. Baselga, *Epidermal Growth Factor: A Rational Target for Cancer Therapy*, American Society of Clinical Oncology)ASCO) (2003) (presentation available online at www. Egfr-info.com.

26. Normanno, *Cooperative inhibitory effect of ZD1839 (Iressa) in combination with trastuzumab (Herceptin) on human breast cancer cell growth,* Annals of Oncology 13:65-72, 2002.

27. Ranson, ZD1839 (IressaTM): *For More Than Just Non-Small Cell Lung Cancer,* The Oncologist, Vol. 7, Suppl 4, 16-24, August 15, 2002.

28. Slamon, *Use of Chemotherapy plus a Monoclonal Antibody against HER2 for Metastatic Breast Cancer That Overexpresses HER2,* New England Journal of Medicine, Volume 344:783-792, March 15, 2001, number 11.

29. HER-2 diagnostics, Magy Onkol 2002;46(1):11-5 (2002).

30. Potti, *Predictive role of HER-2/neu overexpression and clinical features at initial presentation in patients with extensive stage small cell lung carcinoma*, Lung Cancer 2002 Jun;36(3):257-61.

31. www.NCI.org.

32. Steinberg, *Closing in on Multiple Cancer Targets*, The Scientist 16[7]:29, Apr. 1, 2002._

33. *A phase 1 clinical and pharmacokinetic study of oral CI-1033, a pan-erbB tyrosine kinase inhibitor, in patients with advanced solid tumors*, www.asco.org (2002)._

34. *Inhibitors of erbB-1 kinase*, Expert Opinion on Therapeutic Patents, 2002, vol. 12, no. 12, pp. 1903-1907.

35. _ Allen, Potential benefits of the irreversible pan-erbB inhibitor, CI-1033, in the treatment of breast cancer, Semin Oncol 2002 Jun;29(3 Suppl 11):11-21.

36. www.brittanica.com Growth Factors._

37. Lipton, *Mollecular Profiling of an Individual Patient's Tumor: is this the Future of Cancer Treatment*, Signal, Volume 3, Issue 4, 2-3, 21, available online at www.egfr-info.com.

38. Hynes, *Tyrosine Kinase Signalling in Breast Cancer*, Breast Cancer Res 2000, 2:154-157, http://breast-cancer-research.com/content/2/3/154.__

39. Satoh, *Regulation of the Expression of Epidermal Growth Factor Receptor MRNA* . . . ,Yomago Acta medica 1997;40:133-36 http://lib.med.tottori-u.ac.jp/yam/bef_41/yam40(3)/sato.pdf.

40. _ Albanell, *Unraveling Resistance to Trastuzumab (Herceptin): Insulin-Like Growth Factor-I Receptor, a New Suspect*, Journal of the National Cancer Institute, Vol. 93, No. 24, 1830-1832, December 19, 2001.

41. Cappuzzo, *Gefitinib in Pretreated Non-Small-Cell Lung Cancer (NSCLC): Analysis of Efficacy and Correlation With HER2 and Epidermal Growth Factor Receptor Expression in Locally Advanced or Metastatic NSCLC*, J Clin Oncol. 2003 Jul 15;21(14):2658-63.

42. Dancey, *Targeting epidermal growth factor receptor—are we missing the mark*, Lancet. 2003 Jul 5;362(9377): 62-4.

43. Talbot, *The Epidermal Growth Factor (EGF) Family*, (Gropep advertisement for EGF gene products)._

44. Janmaat, *Response to Epidermal Growth Factor Receptor Inhibitors*

in Non-Small Cell Lung Cancer Cells: Limited Antiproliferative Effects and Absence of Apoptosis Associated with Persistent Activity of Extracellular Signal-regulated Kinase or Akt Kinase Pathways. Clin Cancer Res. 2003 Jun;9(6):2316-26.

45. Funokuora, *Multi-institutional randomized phase II trial of gefitinib for previously treated patients with advanced non-small-cell lung cancer,* J Clin Oncol. 2003 Jun 15;21(12):2237-46. Epub 2003 May 14.

46. Bianco, *Loss of PTEN/MMAC1/TEP in EGF receptor-expressing tumor cells counteracts the antitumor action of EGFR tyrosine kinase inhibitors.,* Oncogene. 2003 May 8;22(18):2812-22.

47. www.fda.gov, Center for Drug Evaluation and Research Approval Package for Application Number 21-399., Medical Review.

48. www.fda.gov, Center for Drug Evaluation and Research Approval Package for Application Number 21-399, Statistical Evaluation. _

49. Klein, *Effect of tyrosine kinase inhibition on surfactant protein A gene expression during human lung development,* Am J Physiol Lung Cell Mol Physiol 274: L542-L551, 1998.

50. World Conference on Lung Cancer, webcast, *Mollecular Targeted Lung Cancer 1 Epdimeral Growth Factor Tyrosine Kinase Inhibitors._*

51. Miller, *Bronchioloalveolar pathologic subtype and smoking history predict sensitivity to gefitinib in advanced non-small-cell lung cancer,.* J. Clin Oncol. 2004 Mar 15;22(6):1103-9.

52. Gelibter, *Clinically meaningful response to the EGFR tyrosine kinase inhibitor gefitinib ('Iressa', ZD1839) in non small cell lung cancer,* J Exp Clin Cancer Res. 2003 Sep;22(3):481-5.

53. West, *Gefitinib (ZD1839) therapy for advanced bronchioloalveolar lung cancer (BAC):* Southwest Oncology Group (SWOG) Study S0126, Abstract 7014, 2004 Asco Annual Meeting, asco.com.

54. Tortora, *Combination of a Selective Cyclooxygenase-2 Inhibitor with Epidermal Growth Factor Receptor Tyrosine Kinase Inhibitor ZD1839 and Protein Kinase A Antisense Causes Cooperative Antitumor and Antiangiogenic Effect,* Clinical Cancer Research Vol. 9, 1566-1572, April 2003.

55. Lynch, T. J. *Specific Activating Mutations in the Epidermal Growth Factor Receptor Underlying Responsiveness of Non-Small-Cell Lung Cancer to Gefitinib. The New England Journal of Medicine* (online April 29, 2004).

56. Paez, J. G. *EGFR Mutations in Lung Cancer: Correlation with Clinical Response to Gefitinib Therapy*. Science (Published online April 29, 2004).

57. Matar, *Combined Epidermal Growth Factor Receptor Targeting with the Tyrosine Kinase Inhibitor Gefitinib (ZD1839) and the Monoclonal Antibody Cetuximab (IMC-C225)*, Clinical Cancer Research Vol. 10, 6487-6501, October 1, 2004.

58. Cunningham, *Cetuximab Monotherapy and Cetuximab plus Irinotecan in Irinotecan-Refractory Metastatic Colorectal Cancer*, Volume 351:337-345. July 22, 2004, No. 4.

59. Perez-soler, *Determinants of tumor response and survival with erlotinib in patients with non-small-cell lung cancer*, J Clin Oncol. 2004 Aug 15;22(16):3238-47.

60. www.drugdevelopment-technology.com/projects/tarceva/.

61. www.roche.com.

62. Pao, *EGF receptor gene mutations are common in lung cancers from "never smokers" and are associated with sensitivity of tumors to gefitinib and erlotinib*, PNAS | September 7, 2004 | vol. 101 | no. 36 | 13306-13311.

63. www.asco.org.

64. *Cancer pathology & tyrosine phosphorylation*, www.bio.ilstu.edu/Edwards/sigcanc.html.

65. *New Agents Regulating Tyrosine Kinase Can Be Used Against Several Cancers*, www.managedcaremag.com/archives/0405/0405.biotech.html.

66. *Molecular test helps guide treatment for lung cancer*, www.partners.org/Pharma_Testing_Popup.html.

67. Research continues. One study found EGFR positive cells,

"in 51% of tumor tissues. We found an inverse correlation between pEGFR, and both tumor size and the degree of tobacco smoking. In addition, we found a trend in which pEGFR expression was inversely correlated with disease stage (IA higher than IB). There was no correlation with sex, histology, or disease-free or OS. CONCLUSIONS: Our results suggest that pEGFR levels are present in early-stage NSCLC, especially in patients with small tumors and in those with short smoking histories, but there is no prognostic impact on a patient's disease course. Targeting

EGFR may therefore have more promise in chemoprevention or in patients with smaller early-stage NSCLCs compared with those with more advanced disease." *Small Tumor Size and Limited Smoking History Predicts Activated Growth Factor Receptor in Early Stage (NSCLC)*, Chest. 2005 Jul;128(1):308-16.

CHAPTER 16

ANTI-ANGIOGENESIS DRUGS

16.1 ANGIOGENESIS

Metastasis remains the most serious danger of lung cancer. While considerable progress has been made in understanding cancer, that has not translated to success in treating metastatic cancer.

16.11 What is Angiogenesis?

Angiogenesis is the disturbing ability of cancer cells to form new sources of blood supply to facilitate their expansion into other organs.

"Angiogenesis is the term for the growth of new blood vessels in the body. In a healthy body, angiogenesis produces blood vessels to heal wounds and restore blood flow to tissues after injury. In females, angiogenesis occurs during the monthly reproductive cycle (to rebuild the uterus lining, to mature the egg during ovulation) and during pregnancy (to build the placenta, the circulation between mother and fetus). A healthy body controls blood vessel development through a process of stimulating or inhibiting angiogenesis. Normally, the inhibitors dominate the stimulators so angiogenesis does not occur. When the body loses control over angiogenesis, serious diseases may take over. Excessive angiogenesis is noted in cancer, but also such diseases as diabetic blindness, rheumatoid arthritis, and psoriasis. The new blood vessels feed the diseased tissues and destroy normal tissue because the diseased cells produce abnormal amounts of angiogenic stimulants or growth factors, overwhelming the natural inhibitors. These new blood vessels also allow tumor cells to escape into the circulatory system and find their way to other organs. This migration is known as tumor metastases.: Biopulse (1).

The National Cancer Institute provided this summary:

"Angiogenesis is a process controlled by certain chemicals produced in the body which stimulate cells to repair damaged blood vessels or form new ones . . . Angiogenesis plays an important role in the growth and spread of cancer. New blood vessels "feed" the cancer cells with oxygen and nutrients, allowing these cells to grow, invade nearby tissue, spread to other parts of the body, and form new colonies of cancer cells. Because cancer cannot grow or spread without the formation of new blood vessels, scientists are trying to find ways to stop angiogenesis. They are studying natural and synthetic angiogenesis inhibitors, also called anti-angiogenesis agents, in the hope that these chemicals will prevent the growth of cancer by blocking the formation of new blood vessels. In animal studies, angiogenesis inhibitors have successfully stopped the formation of new blood vessels, causing the cancer to shrink and die." http//cancernet.nci.nih.gov/

16.12 Size and Angiogenesis

The process of angiogenesis is necessary for tumors to survive, and conversely, shutting off or inhibiting the process may limit the spread of the cancer or even reduce the size of the tumor itself:

"One promising avenue of cancer research is the study of a group of compounds called angiogenesis inhibitors. These are drugs that block angiogenesis, the development of new blood vessels. Solid tumors cannot grow beyond the size of a pinhead (1 to 2 cubic millimeters) without inducing the formation of new blood vessels to supply the nutritional needs of the tumor. By blocking the development of new blood vessels, researchers are hoping to cut off the tumor's supply of oxygen and nutrients, and therefore its continued growth and spread to other parts of the body." Lycos.com, Angiogenesis.

In proceedings from a National Cancer Institute conference, a speaker explains the angiogenesis process.

"The process that we are talking about is angiogenesis. As we all know, in order for tumors to grow beyond the size of 2 cubic millimeters in volume, they must develop a vasculature so that, as the tumor cell population grows, the malignant cells secrete angiogenic factors which stimulate nearby vasculature endothelial cells to proliferate and to form tubes and capillaries to promote the continued growth and expansion of the tumor."

"This new blood vessel formation also allows tumor cells to extravasate into the bloodstream, travel through the bloodstream, establish colonies again at distal sites, and grow metastatic disease and establish a vasculature once again." Teicher, Angiogenesis as a Target for CancerTherapy www.conference-cast.com/webtie/sots/lung/transcripts/teichertran.htm

Thus, if this process can be eliminated, or even delayed, the prospect for long-term survival would dramatically increase. Chemicals called angiogenesis inhibitors signal the process to stop. Squamous cell and adenocarcinoma are two types of non-small cell lung cancer. Squamous cell tumors frequently have areas of necrosis, or cell death. Statistically, squamous cell patients seem to survive longer than those with adenocarcinoma. We could hypothesize that adenocarcinomas produce angiogenesis more effectively than squamous cell tumors, enabling the adenocarcinomas tumors to spread.

16.13 Practical Difficulties with Anti-Angiogenesis Drugs

Teicher discusses some of the theoretical problems with these drugs and the importance of timing in the drug administration in animal studies:

"We then looked at the antiangiogenic combination, starting therapy very early in the life of the tumor on day 4, when the tumor is just a seed and beginning to explode in its angiogenic activity. We are starting the angiogenic agent combination 3 days later on day 7, when the tumor is actually a fairly well-established nodule. The cytotoxic chemotherapy was administered on days 7-11. So we learned a lesson that cancer researchers learn again and again, and that is the tumor burden is very important. If we started the antiangiogenic therapy early on day 4 and treated at days 4-11 or 4-18, we obtained the greatest enhancement in tumor growth delay, but even if we had to limit the antiangiogenic therapy to the same 5-day period that we gave the cytotoxic therapy, we still had tumor growth delay of 29 days, which was better than cytotoxic chemotherapy alone. It was only when we administered the antiangiogenic therapy for the full 2-week period of days 4-18, which is really the full exponential growth phase of this tumor, that we obtained the greatest tumor response and with this therapeutic regimen forty to fifty percent of the animals were cured of the Lewis lung carcinoma." Cancer Therapy. (22)

16.2 SUMMARY OF ANTI-ANGIOGENESIS DRUGS

16.21 Overview

Newer therapy attempts are being made to frustrate cancer spread through molecular therapy. The task is to identify agent with tumor specificity and low toxicity. More specifically, we want to identify a molecular target

1. which drives tumor growth and or cancer progression,
2. which can be measured,
3. whose function can be reversed or altered significantly,
4. inhibition of that molecule will not alter normal body functions. Kelly (23).

Stating goals is easier than meeting them. A May 21, 2002 article provides a summary of anti-angiogenic agents:

"Like many experimental therapies, results from initial lab studies of antiangiogenic agents have appeared dramatic. But once they advance to human studies, the bloom tends to fall from the rose. Since 1988, more than 50 experimental antiangiogenesis drugs have been tested in 10,000 patients with few dramatic results . . . . Despite the challenges, antiangiogenesis remains a particularly appealing concept, because it may offer a less toxic alternative to chemotherapy and radiation, or, more likely, it will improve standard treatments when combined with them . . . . Since May 2001, 18 antiangiongenesis compounds have advanced to the phase III stage, which will determine whether a drug merits FDA approval. Seven of the 18 compounds were halted in development because interim results showed no effect or too little effect. Of the 11 remaining drugs, three distinguished themselves with extremely encouraging data, Li says. The front runners are Avastin, by Genentech of San Francisco, Thalidomide, by Calgene Corp, of Warren, and Neovastat, by Aeterna Laboratories." (4)

16.3 CURRENT FORERUNNERS IN ANTI-ANGIOGENESIS

16.31 Neovastat

In laboratory studies, Neovastat was shown to be effective in inhibiting angiogenesis and improved the efficiency of standard chemotherapy drugs:

"A novel naturally occurring antiangiogenic agent isolated from cartilage, referred to as Neovastat (AE-941), was examined for its efficacy against tumor neovascularization and progression. Exposure to Neovastat results in ex ovo antiangiogenic properties in the chorioallantoid membrane of chicken embryo (71% decrease in the angiogenic index as compared to the basic fibroblast growth factor (bFGF) treated control embryos, P < 0.0001). Oral administration of Neovastat inhibits bFGF-induced angiogenesis in the Matrigel mouse model (87.5% decrease in hemoglobin as compared to the bFGF-treated control implants, P < 0.0001). Neovastat also induces a dose response decrease of lung metastases in the Lewis lung carcinoma model (oral administration; 69.1% of inhibition obtained at the maximal dose of 0.5 ml/day, P < 0.0001). Combined with a sub-optimal dose of cisplatinum (2 mg/kg, i.p.), Neovastat (0.5 ml/day) improved the therapeutic index by increasing the antimetastatic efficacy and by exerting a protective activity against cisplatinum-induced body weight loss and myelosuppression. In summary, our experimental data provide evidence of antiangiogenic and antimetastatic properties of Neovastat, following oral administration." Dupont, (5)

Neovastat is derived from cartilage of the dog-fish shark. Shark cartilage was a controversial experimental treatment advocated in the early 90's featured in a book, Sharks Don't Get Cancer.

16.311 Human Studies

There are reports (as indicated above) of favorable human studies. However, as of June, 2002, we were unable to locate these in a recognized medical journal. One article states,

"Neovastat is a complex of naturally occurring anti-angiogenic molecules exhibiting multi-functional mechanisms of action. It has been tested in Phase II clinical trials in non-small cell lung cancer and in renal cell carcinoma .... Several of its activities have been characterized and the antiangiogenic activity of Neovastat can be attributed to inhibition of several key pathways in angiogenesis making it an ideal candidate to test against metastasis formation in highly vascularized bone."

However, the citation is to an article in progress. An intelligent assessment of Neovastat must await published results. Based on the reports, it may be a plausible alternative for patients with advanced cancer.

16.32 Thalidomide

In the 60's, Thalidomide was source of birth defects, as it cut the supply of blood and the development of new vessels in the fetus. It is precisely this characteristic which indicates promise as a potent anti-angiogenic agent.

"In addition to immunomodulatory and cytokine-modulatory properties, thalidomide has antiangiogenic activity. It has been investigated in a number of cancers including multiple myeloma, myelodysplastic syndromes, gliomas, Kaposi's sarcoma, renal cell carcinoma, advanced breast cancer, and colon cancer." Thalidomide (3).

16.33 Endostatin and Angiostatin

If nothing else, the story of Angiostatin and Endostatin is a lesson in the tendency of early clinical results to be given excessive weight, the tendency of news reporters to herald a new cancer cure from limited results in a single animal study, and the interrelationship between corporate goals and scientific research. After numerous early studies on the theory of angiogenesis, Dr. Folkman, a Noble-Prize winning Harvard researcher, reported that tumors in 50% of rats were markedly reduced by administration of Endostatin. The results became national, indeed, world-wide news as the new media profiled the new cancer cure.

Later scientists had difficulty reproducing the results and in any event, the promise was not translated to human studies. Today the future of Endostatin and Angiostatin remain uncertain, and are one of perhaps five hundred anti-cancer drugs which continue to be investigated.

"What is Angiostatin? Endostatin and Angiostatin naturally exist in the body and play an important role in angiogenesis. Angiostatin is a plaminogen fragment produced by MMP's. It is a potent inhibitor of angiogenesis that be isolated from primary tumors, including non-small cell lung carcinomas. (NSCLC) Angiostatin is inversely correlated with VEGF's (vascular endothelial growth factor) and is associated with elevated apoptosis and longer survival. It can maintain the microscopic metastasises in a dormant state known as concomitant resistance . . . ." (Galligioni (2)

However, translating theoretical effectiveness to practical results and getting the drug to where significant results can be achieved has been the difficulty.

16.34 Matrix Metallo Proteinases Inhibitors

Instead of trying to kill the cancer cells, one could try to prevent metastasis or spread to other organs. Recall that cancer cells metastasize because they do not have an enclosing shell and acquire the ability to penetrate the shells or basement membranes of normal cells. Matrix metalloproteinases (MMP) such as collagenase, help break down the extracellular matrix which protects other bodily structures. Some drugs are used to inhibit MMP, and thereby to prevent tissue penetration. We can review some of the recent information about these drugs. However, none have been shown to have proven, clear anti-cancer fighting properties in laboratory experiments and clinical studies. All have a theoretical basis for believing they could be used which are described below.

Experimental data indicate that angiogenesis is crucial for growth and persistence of solid tumor and of their metastasises. Another agent to display anti-angiogenesis properties is suramin. Although suramin has shown, at least in vitro (in cells), to inhibit lung cancer growth (7), clinical studies in NSCLC have yielded negative results. Angiostatin, a component of plasminogen and endostatin, inhibits metastasis by inducing a balance between metastatic and primary tumor cells defined as "dormancy". Both agents are capable of inhibiting tumor growth in vivo in animal models. Although tumors re-grow when anti-angiogenic treatment is discontinued, experimental tumors, remain sensitive to a second cycle of treatment with the same agent. Different from conventional chemotherapeutic agents, no drug-resistance was observed even after multiple repeated cycles of antiangiogenic therapy (9). These agents hold considerable promise for the treatment of a number of tumor types including NSCLC. Other drugs which, in preclinical models, have been found to be angiogenesis inhibitors and that are currently entering clinical trials include TNP-470 (a synthetic fumagillin derivative), thalidomide, vitamin and squalamine.

16.4 COX-2 INHIBITORS

16.41 Cox 1 and 2

There are two cox enzymes appropriately labeled cox1 and 2. (The term cox stands for cyclooxygenase enzymes). Their chemical structures are similar and they belong to the same family, but their functionality varies. Cox-1 is involved with the production of enzymes for hormones, blood platelets, and other normal bodily functions. Cox-1 has been called a house-keeping enzyme present in normal cells throughout the body.

- Cox-1 plays an important role in the stomach and gastro-intestinal tract and older Cox-inhibitors may have caused stomach discomfort and ulcers because they disrupted Cox-1.
- Aspirin inhibits both Cox 1 and 2, and may aggravate stomach problems.

16.411 Cox-2's role in Inflammation and Cancer

While Cox-1's role helps regulate many normal bodily functions and is present in normal tissues. Cox-2's role is more specialized. Cox-2 is produced in response to injury and is associated with inflammatory processes involving repair. Cox-2 is frequently undetectable in normal tissue, but is induced by cytokines, growth factors, and chemical carcinogens, and intercellular signals indicating cell damage. Cox-2 is present in many cancer cells of various types, and is specifically associated with various carcininogenic behaviors. Overexpression of tumor Cox-2 may be important in angiogenesis, resistance to apoptosis, suppression of host immunity. "Moderate to strong Cox-2 expression was detected in approximately 40%-80% of the total neoplastic (cancer) cells in most tumors. In addition to expression of Cox-2 within neoplastic cells per se, Cox-2 was also detected in the angiogenic vasculature present within the tumors and preexisting vasculature adjacent to cancer lesions. Cox-2 was observed in the angiogenic vessels in most of the human cancers analyzed thus far, including head and neck and pancreas" Maspherer (17). A 2004 study suggests Cox-2 induces VEGF (see below) and Erb 2 production. (14).

16.42 The Role of Cox-2 in Lung Cancer

Cox-2 is involved with the development and spread of lung cancer.

"Increased expression of cyclooxygenase-2 (COX-2) significantly enhances carcinogenesis and inflammatory reactions.

Regulation of COX-2 overexpression may be a reasonable target for cancer chemoprevention. We have tested the hypothesis that levels of COX-2 expression determine the growth of human lung cancer cells in nude mice . . . . levels of COX-2 expression determine the extent of human lung tumor growth in athymic mice. Therefore, inhibition of COX-2 expression by agents such as p-XSC provides a strong rationale for the development of future clinical prevention trials." (6).

One study found Cox 2 expressed in over 90% of adenocarcinomas, a type of non-small lung cancer. That study found that tumors that overexpressed p53 (mutant or disfunctional form) had higher levels of Cox-2." (6). Cox-2 inhibitors have shown success in a laboratory setting:

"The COX-2 selective inhibitor nimesulide can inhibit proliferation of NSCLC cell lines in vitro. Similar findings have been reported showing sensitivity of lung cancer cells to nonselective, nonsteroidal anti-inflammatory drugs such as sulindac and sulindac sulfone, which inhibit both COX-1 and COX-2. Importantly, the results present here show for the first time that selective inhibition of COX-2 by nimesulide can induce apoptosis even at clinically achievable low concentrations and that the level of COX-2 expression in NSCLC cells may affect their responsiveness to COX-2 inhibitors. Previous studies of ours indicate that a significantly increased COX-2 expression is present in up to 70% of adenocarcinoma cases, showing its potential association with tumor progression. It is, therefore, possible that a significant proportion of adenocarcinomas in vivo may be sensitive to COX-2 inhibitors." (20).

16.43 Success of Cox-2 Inhibitors

Developing a new drug poses two important challenges. First, how does one deliver the drug to the relevant area. This is where many anti-angiogenic drugs have failed; in cells tests, the drug suppresses cancer cells in the laboratory or in large quantities upon an animal, but in the complexity of the human body, little impact is seen. Secondly, how do we avoid disruption of normal cells and bodily functions, the obstacle facing many chemotherapy drugs. These problems have been solved to some extent with Celebrex and other drugs.

Celebrex has been able to reduce the inflamation associated with arthritis for many people, displaying few side effects. "NSAID's have been widely used with comparatively few side effects. Nonsteroidal anti-inflammatory drugs (NSAIDs) annually account for 70 million prescriptions and 30 billion over-the-counter (OTC) medications sold in the United States alone." The side effects appear limited compared with traditional forms of chemotherapy. 1.Cox-2 inhibitors represent a promising alternative in treatment with established impact and limited side effects.

16.44 Celebrex

Maspherer (17) showed that Celebrex suppressed growth of lung and colon tumors in mice, "Celecoxib supplied in the diet continuously from date of implant at doses between 160-3200 pip significantly retarded the growth of these primary tumors. The inhibitory effect of celecoxixib was dose dependent and ranged from 48% to 85% when compared with untreated tumors."

16.45 Side Effects

NSAID's have been used for the past decade with comparatively few side effects. Nonsteroidal anti-inflammatory drugs (NSAIDs) accounted for 70 million prescriptions and 30 billion over-the-counter (OTC) medications sold in the United States. Nonetheless, in 2004, heart problems were seen with both Cox-2 inhibitors, Vioxx, and Celebrex. In a placebo trial for early stage colon cancer, users of Vioxx had almost twice the risk of serious heart disease:

> "In 2600 patients, rofecoxib 25 (Vioxx) mg was compared with placebo in the prevention of the recurrence of adenomatous polyps of the large bowel in patients with a history of colorectal adenomas. The study included patients aged 40-96; approximately 62% male. In total, 25 patients receiving placebo and 45 receiving rofecoxib demonstrated thromboembolic

events. There were three absolute event rates per 400 patient years in the placebo group versus six events per 400 patient years in the rofecoxib treatment group. These increased risk of confirmed serious thromboembolic events including heart attack and stroke appeared statistically evident at 18 months of chronic dosing. Preliminary data released showed that five people died out of the 1,287 taking rofecoxib during the almost three-year study, one from a heart attack and three from sudden cardiac death (i.e. conduction problems with the heart). One death was unrelated to the study. Among the 1,299 participants given a placebo, there were also five deaths—three from heart attacks, one from sudden cardiac death and one from another cause. There were no stroke deaths, although patients on rofecoxib had double the number of strokes as compared with those in the non-drug group. Although the number of deaths was equal in both groups, those on placebo had only 25 cardiovascular problems, compared to the 45 among those administered rofecoxib once a day. These findings, observed just two weeks from the end of the trial, suggested that rofecoxib doubled the risk of heart attack or stroke." Davies (22)

Vioxx was recalled because a clinical trial identified a substantial increase in heart attack or stroke. These findings were significant for the target group, healthy primarily middle aged patients with arthritis but in otherwise decent health.

Different considerations would apply to the use as an anti-cancer drug, particularly among stage 4 patients. Many stage 4 lung cancer patients would expire from cancer causes during a three year study period. If the drug increased life expectancy, a small increase in cardiac events might not preclude the use of the drug in a high-risk population. The above trial compared the drug with placebo, if compared with powerful chemotherapy drugs, the cox-2 inhibitors might well be less. Clinical trials are needed to test Vioxx and other drugs in stage 4 patients.

16.46 Celebrex

Initially some thought the adverse risks were limited to Vioxx. In late December, 2004, a clinical trial reported similar hazards from

Celebrex. "The Food and Drug Administration on Friday warned physicians to consider alternatives to the popular arthritis drug Celebrex because of new evidence that, like the similar drug Vioxx, removed from the market in September, it doubles the chances of heart attacks and strokes." (25 FDA Warns of Health Risk).

16.47 Assessing the Risks of NSAID's

Why do it? Why risk it? He didn't die from the cancer, it was the drug they gave him that killed him, some family members will say while considering legal action. Indeed, as lawsuits against Pfizer and Merck (makers of Celebrex and Vioxx) are being readied, some of those lawsuits will include claims against physicians who failed to investigate risks, failed to notify patients, and are otherwise liable for adverse events connected with the drugs. Most physicians will not want to risk years of litigation and potential liability to provide a drug whose efficacy is debated.

Celebrex's availability may be limited to clinical trials, or university settings where warnings of adverse events are prominently displayed, and use is carefully circumscribed.

16.472 Considerations for the Patient

For the stage 4 lung cancer patient, Celebrex may still be an option. The course of the disease presents serious risks, chemotherapy is not a permanent cure, and health effects from Celebrex may still be less than those of other drugs. Celebrex does not cause nausea, hair loss, and other discomfort like, for example, the widely used chemotherapy drug Cisplatin. Clinical trials may continue to examine Celebrex's efficacy, alone or with chemotherapy.

16.5 VEGF INHIBITORS

Vascular endothelial growth factor (VEGF) is associated with angiogenesis and metastasis and is thus a target for new drugs. "VEGF stimulates new blood vessel formation, or angiogenesis, by binding to specific receptors on nearby blood vessels to stimulate extensions to existing blood vessels." Gene.com (12)

16.51 The Rationale for VEGF Receptor Drugs

A growth factor comes into contact with a receptor, like a key and lock, and begins a process of cell reproduction and changes. Some newer drugs attempt to prevent the two from connecting. The process is complex since related growth factors and receptors are activated also. As with other forms of gene therapy, targeting the offending protein rather than all cells can reduce harmful side effects. "The high selectivity achieved with neutralizing antibodies, soluble receptors and ribozymes reduces the risk of adverse reactions not related to VEGF inhibition itself." Investigational Drugs (13).

16.52 Flovopirodol

The drug is an analogue of a naturally occurring flavonoid isolated from the stem bark of *Dysoxylum binectariferum*, a plant native to India. Shapiro (10).

> "Preclinical data, both *in vitro* and *in vivo*, have demonstrated antiproliferative activity of Flovopirodol against NSCLC. In cell lines, Flovopirodol causes arrest at both the G_1 and G_2 phases of the cell cycle." Shapiro (10).

Results in a phase 2 trial were modest. No complete or partial responses were observed. Thus, the drug is unlikely to be effective alone. However, a limited impact was seen and toxicity was also limited. Flovopirodol holds some promise as a treatment in conjunction with chemotherapy. See ElSayed (12). Clinical trials comparing chemotherapy with and without the drug can be performed.

16.53 Avastin

Avastin also known as rhuMAb VEGF or bevacizumab, is a promising anti-VEGF drug:

> "VEGF stimulates new blood vessel formation, or angiogenesis, by binding to specific receptors on nearby blood vessels to stimulate extensions to existing blood vessels. Research has shown that

angiogenesis, by supplying blood to tumors, plays an important role in both tumor growth and metastasis . . . . Genentech scientists developed a humanized antibody, rhuMAb-VEGF, that is designed to bind to VEGF preventing it from binding to its receptors and therefore potentially inhibiting tumor growth." (16).

Avastin has shown success with colon cancer, with the manufacturer reporting that Avastin increased survival duration by 30% when combined with first-line chemotherapy. (16). Avastin has recently been approved for treatment of NSCLC, with studies showing a small but discernible benefit when combined with chemotherapy.

Criterion	Chemotherapy Alone	Chemotherapy with Avastin
Response Rate	10%	27%
Progression free survival period	4.5 months	6.4 months
One year Survival Rate	43.7	51.90%

See(23) Anti-Angiogenic Therapy

Some increased side effects were seen with an increase rate of neutropenia and a small increase in hemorrage. Thus patients should be carefully monitored. (14). A prior trial had found squamous cell patients to be particularly at risk. Whether the type is significant or coincidental needs to be determined. Some insurers will not cover the cost of Avastin outside of adenocarcinoma.

16.6-7 RESERVED

16.8 P-53 GENE THERAPY

16.81 P-53's Functions

P-53 is perhaps the most important tumor suppressor gene.

"p53 protein . . . mediates several cellular functions: regulation of the cell division cycle, DNA repair, and programmed cell death. DNA repair, and programmed cell death. In response to various forms of genomic DNA damage . . . the p53 protein can arrest the cell cycle at the G1 to S transition point, thus affording time for DNA repair and preventing duplication of a mutant cell, or alternatively, failing DNA repair, p53 protein can implement programmed cell death (apoptosis). Accordingly, p53 has been dubbed the Aguardian of the genome." *Etiology of Cancer (4)*, see also Lee (1).

Consider its importance in cancer research:

"This protein plays a major role in the transcription ("reading") of DNA, in cell growth and proliferation, and in a number of metabolic processes. Because p53 suppresses abnormal cell proliferation (it acts like an 'emergency brake' in the cell cycle), it may represent an important mechanism for protection against cancer. It also appears to be involved in programmed cell death, or apoptosis. When a mutation in the p53 gene results in the substitution of one amino acid for another, p53 loses its ability to block abnormal cell growth. Indeed, some mutations produce a p53 molecule that actually stimulates cell division and promotes cancer. Almost 50% of human cancers contain a p53 mutation—including cancers of the breast, cervix, colon, lung, liver, prostate, bladder, and skin—and these cancers are more aggressive, . . ." P53 Weitzman (2).

Study of P-53 is important for several reasons. First, P-53 may be an indicator of cancer or carcinogenic processes. Thus P-53 presence might be tested in smokers to determine who is at risk. P-53 may be assessed in patients particularly stage 1 patients whose tumors were removed. Abnormal levels of P-53 might indicate the need for further treatment even where no signs of tumor are apparent on CT or other test. Finally P-53 research holds forth the possibility of improved treatment—a vaccine perhaps—to be used alone or with existing treatments like chemotherapy or radiation.

16.811 Description of P-53

P-53 is a protein of 53 kilodaltons (hence the name). It is located on chromosome 17 (p13). There are two types of P-53. First, we have normal P-53 also called wild-type P-53. This is P-53 in its normal condition, serving various tumor suppression functions outlined above. Mutant P-53 means the gene has been damaged. Not only will the gene not perform its tumor suppressor function, it may even contribute to carcinogenic processes:

> "Mutant p53 loses its original function but may acquire a new potentially oncogenic activity. Conversion of p53 protein from a normal to a mutant phenotype alters its histochemical features; the half-life of the protein is prolonged from 6-20 minutes to several hours. This increases the amount of p53 protein in affected cells, . . . Detection of excessive amounts of p53 protein is useful as a marker of mutation because the amount of wild-type p53 protein is too low to be detected in nonmutant cells." *Gemba, (3) at* 23-31.

P-53 protein is located in the nucleus of cells and is unstable. In a normal person, the body activates P-53, it performs its function of either correcting cell damage or inducing the death of damaged cells, and disintegrates. Malfunctioning or mutant P-53 can maintain itself in cells with the finding of P-53 indicating an abnormality. P-53 damage is seen in approximately 50% of breast colon, stomach, bladder, and non-small cell lung cancers. In non-small cell lung cancer (NSCLC), most series report that 50% to 60% of tumors have identifiable mutations. A 1999 study found that over 50% of small cell patients had traces of P53 in bronchial specimens.

16.812 When Do P-53 Mutations Occur in the Cancer Process?

Scientists have not been able to determine precisely when P-53 mutations occur. Curie suggests P-53 alteration is an early event:

> "p53 alteration is an early event in lung cancer, several years before the clinical diagnosis of the tumor. Recently, p53-Ab were detected in sera of two patients who were heavy smokers without diagnosed lung malignancy. Both of these patients developed invasive squamous lung cancer 5 and 15 months, respectively, after detection of serum p53-Ab . . . . Since p53

alterations represent an early genetic change in lung carcinogenesis, it is suggested that p53-Ab detection represents a new and sensitive tool for detection of preneoplastic and microinvasive bronchial lesions in patients with a high risk of lung cancer, i.e., heavy smokers. This finding was confirmed by Trivers et al. using three types of assays to detect p53-Ab. They were able to find p53-Abs before diagnosis in several patients with Chronic Obstructive Pulmonary disease."

Szak in contrast postulate that P53 mutations occur about midpoint in tumor development, just as damaged tissue becomes cancerous, "Most studies indicate that in the development of squamous cell lung cancer, loss of heterozygosity at 17p (suggesting loss of wild-type p53 function) occurs at the transition of preneoplasia to carcinoma in situ." *(7)*

16.82 P-53 and Patient Prognosis

Determining P-53 impact upon lung cancer prognosis has been unclear:

"For lung cancer, the results diverge as to whether p53 accumulation is related to poor patient prognosis (cf. letter by Mitsudomi and Passlick). As T. Mitsudomi indicates, it is important to establish some level of standardization so that studies of p53 accumulation can be comparable from one series to another. Recent studies have suggested that p53 abnormalities could have a prognostic value for adenocarcinomas whereas there was no significant prognosis factor in NSCLC when all histologic subtypes are combined." Curie, (6).

16.821 Early Stage Lung Tumors

One hypothesis is that even after a tumor has developed, P-53 can play a role in limiting cell proliferation. We know that there is a group of tumors where apoptosis, or cell death, equals proliferation, and those patients have a good prognosis. Under this theory, P-53 mutations would affect survival for early stage patients, but only minimally impact patients with advanced tumors, where P-53 would be limited in its function:

"Horio et al. analyzed resected Japanese lung cancer cases and found adverse prognostic significance, especially in early-stage tumors . . . Damic published on 408 consecutive resected stage 1 NSCLC patients and showed a modest prognostic impact of P53 overexpression." Szak (7), at 126.

Even here, though, results are equivocal. Szak states,

"An even larger study of 515 resected stage NSCLC showed no difference in survival for p53 positive immunostaning . . . the isolated impact of having a mutant p53 or p53 overexpression on time to recurrence or coverall survival in lung cancer is unclear." Szak (7) at 126.

16.83 The Rationale for Treatment

If damage to P-53 could be repaired, then tumor spread could be limited and perhaps P-53 could again perform its function of preventing cell duplication. This type of treatment has worked in a laboratory setting:

"Reintroducing a wild-type p53 gene into lung cancer cells, including Bronchioalveolar lung cancer (BAC), dramatically inhibits tumor cell growth and promotes tumor cell death despite the presence of mutations in multiple other genes." Lee, (1) at 324.

In NSCLC it was initially shown that introduction of a vector containing the wt-53 (wild type) into cell lines, which {had} either a deletion or a missense mutation in p53, markedly reduced cell proliferation and tumorigenicity.

16.84 Studies and Trials Using P-53

Some limited, promising results were seen in phase 1 P-53 clinical trials. In one trial, tumor regression was seen, though it did not affect survival since the patients had advanced metastatic cancer. A recent trial found no impact of P-53 treatment, "There was no difference between the response rate of lesions treated with p53 gene therapy in addition to chemotherapy (52% objective responses) and lesions treated with chemotherapy alone." (1). The treatment cannot be disposed of based upon one clinical trial. In the study, P-53 patients had slightly more favorable results. More importantly, it may be possible to develop more effective methods of delivery.

One strong argument for gene therapy is that the therapy will have limited side effects. Chemotherapy targets or affects different groups of dividing cells, cancerous and normal. On the other hand, gene therapy is designed to create new sources of P-53, and the presence of additional P-53 in the body, or the performance of ordinary functions by P-53, should not involve significant side effects.

16.85 Hurdles to Successful Treatment

It is difficult to repair the gene, the solution being studied is transferring another P-53 gene to the cancer area. Lee writes:

> "The complexities of the three-dimensional structure of the p53 tumor-suppressor gene product and the radical changes in this structure induced by a single point mutation makes it extremely difficult to restore its function with pharmaceuticals. Thus, the basic concept of tumor suppressor gene therapy utilizing p53 is to reintroduce a functionally active copy of the deficient genes in the cancer cell by direct gene transfer to directly induce cell death by apoptosis." Lee, (1) at 324.

Getting enough P-53 to the tumor to have significant results is difficult:

> "In all of these studies, it has been difficult to deliver recombinant virus into solid tumors so as to transduce a significant fraction of the tumor cells, and the effect is limited to the injected nodule, which may be of limited real clinical benefit." Lee, (1) at 324.

16.86 Use in Conjunction with Chemotherapy

The optimal use of P-53 treatment may be to compliment chemotherapy. That type of role must be confirmed in human clinical trials which is one reason why at the time of publication, P-53 was not an FDA approved drug. In one well-known study, that complimentary impact was not demonstrated.

16.9 CONCLUSIONS AND DIRECTIONS FOR FURTHER RESEARCH

The suppression of normal P-53 and expression of its mutated form, expression of Cox-2, the production of epidermal growth factor, expression of VEGF, are steps in the development and spread of lung cancer, with each step a target for research and treatment. Lung cancer has been difficult to cure, probably because so many genes are disrupted, and repair of a small part does not restore normal functioning. Thus future treatment may focus on the use of a variety of drugs, to the extent possible without substantial side effects.

16.91 Impact Upon Treatment at Various Stages

We review treatment by stage in later chapters, but a brief summary is appropriate here. One difficulty with today's treatment is that newer drugs are tested upon the patients with the most advanced illnesses, and thus the toughest to cure. Lung cancer patients tend to enter clinical trials when other forms of treatment have been exhausted.

Unfortunately, the only reliable cure has been surgical removal of tumors in stage 1 patients, and even then here is approximately 30-40% recurrence. Patients may want to consider promising newer forms of treatment at earlier stages. The downside is that the drugs are unproven. The upside is that if the side effects are limited, the patient can benefit at a time when the disease is not advanced.

Drugs like Celebrex present tough choices but may still be an option for stage 4 patients notwithstanding the various side effect. Patients may want to consult with major research facilities and monitor the medical literature for important developments.

REFERENCES

1. www.biopulse.com/anti-angiogenesis.html.
2. Galligioni, *Angiogenesis and Antiangiogenic Agents in Non-Small Cell Lung Cancer*, Lung Cancer 34 (2001) S3-S7.

3. *Thalidomide in Cancer, Potential Uses and Limitations*, BioDrugs 2001;15(3):163-72.

4. Friend, *Starving a Tumor*, May 21, 2002, Daily Record (New Jersey).

5. Dupont, *Antiangiogenic and Antimetastatic Properties of Neovastat (AE-941), an orally active extract derived from cartilage tissue* Clin Exp Metastasis 2002;19(2):145-53.

6. Weber, *The Effect of Neovastat (AE-941) on an Experimental Metastatic Bone Tumor Model, Intl Journal of Oncology*, 20: 299-303, 2002.

7. *Frequent co-localization of Cox-2 and laminin-5 gamma2 chain at the invasive front of early-stage lung adenocarcinomas, Am. J. Pathol*,2002 Mar;160(3):1129-41.

8. El-Bayoumy, *Cyclooxygenase-2 expression Influences the growth of human large and small cell lung carcinoma lines in athymic mice: impact of an organoselenium compound on growth regulation*, Int J Oncol 2002 Mar;20(3):557-61.

9. Pyo, Selective cyclooxygenase-2 inhibitor, NS-398, enhances the effect of radiation in vitro and in vivo preferentially on the cells that express cyclooxygenase, Clin Cancer Res 2001 Oct;7(10):2998-3005.

10. Shapiro, *A Phase II Trial of the Cyclin-dependent Kinase Inhibitor Flovopirodol in Patients with Previously Untreated Stage IV Non-Small Cell Lung Cancer,*Clinical Cancer Research Vol. 7, 1590-1599, June 2001.

12. Elsayed, *Selected Novel Anticancer Treatments Targeting Cell Signaling Proteins*, The Oncologist, Vol. 6, No. 6, 517-537, December 2001.

13. www.gene.com/gene/pipeline/status/oncology/avastin/index.jsp.

14. Manley, *Therapies directed at Vascular Endothelial Growth Factor*, Expert Opinion on Investigational Drugs 2002, vol. 11, no. 12, pp. 1715-1736.

15. *Phase III Trial With Avastin in Relapsed Metastatic Breast Cancer Does Not Meet Primary Endpoint; Results from Lead Phase III Study in Colorectal Cancer Due in Mid-2003* www.salesandmarketingnetwork.com.

16. www.gene.com/gene/pipeline/status/oncology/avastin/index.jsp (Genentech website).

17. Maspherer, *Antiangiogenic and Antitumor Activities of*

Cyclooxygenase-2 Inhibitors, Cancer Research 60, 1306-1311, March 1, 2000.

18. Su, *Cyclooxygenase-2 Induces EP₁—and HER-2/Neu-Dependent Vascular Endothelial Growth Factor-C Up-Regulation, a Novel Mechanism of Lymphangiogenesis in Lung Adenocarcinoma* Cancer Research 64: 554-564 Jan. 15, 2004.

19. Ferrario, *Cyclooxygenase-2 Inhibitor Treatment Enhances Photodynamic Therapy-mediated Tumor Response*, Cancer Research 62, 3956-3961, July 15, 2002.

20. Hida, *Cyclooxygenase-2 Inhibitor Induces Apoptosis and Enhances Cytotoxicity of Various Anticancer Agents in Non-Small Cell Lung Cancer Cell Lines*, Clinical Cancer Research Vol. 6, 2006-2011, May 2000.

21. Kelly, *Molecular Biology and Targeted Therapies in Lung Cancer*, Asco Virtual Meeting, *www.asco.org*.

22. Cancer Therapy,www.conference-cast.com/ webtie/sots/lung/transcripts/teichertran.htm

23. *Anti-Angionenic Therapy for Advanced NCSLC*, www.professional.cancerconsultants.com

REFERENCES TO P-53 SECTION

1. Lee, *Gene Therapy*, in Pass, Lung Cancer: Principles and Practice (Lippincott 2000).

2. P53 http://bioinformatics.weizmann.ac.il/hotmolecbase/entries/p53.htm.

3. Gemba, *Immunohitochemical Detection of Mutant P53 protein in Small Cell Lung Cancer: Relationship to Treatment Outcome*, Lung Cancer, vol 29 (1) (2000) pp. 23-31.

4. Etiology of Cancer: Carcinogenesis:http:/edcenter.med.cornell.edu./CUMC_PathNotes/Neoplasia/Neoplasia_04.html.(6).

5. Schuler, *Adenovirus-mediated wild-type p53 gene transfer in patients receiving chemotherapy for advanced non-small-cell lung cancer: results of a multicenter phase II study*, J Clin Oncol 2001 Mar 15;19(6):1750-8.

6. Curie, *P-53 Mutation in Lung Cancer* http://perso.curie.fr/Thierry.Soussi/p53_mutation_in_%20lung.html #Bronchopulmonary%20cancers.

7. Szak, *Gene Therapy*, in Pass, Lung Cancer: Principles and Practice (Lippincott 2000).

8. Nishihaki, *Synergistic inhibition of human lung cancer cell growth by adenovirus-mediated wild-type p53 gene transfer in combination with docetaxel and radiation therapeutics in vitro and in vivo.* Clin Cancer Res 2001 Sep;7(9):2887-97.

CHAPTER 17

TREATING NON-SMALL CELL LUNG CANCER—STAGE 1

17.0 OVERVIEW

In the next four chapters, we take our knowledge of lung anatomy, chemotherapy, surgery, and radiation, and apply it to non-small cell lung cancer, the most common form of lung cancer. Treatment is divided by stage, with each chapter reviewing treatment of a particular stage. The material can still be challenging, though I believe a good knowledge of this will be important for the patient or family member seeking to understand the nature of treatment and any options presented.

17.01 Suggestions to Make the Material Easier

Try to read each section, consult the definitions at the end of the book, and have a medical dictionary on hand. If you become confused about different stages, review the discussion of different stages. If you are able to digest the information here, you may be able to reduce the general information which takes up time in doctor-patient conferences, better understand your condition and the treatment which is proposed, and be able to ask your physician knowledgeable questions about treatment procedures and alternatives.

17.02 Division into Stages 0, 1a, 1B

Scientists divide stage 1 cancer into three substages: occult, also called stage 0, the very earliest type of tumor, stage 1A, a small discrete tumor with no involvement of the main bronchus or adjoining areas, and 1B, a tumor with no lymph node involvement or metastasis, but which is larger than 3cm, had made contact with the main bronchus, visceral pleura, or is associated with pneumonia or ateclasis.

STAGE	TUMOR SIZE	POSITIVE NODES	FIVE YEAR
Occult Tumor	Not visible on x-ray microscopic	0	75-85%
Stage 1A	3 cms or less, no involvement with adjoining areas	0	65-75%
Stage 1B	More than 3cm or invasion to main bronchus or visceral pleura,	0	55-65%

As the tumor increases in size, the patient's long-term survival prospects decrease though they still remain excellent throughout stage 1. The division into three stages reflects increasing specificity and sophistication in the treatment of these early stage tumors. For all stages, surgery will be recommended if the patient is in good health, and specifically, has sufficient pulmonary reserve—enough breathing capacity to survive the removal of a sufficient part of the lung. The hot topic today is whether some type of treatment before or after surgery should be recommended before a recurrence is seen and to improve the patient's prospects. Clinical trials are investigating whether chemotherapy before or after surgery should be prescribed, and before any evidence of spread of the tumor is observed.

Additionally, scientists are investigating whether molecular markers can detect a subset of patients whose tumors are likely to spread, and to prescribe therapy for those patients before the tumor does spread. Because these approaches are experimental, they are likely to be utilized only in a university setting.

17.1 OCCULT TUMORS

An occult cancer is a microscopic tumor which cannot be seen on a chest x-ray. Tumors discovered in this fashion are very early stage and given their limited area and lack of metastasis, usually cured by surgery.

17.11 Why Most Occult Tumors are Squamous Cell

One text states, "90% of occult lung cancers are squamous carcinomas, and 10% are either adenocarcinomas or large cell carcinomas." Martini, (1). Squamous cell tumors are usually in the main bronchus. Sputum cytology is gathering sputum from a cough. These small central tumors can sometimes be detected during an analysis of cells from a cough while deeper tumors in the smaller airways are not so easily found. The 90% figure means that of early cancers diagnosed, 90% are squamous cell, not that 90% of all tumors are squamous cell.

17.12 Sputum Cytology as a Tool for Early Detection

Diagnostic tools like sputum cytology need to be used more often, so we can treat certain lung cancer in its early stage when treatment is most effective. Since sputum cytology is less effective at revealing adenocarcinomas, it is not an all-inclusive diagnostic tool. Nonetheless with a cost of less than $100.00 per administration and date of detection critical, it needs to be utilized more frequently.

17.13 Treatment Similarities to Stage 1a Tumors

An occult tumor detected by sputum cytology, and a small tumor detected on a CT Scan which has not metastasises to a lymph node and has a limited area, are generally treated in the same fashion. If the patient is in good enough shape for surgery, the tumor is surgically removed and the patient has an excellent prognosis, with five year survival rates ranging from 70-85%, depending upon the study.

17.14 Phototherapy

Phototherapy is an alternative to surgical resection in certain patients. This investigational treatment seems to be most effective for very early central tumors. A recent article discusses photodynamic therapy and its use with Stage 0 patients:

> "Photodynamic therapy uses a photosensitizing agent, which becomes activated when exposed to light of the appropriate wavelength (1) and produces toxic oxygen radicals, resulting in cell death . . . . Tissue penetration is limited to a few millimeters in this method. This fact and the relatively low power prohibit complete eradication of large airway obstructing lesions. However, successful eradication of superficial (penetration less than 5 millimeters) bronchial wall tumors has been demonstrated. Superficial tumors are usually squamous cell carcinomas that are radiographically occult. They are often detected through cytological examination of sputum." Edell (2)

Surgical resection remains the best treatment for early-stage lung cancer. However, photodynamic therapy may be considered for some operable cancers, for cancers that are inoperable because of high surgical risk or limited pulmonary function or because they are multi centric, and for cancer in patient who refuse surgery. To be a candidate for photodynamic therapy, a patients must have a superficial stage 1 lesion (I/e. no evidence of nodal metastasis) that has a surface area estimated to be less than 3cm. Midthun (3).

Note that this photodynamic surgery is generally an option only for those patients who cannot tolerate surgery. For example, if an 84 year old man with previous heart problems and poor health were diagnosed with in-situ lung cancer, photodynamic therapy could be used. For others, given the overall good results achieved through surgery, that is the preferred form of treatment.

17.2 SURGERY AND STAGE I NON-SMALL CELL LUNG CANCER

17.21 Surgery is the Preferred Option Leading to Impressive Five Year Survival Prospects

Surgery, specifically a lobectomy—removal of the affected lobe of the lung and surrounding tissue, is the preferred option for stage 1 patients. Stage 1 patients whose tumors have been surgically removed have an excellent prognosis, with five year survival rates ranging from 55% to 85%, depending upon the study. (Since the occult tumors are even smaller, the survival rate is even higher).

17.22 Surgery and Pulmonary Reserve

The main consideration for surgery is whether the patient has sufficient pulmonary reserve. That is, can his pulmonary or respiratory system tolerate the removal of substantial parts of a lung. Surgery involves removal of not only the tumor, but surrounding tissue. For the average person, removal of a part of one lung would not present significant problems. However, if a patient's lungs have been damaged not only by cancer but diseases such as emphysema, a physician may decide against surgery. Pulmonary function tests assess the patient's breathing capacity in various contexts.

> "The objective is to establish that after surgical resection of the lung for a tumor, there will be sufficient pulmonary reserve to keep the patient comfortable, and he will not become a respiratory cripple. You should always evaluate the patient to determine whether he could withstand pneumonectomy even if radiologically only a lobectomy or limited resection is contemplated. On thoracotomy, a surgeon may be forced to do pneumonectomy because of an unexpected node over the pulmonary artery. If you have decided the patient cannot withstand pneumonectomy, this should be addressed with the surgeon ahead of thoracotomy."

Step 1: Routine PFTs. If the patient meets the following criteria, no further workup is necessary:

FEV1   > 2 liters
FEV1/FVC > 50%
MVV   > 50% of predicted
RV/TLC   < 50%"

17.23 Radiation for Stage 1 Patients with Diminished Pulmonary Reserve

NCI states,

> "Patients with stage I disease for whom surgery is deemed inappropriate may be considered for radiation therapy with curative intent. In one report of patients older than 70 years of age who had resectable lesions smaller than 4 centimeters but who were medically inoperable or who refused surgery, survival at 5 years following radiation therapy with curative intent was comparable to a historical control group of patients of similar age resected with curative intent. In the two largest retrospective radiation therapy series, inoperable patients treated with definitive radiation therapy achieved 5-year survival rates of 10% and 27%. Both series found that patients with T1, N0 tumors had better outcomes, with 5-year survival rates of 60% and 32% in this subgroup . . . . Careful treatment planning with precise definition of target volume and avoidance of critical normal structures to the extent possible is needed for optimal results and requires the use of a simulator." NCI (3).

17.3 POST SURGICAL CHEMOTHERAPY FOR STAGE 1 TUMORS

17.31 The Argument for Chemotherapy and or Radiation Following Surgery

Even though stage 1 patients have a good prognosis with the surgery having apparently removed the tumor, approximately 40% of patients will develop metastasises to lymph nodes and other organs. As the tumor spreads, it becomes increasingly more difficult to treat. Would it not make sense to provide some type of prophylactic chemotherapy or radiation designed to kill any cancer cells not visible to the human eye to prevent relapse? That is the question scientists are confronting.

With occult tumors and stage 1A tumors, one may argue that the patient should not be put through the stress and physical changes chemotherapy or radiation may entail. However, by stage 1B, the long-term survival chances are just above 50%. Thus, there is a substantial group of patients whose tumors will recur.

17.32 The Argument Against Post-Surgical Chemotherapy or Radiation

Chemotherapy is a serious treatment which causes side effects based upon its impact upon normal cells. A physician should not begin damaging normal tissue without clear medical justification.

17.33 Adjuvant Chemotherapy

Chemotherapy following surgery is called *adjuvant chemotherapy*. If adjuvant chemotherapy was given to a patient, that means that surgery was first performed and chemotherapy later given. Giving chemotherapy first to reduce tumor size, and then performing surgery is called *neoadjuvant chemotherapy*.

17.34 1970's and 1980's Studies Did not Show a Survival Increase for Adjuvant Chemotherapy

The book Lung Cancer reports that studies in the 70's and 80's showed little benefit to adjuvant chemotherapy:

> "The Veterans Administration Surgical Adjuvant Group conducted a series of adjuvant chemotherapy studies . . . long-term follow-up revealed no benefit in overall survival . . . . Data from the Swiss Group for Clinical Cancer Research . . . . concluded that treatment with intermittent courses of cyclophosphamide over a two year period seemed to increase the recurrence and death rates . . . . In 1985, Gerling reported that prolonged cytoxic chemotherapy . . . did not improve survival over surgery alone."
> Pisters (4) Girling (5).

The National Cancer Institute states, "Trials of adjuvant chemotherapy regimens have failed to demonstrate a consistent benefit."

NCI.net. (3). Thus, most physicians do not prescribe chemotherapy for stage 1 patients whose tumors have been successfully removed and no evidence of cancer is seen on x-ray or other tests.

17.35 Recent Studies of Adjuvant Chemotherapy

Some studies in the 80's and 90's, using more effective forms of chemotherapy have shown a benefit to chemotherapy. In a Finnish study, "survival in the chemotherapy arm was significantly better than control (61% versus 48%)." A recent study said the following:

> "The trial was designed as a randomized, two-group study with postoperative adjuvant chemotherapy versus surgery alone as control group. All patients had stage IB disease (pT2N0) assessed after a radical surgical procedure. Chemotherapy consisted of treatment with cisplatin (100mg/m(2) on day 1) and etopiside (120mg/m(2) on days 1-3) for a total of six cycles. Results: Between January 1988 and December 1994, 66 patients were included in the study. Thirty-three belonged to the adjuvant chemotherapy group and 33 to the control group. Patients were followed for a minimum period of 5 years . . . . The rates of locoregional recurrence and distant metastasizes were 18 and 30%, respectively, in the adjuvant chemotherapy group and 24 and 43%, respectively, in the control group. The 5-year disease-free survival rates were 59% in the adjuvant group and 30% in the control group (P=0.02) . . . Conclusions: Our results suggest that adjuvant chemotherapy may reduce recurrences and prolong overall survival in patients at stage IB NSCLC deemed radically operated. Despite being difficult to accept, the use of adjuvant chemotherapy might have better long-term results." Mineo (5).

Distinguishing the successful results here from prior studies is not easy. Taxol and Carboplatin were used here, which many believe to be the optimal combination. Did prior studies fail to utilize the optimum chemotherapy mix? Or is the fact that this subgroup was stage 1B patients, with a higher potential for metastasis the decisive factor? Another recent study showed a slight survival advantage for chemotherapy, using different chemotherapy drugs, 76% in the chemotherapy and surgery group versus 71% in the surgery group alone. Wada (8).

17.36 Why Doctors Do Not Always Consider New Forms of Treatment

There is some recent evidence that chemotherapy does provide a survival benefit. Putting aside the issue of side effects, why wouldn't doctors utilize the latest research in their treatment? Is my doctor unaware of the latest research? The issue is more complex than that.

There is a maxim in medicine, first do no harm. That is, the physician's intervention should not do damage to the patient. Without a sound medical foundation, most physicians are reluctant to undertake new forms of treatment until they have become generally accepted in a particular area of practice. At this point, while some studies are favorable, they are not sufficiently widely accepted to constitute the standard of care or accepted practice. Most physicians would still consider adjuvant chemotherapy experimental.

Another reason is the concern about professional liability claims. From my perspective, that is unreasonable; the number of chemotherapy-related claims is rather low. When physicians are diagnosing many patients at advanced stages, it would seem the real danger is delayed diagnosis. Nonetheless, there is a concern, realistic or not, about using new treatments, finding out they went beyond the standard of care, and even with the best of intentions, that physician would face liability.

17.37 Accessibility to New Forms of Treatment

Where does the patient go to obtain new forms of treatment, or more accurately, known treatment given in a new context? First, there are clinical trials which assess and evaluate new forms of treatment. (Clinical trials are the subject of another chapter). Many university hospitals where clinical trials are being given may be somewhat more aggressive in providing new forms of treatment even outside the context of a clinical trial.

17.38 Differences between Stage 1A and 1B treatments

Medicine is moving towards some type of prophylactic treatment of stage 1B patients. The larger size of the tumor, and the number of patients who will have ultimately metastasises, between 40 and 50%, means that the risk of spread is real and substantial.

17.4 POST-OPERATIVE RADIATION FOR STAGE 1 TUMORS

A 1999 article in the journal Lung Cancer states, "There is no place for routine postoperative thoracic radiotherapy after complete resection of a stage 1 tumor." Another article suggested:

> "The Port meta-analysis found a detrimental effect of postoperative radiotherapy particularly for patients with stage 1/ II disease. At present, the use of postoperative radiotherapy should be restricted to those patients with incompletely resected disease (positive surgical margins or residual local disease) or selected patients with multiple lymph nodes involved at surgery." Pisters, (6).

Yet investigation continues. An Italian study found beneficial results:

> "Background and purpose: To evaluate the benefits and the drawbacks of post-operative radiotherapy in completely resected Stage I (a and b) non-small cell lung cancer . . . Overall 5-year survival (Kaplan-Meier) showed a positive trend in the treated group: 67 versus 58% (P=0.048). Regarding toxicity in G1, six patients experienced a grade 1 acute toxicity . . . ."
>
> "Radiological evidence of long-term lung toxicity, with no significant impairment of the respiratory function, has been detected in 18 of the 19 patients who have been diagnosed as having a post-radiation lung fibrosis. Conclusions: Adjuvant radiotherapy gave good results in terms of local control in patients with completely resected NSCLC with pathological Stage I. Overall 5-year survival and disease-free survival showed a promising

trend. Treatment-related toxicity is acceptable." *Adjuvant therapy (10)*.

Whether radiation is effective for stage 1 patients continues to be debated. Absent clear proof of its benefits, few physicians will utilize it because of its effects and radiation for stage 1 patients is now reserved for clinical trials or other investigational settings. In the future, molecular markers may help us target a subgroup of stage 1 patients who would benefit from radiation or chemotherapy.

17.5 POST SURGICAL DIAGNOSTIC TECHNIQUES

One could also conclude that *routine* use of chemotherapy should not be recommended for stage 1 patients, but that they should be intensively watched so that any signs of spread or metastasis can be timely treated. That is not what occurs today. Most physicians prescribe a yearly or bi-yearly chest x-ray and wait until tumor spread manifests itself on such an x-ray before recommending additional treatment. The difficulty here is that the chest-ray is an imprecise tool, detecting tumors of usually at least a centimeter, and the tumor has spread before it is identified.

17.51 Ct Scan

One plausible alternative is the use of post-operative Ct Scans. The CT is significantly more accurate than the chest x-ray in detecting small tumors. Low dose Ct (Ct designed to minimize exposure presents limited risk of exposure. One difficulty is that this does not yet represent the standard of care. Therefore, some insurers might balk at paying for such CT's if they were regarded as experimental.

17.511 Studies of Ct Scan for Post-Surgical Stage 1 Patients

A recent study compared post-surgical evaluation with Ct Scan and x-ray. Seven smaller nodules were identified on Ct Scan while only the four larger nodules were seen on x-ray. Ray, *(15)*.

17.6 DEFINING SUBGROUPS OF STAGE 1 PATIENTS WHO WOULD BENEFIT FROM CHEMOTHERAPY

While most stage 1 patients are cured, some are not. Scientists today are attempting to identify risk factors with stage 1 patients.

17.61 Micro-Vessel Density

Angiogenesis is the formation of new blood vessels. While it is a normal process in wound healing and other areas, in cancer, it is the primary way that metastasis occurs and the cancer spread:

> "Angiogenesis is a complex regulated process, forming new blood vessels from pre-existing vessels . . . . The determination of microvessel density constitutes a measure for tumor angiogenesis. According to investigations by Fontanini et. al. high vessel density is a negative prognostic factor for the overall survival of patients suffering non-small cell lung cancer. In these tumors, increased microvessel density was also associated with a higher incident of lymph node metastasises and distant metastasises. In their study on 227 patients with surgically treated stage I non-small cell lung cancers, Lucchi et. al. confirmed the prognostic significance of microvessel count regarding both overall and disease-free survival." Junker, (3).

The theory is not free from challenge. One study of "69 stage I-II non small lung cancers failed to demonstrate the prognostic relevance of microvessel density." Junker (9) (10).

17.611 Micro-Metastases

Stage 1 patients have no lymph node metastases measured by conventional diagnostic tools. However, a Japanese study measured micro-metastases, which would be undetected by conventional means. Not surprisingly, the extent of such metastases in the lymph nodes negatively impacted long-term survival. Osaki, (16). Similar findings were made in a 1996 study:

"Among the 67 patients available for follow-up with a histopathologic nodal stage of N0, 51 patients had disease classified without nodal micrometastases by our immunohistochemical assay. Their mean relapse-free survival and cancer-related survival were 41.1 months and 44.6 months, respectively. For the 16 patients with nodal micrometastases, the mean relapse-free survival and cancer-related survival were 29.0 months and 36.5 months, respectively. Patients with histopathologic stage N1 disease without further nodal micrometastases (n = 11) exhibited mean relapse-free survival of 34.8 months and cancer-related survival of 38.2 months, compared with six patients with nodal micrometastases who had mean relapse-free and cancer-related survivals of 18.0 months and 23.5 months, respectively." Izbicki (17)

Measurement of nodal micro-metastases has a clear factual basis. We know the extent of metastasis directly impacts survival. Micro-vessel density, a similar marker, is also reliable. Other chemical markers are showing promise but a consensus is not seen as to which is most reliable or the best predictor. Measuring micro-metastases and micro-vessel density makes sense and should be tested in clinical trials.

17.62 VEGF Factor

Microvessel density measures preliminary indications of metastasis. The metastatic process involves production of VEGF, (vascular endothelial growth factor). Some scientists suggest measuring VEGF levels, and there is some correlation with VEGF levels and later metastasis. Again, patients could be measured following surgery, and consideration given to providing chemotherapy to those patients with high microvessel density and/or VEGF levels. Because there has been some variation in the studies, some scientists would like to see consistent results or some consensus within the medical community about what to measure before providing any recommendation.

17.621 P-53

P-53 is a potent tumor suppressor which has been measured with conflicting results:

"Interestingly, we found no evidence for an effect of P53 expression level on prognosis. While some investigators have reported that P53 protein expression was a significant factor for poor prognosis in patients with lung cancer, other studies found that P53 expression had no impact on clinical outcome." Minami (14).

17.622 Combination of VEGF and P-53 Measurement

One study found the prognostic value of either VEGF or P-53 to be limited. However, when both were elevated in stage 1 patients, survival rates markedly decreased. Five year survival with VEGF and P-53 negative was 64% compared with 38% in patients with both factors positive. That makes sense. The activation of VEGF combined with the suppression of P-53 means that a critical factor leading to metastasis is present while a critical regulator is absent. Research is continuing but it would make sense for patients in the dual positive group to consider post-surgical treatment.

17.63 BCL-2

Tumor cells manage to escape apoptosis, or cell death. Where cells are damaged or deficient, apoptosis generally occurs. That process is circumvented in cancer. BCL-2 protects cells from cell death and is therefore associated with various cancers, with its role in lung cancer being researched:

"We found Bcl-2-protein expression with statistically significant association with histology and clinical outcome in 30% of the tumors of this series. These results are in agreement with previous reports 10 and 11 showing that SCCs express Bcl-2 more frequently than adenocarcinomas. We also found in multivariate analysis that Bcl-2 protein expression emerged as a significant marker of poor long-term prognosis; only 7 of 37 patients with Bcl-2Bnegative tumors had recurrence. Moreover, Bcl-2 also appeared as a prognostic factor on univariate analysis regardless of the histopathologic type and stage subcategories. Bcl-2 is a human proto-oncogene located on chromosome 18 that encodes inhibitors of apoptosis and can act as oncogene by reducing the rate of cell death." II.

17.64 Cell Death or Apoptosis

A properly working system in the body provides for cell death, and this is one way of preventing unlimited proliferation. One study measured rates of apoptosis and found that the measurement did impact the patient's prognosis. This measurement may show at an earliest stage where the cancer is reoccurring, and direct us to early intervention for those patients with a poorer prognosis. Junker (3).

17.65 Other Measurements

17.651 Cyclin B

Cyclin B1 is a key molecule for G_2-M-phase transition during the cell cycle and is overexpressed in various tumor types. Soria (19). One can hypothesize that its presence indicates that cell duplication is occuring and at elevated levels are an indicator of cancer. Soria found:

> "Patients with tumors that overexpressed cyclin B1 had significantly shorter survival times than patients with tumors that displayed low levels of cyclin B1 ($P = 0.02$, log-rank test). About 60% of the patients whose tumors had a low cyclin B1 expression were alive at 5 years compared with only 30% of the patients whose tumors had high cyclin B1 expression" Soria (18).

Similar findings were made with other types of tumors.

17.652 Glut-1

One study found rates of glucose (sugar) metabolism (Glut-1) of the resected tumor relevant in determining the patient's survival. Minami (14).

> "The appearance of Glut-1 positive clones was associated with aggressive tumor behavior and Glut-1 was significant indicator

of poor prognosis in cases of NSCLC." Minami (14) at 56. Minami reports that "the state of Glut-1 may reflect the biologic behavior of tumor cells . . . . Brown reported that Glut-1 was the major glucose transporter expressed in NSCLC." Minami (14) at 56.

17.653 CEA

CEA (Carinoembryonic antigen) is a commonly used tumor marker. Unlike many of the items above, CEA is easily and quickly tested. A recent study found:

"We studied 118 consecutive NSCLC patients who were clinically judged operable and were eventually operated upon . . . In tumors pathologically classified in stage Ia to IIb, a preoperative CEA level higher than 10 ng/mL was associated with a 67% probability of tumor relapse. In the same stages of disease, a CEA level less than 10 ng/mL increased the baseline probability of no recurrence from 80% to 88%. CONCLUSIONS: In operable patients with NSCLC the frequency of abnormal serum concentrations of CEA is low (17% in our series). However, it is important to identify such a small group of high-risk patients as many of them (in our study, 55% and 70% of those with a CEA value in excess of, respectively, 5 and 10 ng/mL) will develop an early postoperative recurrence. Such patients should be investigated preoperatively by mediastinoscopy or positron emission tomography in even in the absence of suspicious symptoms and signs. Then after an apparently successful operation, they should be carefully followed up. These patients could represent a suitable target for neoadjuvant clinical trials of selected high-risk groups." Buccheri (18)

17.654 Cox 2 Levels

One oncologist writes, "If you look at all stage I cases there is a clear survival difference for stage I lung cancers for overexpression of COX-2 cases versus those that have negative expression." Thus, it may make sense to test cox-2 and provide cox-2 inhibitors and other treatment to those with cox-2 positive tumors.

17.66 Conclusion

Various cell characteristics indicate whether the patient was cured by surgery or whether carcinogenic type processes are still occuring. Using one or more of these indicators, we can identify patients at enhanced risk and prescribe some type of post-surgical treatment. However, while many studies have and will be conducted, this analysis remains experimental as scientists struggle to identify which factors are most important and attempt to duplicate results in subsequent tests. One would not be surprised to see multi-faceted tests incorporating multiple factors since cancer itself involves multiple genetic changes.

17.7 POST-SURGICAL GENE THERAPY IRESSA

17.71 Response to Iressa

In a separate chapter, I review Iressa and epidermal growth factor (EGF) inhibitors. EGF is associated with the spread of lung cancer and worse prognosis. In 2004, scientists identified a subgroup of patients who responded particularly well to an anti-EGF drug called Iressa. EGF meets a receptor (EGFR) to create binding and then chemical changes in the tyrosine kinase portion of the cell. Iressa inhibits those chemical changes called.

Scientists found that patients with defects in the tyrosine portion of the EGFR responded particularly well to Iressa. Response rates in some studies exceeded 35% in particular subgroups. Iressa has limited side effects, generally significantly less than chemotherapy, because Iressa impacts only a specific cell, not a large group of dividing cells.

Thus it may make sense to test individuals for this defect and if the testing is positive prescribe Iressa to prevent possible spread of the tumor.

17.72 Who Should be Tested

Not all patients are likely to have this defect. Studies found that non-smokers and very light former smokers with adenocarcinoma or bronchoalveolar cancer were likely to have the defect. Certainly there is a strong argument for testing patients in this subgroup.

For others testing might make sense if only to exclude some patients. Those with normal (called wild) type EGFR are less likely to benefit. Those with some defects though not fitting the precise pattern of responders might still consider some treatment. EGFR treatment is evolving, and more is being learned each month.

17.73 Testing Cost and Procedure

Today EGFR testing can be performed at Harvard's Center for Genetics and Genomics, in Cambridge, Massachusetts. The current cost if $850. As testing becomes effective, more testing laboratories will offer it, reductions will be negotiated by HMO's and hospitals, and procedures will develop. Whether today's insurance carriers will pay the cost remains unclear. Since most stage 1 patients have had surgery, obtaining samples for testing should be easy.

CONCLUSION

In the upcoming years, the stage 1 patient will be followed more closely at the major hospitals, with new forms of genetic testing used to identify potential recurrence or spread at early stages. Some of these institutions will begin utilizing newer drugs like Iressa for post-surgical treatment to inhibit the spread of tumors and improve the long-term survival of stage 1 patients.

REFERENCES

1. Martini, *Treatment of Stage 1 and II Disease* 339 in Aisner, *Comprehensive Textbook of Thoracic Oncology* (Williams & Wilkins 1996).
2. Edell ES, Cortese DA: *Photodynamic Therapy in the Management of Early Superficial Squamous Cell Carcinoma as an Alternative to Surgical Resection*, Chest 102(5): 1319-1322, 1992.
3. Midthun, *Endobronchial Techniques in Lung Cancer, Options for Nonsurgical Care*. Vol. 101, No. 3, March 1997 Postgraduate Medicine.
4. NCI.org.
5. Pisters, *Surgery and Chemotherapy*, 770, in Pass, Lung Cancer (2000).

6. Girling, *Fifteen-year Follow-up of all patients in a study of postoperative chemotherapy for bronchial carcinoma,*" Br. J. Cancer 1985; 52:867.

7. Mineo, *Postoperative adjuvant therapy for stage IB non-small-cell lung cancer,* Eur J Cardiothorac Surg 2001 Aug;20(2): 378-84.

8. Wada, *Postoperative adjuvant Chemotherapy with PVM . . .* Eur J Cardiothorac Surg 1999 Apr;15(4):438-43.

8. Furuse K, Fukuoka M, Kato H, et al.: *A prospective phase II study on photodynamic therapy with photofrin II for centrally located early-stage lung cancer.* Journal of Clinical Oncology 11(10): 1852-1857, 1993.

9. Junker, *Prognostic Factors in Stage 1/II Non-Small Cell Lung Cancer,* Lung Cancer Suppl. 1 (2001) S17-24.

10. Decaussin, *Expression of Vascular Endothelial Growth Factor and its two receptors in Non-Small Cell Lung Carcinomas . . .* J. Pathol 1999; 188: 369-77.

11 *Adjuvant radiotherapy in non-small cell lung cancer with pathological stage I: definitive results of a phase III randomized trial,* Radiother Oncol 2002 Jan;62(1):11-19.

12. Fontanini, *Microvessel Count Predicts Metastatic Disease and Survival in Non-Small Cell Lung Cancer,* J Pathol 1995; 177: 57-63.

13. Lucchi, et. al, Tumor *Angiogeneis and Biologic Markers in Resected Stage I NSCLC,* Eur J. Cardiothorac Surg, 1997; 12: 535-41.

14. Minami, *Prognostic Significance of p53, Ki-67, VEGF and Glut 1 in resected Stage 1 Adenocarcinoma of the Lung,* Lung Cancer 38 (2002) 51-57.

15. Ray, *Monitoring Stage 1 and II Lung Cancer Patients Post-Thoracotomy Using Low Dose Spiral CT,* Lung Cancer 34 (Suppl. 1 S1-S76, S 41).

16. Osaki, Prognostic Impact of Micrometastatic Tumor Cells in the Lymph Nodes and Bone Marrow of Patients With Completely Resected Stage I NonBSmall-Cell Lung Cancer Journal of Clinical Oncology, Vol 20, Issue 13 (July), 2002: 2930-2936.

17. Izbicki, Mode of spread in the early phase of phymmphatic metastases in non-small cell lung cancer: significance of nodal miscrometastases. J Thorac Cardiovasc Surg 1996;112:623-630

18. Buccheri, Identifying patients at risk of early postoperative recurrence of lung cancer: a new use of the old CEA test. Ann Thorac Surg. 2003 Mar;75(3):973-80.

19. Soria, *Overexpression of Cyclin B1 in Early-Stage Non-Small Cell Lung Cancer and Its Clinical Implication,*Cancer Res. 2000 Aug 1;60(15):4000-4.

20. Hassan, *Clinical Significance of Cyclin B1 Protein Expression in Squamous Cell Carcinoma of the Tongue,* Clinical Cancer Research Vol. 7, 2458-2462, August 2001.

21 Liao, *Vascular Endothelial Growth Factor and Other Biological Predictors Related to the Postoperative Survival Rate on Non-Small Cell Lung Cancer,* Lung Cancer, Vol. 33 (2-3) (2201) 125-132.

22. The gene was discovered as the translocated locus in a B-cell Leukemia and thereby acquired its name. The gene has also been associated with B-cell lymphoma.

23. The mammalian Bcl-2 protein family comprises at least 24 members encoded by 20 genes.The various members function as sensors of cellular stress and they receive input from various sources including . . . the cytoskeleton, the nucleus and the mitochondria The archetypal family member called Bcl-2 and its pro-survival homologues process most of the information collected by these sensors. Bcl-2 was the first member to be discovered when the encoding gene was found to be translocated in human follicular lymphoma. Bcl-2 protects cells from growth factor deprivation or against exposure to cytotoxic drugs, taxol, cisplatin, glucocorticoids or ionising radiation.

24. *Lung Cancer Targeted Therapies, Cox-2 Inhibitors, Retinoids and Aerosolized Delivery,* www.webtie.org/sots/Meetings/Lung/June192001/lectures/Transcripts/Dmitrovsky/transcript.htmwww.webtie.org/sots/Meetings/Lung/June192001.

25. Driscolle, Lung Cancer Mollecular Pathology and Methods, (Humana Press, 2002), available online at no charge on Google books.

CHAPTER 18

STAGE 2 NON-SMALL CELL CANCER

18.1 TREATMENT OVERVIEW

18.10 Classification

Stage 2 comprises a diverse group:

> "Patients with stage II NSCLC represent a heterogeneous group, since stage II consists of patients with T1-2N1 or T3N0 tumors. By definition, patients with tumors invading the chest wall apex, mediastinum, diaphragm, or even the mainstem bronchus may all have T3 tumors. The extent of the data available regarding treatment of each of these different groups is therefore limited." Scott (8).

18.11 Surgery as the Preferred Option

Surgery is the treatment of choice for stage II patients. As with stage 1, careful consideration of pulmonary reserve is required for major surgery. Mortality rates tend to be age related, and in the 3%-5% area. A 78 year former smoker with pulmonary abnormalities is more likely to suffer an adverse result than a 50 year old in otherwise good health.

18.12 Radiation

Stage II patients who are not recommended for surgery may undergo radiation with curative intent. (NCI 6). Among patients with excellent performance status, a 20% 3-year survival rate may be expected with a completed course of radiation. In one study, an overall 5 year survival rate of 10% was reported, but patients with small T1 tumors had a substantially higher rate.

18.13 Survival Rates

A 1999 article in the journal Lung Cancer states,

> "For the 98 patients with postoperative lobar or hilar node metastasises, overall survival rates at 3 and 5 years of 45.2 and 37.3% were found. Fifteen (15.3% showed a local failure within the radiation field as a first failure relapse. Distant metastasises as first failure were noted in 38 patients (39%) with 12/38 brain metastasises . . . . At 5 years, a local progression free survival rate of 79% and a distant metastasis free survival rate of 52% was noted." Rodrigues (5).

Another found survival rates as follows: 1 year 70%, 3 year 50%, 5 year, 30%.

18.131 Survival Rate Differences Between Adenocarcinoma and Squamous Cell

Some studies have reported differences in survival rate for stage 2 based on type:

> "For the 71 stage II patients with a squamous histology, a 5-year survival rate of 44% was noted as opposed to 14% for patients with a large cell or adenocarcinoma. Although the local failure was not different (the term local failure meaning reappearance of the tumor in the area of radiation or where the tumor was removed) 17% for squamous, 11% for non-squamous, the non-squamous group failed more often at distant sites. From

the 27 patients, 18 developed metastasises as a first failure with 8/27 (30%) brain metastasises. For the squamous group, 20/71 (28%) developed distant metastasises, with 5/71 brain (metastasises)." Rodrigues, (5).

18.2 CHEMOTHERAPY

18.21 An Uncertain Area

Recall that stage 2 means that the tumor has penetrating adjoining lymph nodes. Thus the potential for dissemination of the cancer is greater and the chance that surgery can remove the entire tumor less. Combining surgery with some type of post-surgical treatment for eradicating any remaining tumor cells makes logical sense. However, precisely what should be done and what benefits can be realized continues to be debated.

With lymph node involvement at stage 2, the possibility of recurrence or metastasis increases. One may reason that in addition to radiating the area of the tumor to kill any cancer cells missed at surgery, why not add chemotherapy to attack any cells in that or other areas? While the approach carries with it some logic, clinical studies have not shown success, and many physicians reason that patients should not be required to deal with chemotherapy treatment until definitive benefits are not shown. Here are results from one study.

A presentation at the 2000 World Conference on Lung Cancer summarizes the results: "This large, well-conducted, multicenter study suggests no clinical advantage at all for adding chemotherapy to radiation therapy in the management of resectable lung cancer. While newer chemotherapy agents are available, it is not clear that these drugs would change the fundamental outcome compared with the widely used platinum-based regimen used in this study. It is fair to say that the use of chemotherapy in the adjuvant setting of stage 2 or 3A NSCLC remains investigational." Burstein(1), see also (2)(3).

Others have reached different conclusions, "Chemotherapy used alone or in combination with radiation therapy postoperatively resulted in prolonged time to disease progression and a modest improvement in survival. However, long-term survival was not affected. The precise role of adjuvant chemotherapy and/or radiation therapy in patients with stage II NSCLC remains to be determined. Investigators are also exploring the use of preoperative and postoperative paclitaxel and carboplatin chemotherapy in patients with stages Ib, IIa, IIb, and IIIa NSCLC." (4) (U.S. Pharmacist).

18.3 GENE THERAPY FOR STAGE 2

18.31 Rationale for Stage 2 Gene Therapy

Gene therapy probably makes the most sense at this stage, but interestingly has been tested the least. With stage 4 disseminated cancer, the possibility of reworking cell-signaling is limited, and at stage 1, why apply therapy to patients who likely have been cured. At stage 2, we have patients with relatively early disease, but the existence of lymph node involvement means that the possibility of cure with surgery is less than 50%. Unfortunately, there have been relatively few trials directed at stage 2 patients.

18.32 Epidermal Growth Factor Receptor Therapy

We discuss Iressa in our chapter on epidermal growth factor inhibitors. Patients with adenocarcinoma, BAC, non-smokers and light smokers are more likely to have lung tumors involving damage to the tyrosine kinase portion of the EGFR. Since Iressa which is a tyrosine kinase inhibitor, it is highly effective with this group. Tests have been developed to identify tyrosine kinase damage, and patients may wish to take it to assess treatment options.

REFERENCES

1. *Adjuvant Chemotherapy for Lung Cancer: Still No Benefit*, World Conference on Lung Cancer (2000), www.medscape.com.
2. Non-Small Cell Lung Cancer Collaborative Group. *Chemotherapy in non-small cell lung cancer: a meta-analysis using updated data on individual patients from 52 randomized clinical trials.* BMJ. 1995;311:899-909.
3. *Burstein*, SM, Adak S, Wagner H, et al. *A randomized trial of postoperative adjuvant therapy in patients with completely resected stage II or IIIA non-small-cell lung cancer.* N Engl J Med. 2000;343:1217-1222.

4. www.uspharmacist.com current Treatment of Non-Small Cell Lung Cancer, (US Pharmacist Continuing Education).

5. Rodrigues, *The Impact of Surgical Adjuvant Thoracic Radiation for different Stages of Non Small Cell Lung Cancer: the Experience from a Single Institution*, Lung Cancer 23 (1999) 11-17.

6. NCI.org.

7. Riantawan, *Survival analysis of Thai patients with non-small-cell lung cancer undergoing surgical resection*, J Med Assoc Thai. 1999 Jun;82(6): 552-7.

8. Scott, *Treatment of Stage II Non-small Cell Lung Cancer*, Chest. 2003;123:188S-201S.

CHAPTER 19

STAGE 3 NON-SMALL CELL LUNG CANCER

19.1 STAGE 3 IS DIVIDED INTO 3A AND 3B

One website explains how stage 3 non-small cell cancer came to be subdivided into two categories:

> "Stage III lung cancer originally included patients with locally advanced disease, without distant metastasises. In 1986, the International Staging System for Lung Cancer further divided this group into two subgroups C IIIA and IIIB.[4] These subgroups attempted to separate patients with tumors that were potentially resectable (stage IIIA) from patients with tumors clearly beyond the scope of surgical extirpation (stage IIIB). Stage IIIA originally included tumors of any size within the lung with limited extension of the primary site to the pericardium, mediastinal pleura or fat, or chest wall and without lymph node metastasises or with lymph node metastasises confined to the ipsilateral mediastinal lymph nodes. Experience has demonstrated that patients with this classification form a very heterogeneous group, with a long-term survival following surgical resection that ranges from 10 to 50%. Consequently, this classification has recently been modified."
> Chestnut (1)

One of the main differences between stage 3 A and B non-small cell cancer is that surgery is part of 3A treatment. Surgery in stage 1 patients is designed to remove all of the tumor. In stage 3A, while that may not be the goal, it can at least remove enough tumor to make the risks of surgery and reduction of lung capacity make sense. In stage 3B where the tumor has extended beyond the immediate area into the mediastinum and adjoining structures, it is felt that the risk does not make sense. Since one group with different treatment plans is confusing, the groups are divided into 3A and 3B. Note that within each category are tumors with different characteristics, but the intra-category treatments are essentially the same.

19.2 CHEMOTHERAPY, RADIATION AND SURGERY IS STANDARD TREATMENT WITH THE BEST MIX STILL UNDER INVESTIGATION

A pharmaceutical site provides a good overview of Stage 3 A treatment:

"Historically, patients with stage III NSCLC (locally advanced disease) were managed with radiation therapy, but long-term survival was poor (5%B10%). The development of active chemotherapy regimens for NSCLC has led to the use of combined modality therapy for the management of stage III disease. Surgery and radiation are effective at controlling local disease, while chemotherapy works to control distant metastatic disease. Any two of these modalities or all three could be combined to treat stage III disease. However, patients with stage IIIb disease are generally not candidates for surgical resection and will most commonly receive combination chemotherapy, plus or minus radiation therapy."

"Numerous trials comparing combined chemotherapy/radiation to radiation alone have been conducted in patients with stage III NSCLC. The chemotherapy regimens and radiation schedules have varied greatly among the studies, and conflicting results have emerged . . . . When two different meta-analyses were conducted with the data from all of the published randomized trials comparing chemotherapy/radiation with radiation alone, a small improvement in survival was reported for combined modality therapy. All of these studies utilized the older generation of chemotherapy regimens (cisplatin or cisplatin-based) in combination with radiotherapy. The improved activity of the newer combination chemotherapy regimens used in stage IV disease could lead to improved results when combined with radiation for the treatment of stage III disease." USPharmasist (2).

19.21 Chemotherapy Before Surgery or NeoAdjuvant Surgery

Chemotherapy and radiation are also, with research continuing as to what combination of these three forms of treatment will achieve the best results. Recall that Stage III A tumors involve either large T2 or 3 tumors or situations of significant lymph node involvement. Many physicians believe in chemotherapy before surgery:

"Neoadjuvant chemotherapy with or without radiation therapy followed by surgery is another combined modality treatment for stage III (primarily stage IIIa) disease that is under investigation. Neoadjuvant chemotherapy is administered to patients with bulky disease prior to surgery in an attempt to decrease tumor size and increase surgical resectability. Two randomized studies have {favorably} compared chemotherapy followed by surgery with surgery alone." U.S. Pharmacist (2).

A recent article discusses the purposes of neoadjuvant chemotherapy:

"The purpose of neoadjuvant chemotherapy is the eradication of micrometastatic disease, which is almost invariably manifest when ipsilateral mediastinal or subcarinal lymph nodes (N2) are involved. A chest computed tomography (CT) imaging study may show lymph nodes extending throughout many mediastinum regions, including the aortopulmonic window, the paratracheal region, and the precarinal and subcarinal areas . . . . Three randomized phase III trials reported that administering cisplatin-based chemotherapy before surgery to patients with resectable stage IIIA lung cancer improved survival results over those obtained with surgery alone or surgery plus radiotherapy. The MD Anderson investigators have recently updated the long-term follow-up of a selected high-risk population of patients with advanced but still resectable non-small cell lung cancer (NSCLC), T1-3N2M0 or T3-4N0M0 . . . . This study shows that a preresectional chemotherapy regimen of cisplatin in combination with ifosfamide and mitomycin does improve the clinical outcome in comparison with surgery alone." Rosell (3).

19.3 STAGE IIIB NON-SMALL CELL LUNG CANCER

Chemotherapy is the primary treatment for Stage 3B and Stage 4 non small cell lung cancer. We can note the following:

1. In the 80's and early 90's, there was some debate about whether chemotherapy improved survival, and whether multiple agents helped. That debate has probably ended. **Studies have demonstrated a consistent (if relatively modest) benefit to chemotherapy over other treatments,** and have also shown that multi-modal chemotherapy is better than single agent. If different drugs can fight cancer and work in different ways, it would make sense that a combination would achieve better results so long as significant side effects were not created.

2. **No one combination has demonstrated markedly better results throughout different clinical trials than others.** Clinical trials continue to test various combinations against one other to determine rates of tumor diminution, partial and complete response rate (partial meaning at least 50% reduction of the tumor and complete meaning no visible tumor at a certain point in time), survival rates, and side effects. To call such clinical trials "experimental" is a little misleading. The clinical trials are generally using the same drug combinations that practitioners use, only in a defined clinical setting.

3. The term non-small cell lung cancer includes adenocarcinoma, squamous cell, and large cell cancers. While we have grouped these three types together, it is possible that each type acts a

little differently. Conceivably, one drug could be better for squamous and another for large cell. **The fact that people with different types of tumors are grouped together, and different ages and health has made it more difficult to distinguish which drug is most effective.**

4. **The platinum-drugs, cisplatin and carboplatin have been the mainstays of chemotherapy for stage 3B patients,** with the above list concentrating on platinum drug combinations. Taxol and Carboplatin appear in practice to be the most frequently used combination, though the literature does not clearly indicate better results with this combination.

5. Gemcitabine and Gemcitabine combinations have been showing results almost comparable to these platinum combinations, with **Gemcitabine sometimes reported to have fewer side effects—** "Kosimidis showed that a nonplatinum-containing regimen was equivalent to standard carboplatin/paclitaxel for the treatment of advanced disease. The results of this study are also consistent with the recent South West Oncology Group (SWOG) and Eastern Cooperative Oncology Group (ECOG) studies presented at the American Society for Clinical Oncology (ASCO) over the past 2 years." Kosmidis (4).

6. Gene and angiogenic therapy is debated and investigated. **Tarceva and Iressa appear to benefit non-smokers and light former smokers with adenocarcinoma and its subtypes.** Initial studies indicate Avastin provides a modest benefit in survival though side effects are increased.

There are difficult issues of medical choice which might ultimately have to be made by the patients themselves. Is a slightly longer projected life-span worth additional side effects. Chemotherapy presents the problem of killing cancer cells, while preserving normal cells and bodily functions. How do we eliminate the rapidly dividing cells we call cancer, but preserve the other rapidly dividing cells necessary for different life functions?

19.31 Stage 3 B Chemotherapy and Radiation

NCI states,

"Patients with stage IIIb non-small cell lung cancer (NSCLC) do not benefit from surgery alone and are best managed by initial chemotherapy, chemotherapy plus radiation therapy, or radiation therapy alone, depending on sites of tumor involvement and performance status. [6].

For a subgroup, adenocarcinoma patients who are nonsmokers or former light smokers, EGFR drugs Tarcev and Iressa appear to provide a benefit. These patients' tumors appear to be driven at least in part by a malfunctioning EGFR tyrosine kinase which can be identified in a recent EGFR test. (See 15.7. Harvard Laboratories Gene Test). For others, Avastin is showing promise, and cox-2 inhibitors like Celebrex are being evaluated.

REFERENCES

1. www.chestnet.org/education/pccu/vol12/lesson18.html.
2. Current Treatment of Non-Small Cell Lung Cancer, U.S. Pharmacist Continuing Education, www.uspharmacist.com.
3. Rosell, *Preresectional chemotherapy in stage IIIA non-small-cell lung cancer: a 7-year assessment of a randomized controlled trial* Lung Cancer, Vol. 26 (1) (1999) pp. 7-14.
4. Kosmidis (4) *A randomized phase III trial of paclitaxel plus carboplatin versus paclitaxel plus gemcitabine in advanced non-small cell lung cancer (NSCLC): a preliminary analysis.* Lung Cancer. 2000;29(Suppl 2):147, cited in Lynch, 9th World Conference on Lung Cancer, Presidential Symposium, (2000), www.medscape.com.

CHAPTER 20

STAGE 4 NON-SMALL CELL LUNG CANCER

20.1 SUMMARY OF STAGE 4 TREATMENT

20.11 Overview

Stage 4 means the tumor has metastasized to another organ and surgery is not an option. Removal of a usually large tumor in the lung will not eradicate the cancer (since there is a metastasis), and current science reasons that the limited benefit is not worth the risk such surgery entails. The focus in stage 4 treatment is on chemotherapy, radiation to diminish tumor size in the lung and improve quality of life, and newer forms of gene therapy such as Tarceva.

Stage 4 treatment is generally not curative, though there are a few reports of complete remissions and more of partial remission and 2,3, and even 5 year survival. Many cancer groups and patients living with stage 4 tumors will counsel others to live one day at a time, and aggressively seek the best treatment.

Palliation, preventing pain and maintaining quality of life becomes significant. See Bianco (4) (Improvement in quality of life of elderly patients seen after three cycles of Gemcitabine chemotherapy).

Radiation is designed to reduce tumor volume and may provide pain and symptom relief as well as extend life. Since radiation provides few side effects and only limited discomfort, it is a standard treatment for stage 4 patients. Most oncologists would not regard radiation as curative since they cannot eliminate the entire tumor nor prevent metastasis. Since a substantial amount of tumor is eliminated through radiation, survival should be improved, though that is difficult to establish since there are relatively few clinical trials comparing radiation to best supportive care with the absence of any radiation or chemotherapy.

Current forms of chemotherapy are also not curative though they have the potential to reach different parts of the body including areas of metastasis. Since they have that potential, there are periodic reports of patients with 3 and 5 year survivals after chemotherapy, and clinical trials will report instances of complete response. A typical clinical trial report of 200-300 people will report an individual with a complete response. Studies show a modest or reasonable increase in survival times from chemotherapy though one year survival rates are less than 50% even in favorable studies.

Studies report pain relief and improvement of quality of life from chemotherapy. One must be careful in generalizing about chemotherapy or using another patient's experience as a guide; the drugs have gotten better and are causing fewer side effects. Additionally, there is a greater sensitivity to chemotherapy side effects, with many physicians are recommending other drugs to reduce stomach discomfort or other side effects. Nonetheless, a drug which impacts many types of dividing cells, not just cancerous ones, is likely to have an impact upon the body. Improvement in quality of life exists simply because the side effects of chemotherapy are less than the consequences of an untreated disease.

Gene therapy is looked at in both curative and palliative ways. A small subgroup of stage 4 patients showed tremendous improvement from Iressa, while stabilization for a modest period and some symptom improvement was seen in more. Genetic testing is coming into play as we enter the 21st century and major research centers will be beginning to tailor treatment to what cellular studies show. With the first test of epidermal growth factor receptor available, such testing will become part of mainstream treatment at University hospitals, giving more hope to patients. The FDA has already approved one drug for third line treatment of lung cancer at stage 4, and more approvals and use of targeted gene therapy can be expected this decade.

20.12 The Broad Scope of the Stage 4 Category

Stage 4 has many variations since the number of organs, the extent of metastasis, and other factors impact the period of survival and chances for cure. Stage 4 would include an elderly patient with extensive COPD (chronic obstructive pulmonary disorder) and extensive metastasises as well as a middle-aged patient with a single metastasis and otherwise good health. Given the variation in disease type, patient status, and extent of metastasis, one must be careful with general assessments of stage 4 patients.

New research is showing that patients respond differently based upon their subtype. Adenocarcinoma and BAC patients who did not smoke or smoked little had over 35% response rates to Iressa and Tarceva in several recent studies. (A separate chapter is devoted to epidermal growth factor inhibitors so I will only summarize findings here.)

20.13 Varying Survival Statistics for Stage 4

Survival reports differ. Some are favorable: "The 5-year cumulative survival rate was 88.0% for patients in stage IA, 53.9% in stage IB, 33.5% in stage II, 14.7% in stage IIIA, 5.5% in stage IIIB and 7.0% in stage IV." Wu (1). AThe 5-year survival rates for these patients were as follows: stage I, 68.5%; stage II, 46.9%; stage IIIA, 26.1%; stage IIIB, 9.0%; and stage IV, 11.2%." Naruke (2). Others are dim, reporting survival rates of 20-30 weeks in clinical trials, even those receiving chemotherapy.

It may well be the status of the patient, since we know that the overall health or performance status, as well as the number of lymph nodes involved and other factors influence survival. A 45 year patient with a small area of metastasis in otherwise good health should do better than an older patient with COPD and multiple metastases. Those looking for hope can legitimately find it, not in bizarre reports from other countries, but legitimate clinical trials. Those looking for stark reality may find that the prospects of overall cure are limited.

20.14 Mental Attitude

Some would suggest attitude can play a role and that the willingness to fight and undergo treatment can extend life. The author of The Cancer

Patients Handbook wrote the book while 3 years post-diagnosis for stage 4 NSCLC.

A patient in a support group wrote:

> "I was diagnosed 7/99 with stage 4 NSCLC and chose to have chemo (taxol and carboplatin). Over three years later I am in remission and still enjoying life. I grant you that it is not life as I knew it before, but it is still quite enjoyable. So please, everyone who has lung cancer, don't think there isn't any use to fight it. I am living proof that for some, the outcome is NOT always the same and there is a possibility of living much longer than the statistics say." Acor.org support group.

20.2 CHEMOTHERAPY

20.21 Chemotherapy Is Standard

Chemotherapy is the primary form of treatment for stage 4 and serves to extend life and frequently reduce cancer-related symptomlogy. While there is near agreement that chemotherapy is beneficial, the exact form of chemotherapy which should be used remains unclear, though the combination of Taxol and Carboplatin is generally given today (March, 2002). Carboplatin, vinorelbine, taxol, gemcitabine and other forms of chemotherapy have displayed benefits, but the optimal mix of drugs remains unclear since clinical trials have reached varying results. There is detailed information on the Internet about clinical trials with different chemotherapy combinations. One must be careful not to place undue emphasis on the result of a single trial, for it is only consistent results which can create a standard of care. There is an emerging consensus that multi-modal chemotherapy is preferable to single agent, though scientists may struggle to minimize side effects.

The National Cancer Institute states,

> "Cisplatin-containing and carboplatin-containing combination chemotherapy regimens produce objective response rates (including a few complete responses) that are higher than those achieved with single-agent chemotherapy. Although toxic effects may vary, outcome

is similar with most cisplatin-containing regimens . . . Two small phase II studies reported that paclitaxel (Taxol) has single-agent activity in stage IV patients, with response rates in the range of 21%-24%. Reports of paclitaxel combinations have shown relatively high response rates, significant 1 year survival, and palliation of lung cancer symptoms. With the paclitaxel plus carboplatin regimen, response rates have been in the range of 27%-53% with 1-year survival rates of 32%-54%. The combination of cisplatin and paclitaxel was shown to have a higher response rate than the combination of cisplatin and etopiside. [8]. Additional clinical studies should better define the role of these newer combination chemotherapy regimens in the treatment of advanced non-small cell lung cancer. Meta-analyses have shown that chemotherapy produces modest benefits in short-term survival compared to supportive care alone in patients with inoperable stages IIIb and IV disease." www.nci.net.

20.22 Carboplatin Compared with Cisplatin

Carboplatin and Cisplatin are both platinum-based chemotherapy drugs. Carboplatin has fewer side effects and essentially the same impact, so it is used more often.

20.23 Physician's Attitudes and Chemotherapy

Many physicians will be familiar with recent favorable developments in treatment for advanced lung cancer. Some may be negative and one writer explains why:

"Early trials in NSCLC (non small cell lung cancer) did not show the improvements in survival with SCLC. Indeed, the earliest regimens, based upon alkylating agents rather than cisplatin, appeared detrimental. Physicians attitudes to chemotherapy for NSCLC were therefore profoundly negative, and have tended to remain so. Subsequent combination chemotherapies have yielded some improvements in survival, as well as symptom relief as described above. Unfortunately, attitudes have not changed despite the now-abundant evidence that chemotherapy is superior to supportive care." Pass (1), at 998.

20.24 The Creation of Multi-Drug Resistance

Chemotherapy has served to extend life and reduce symptoms, but it has unfortunately not served as a cure for most stage 4 lung cancer patients. Even those patients who respond initially to chemotherapy frequently develop multi-drug resistance (MDR). For this reason, attention has focused on gene and other therapies for stage 4 patients.

20.25 Chemotherapy as Improving Quality of Life

There is significant evidence that chemotherapy improves quality of life.

> "There is evidence that most patients either improve or preserve their performance status during treatment. In one report on the MIC (mitomycin C, ifosfamide, cisplatin) regimen, only 9% of patients experienced deterioration in quality of life on treatment, and 30% improved. It is also well documented that improvements in symptoms are not confined to patients with an objective response." Pass (1), at 909.

Devita's well-known cancer treatise states:

> "Disease-related symptoms will improve after chemotherapy, sometimes even in the absence of a measurable tumor response. QOL scores improved with chemotherapy, whereas they declined over the first 6 weeks with best supportive care . . . . Improved survival and QOL were also demonstrated with single agent chemotherapy in a population of patients exceeding the age of 70 years." (Devita 3) at 969.

See Bianco (4) (improvement in quality of life of elderly patients seen after Gemcitabine chemotherapy). However, each individual will need to make determinations of the type of treatment based not only upon statistics but an individualized assessment of the patient's condition.

20.251 Substituting Other Drugs for Cisplatin

Cisplatin was one of the most widely-used chemotherapy for a number of years, and its efficacy has been shown in clinical trials. However, it has been associated with nausea and vomiting. Other drugs are being used to replace Cisplatin with similar effectiveness but without these side effects. Taxol, Carboplatin, and Gemcitabine are three widely used substitutes.

20.26 Multi-Modal Chemotherapy

Combining drugs improve response. Taxol and Carboplatin is the most widely used combination, though any number of combinations have been tried including Cisplatin and Gemcitabine, Carboplatin and Gemcitabine, Cisplatin and Vinorelbine. Whether three drug combinations further improve response is unclear.

20.3 RADIATION

20.31 Local Control and Palliation

Radiation is used to diminish tumor size, reduce pain, and improve breathing ability. Radiation will generally not eradicate the entire tumor, putting aside the areas of metastasis.

20.4 GENE THERAPY

Iressa is discussed in a separate chapter, but I will touch upon recent research and implications for stage 4 patients.

20.41 Clinical trials history

Initial studies showed modest results. FDA.gov. The study group was primarily patients in clinical trials for whom chemotherapy was not working. About 10% in this group had partial responses with about 40% experiencing tumor stabilization. Many patients reported improvement in at least one disease symptom.

20.42 Impressive Results with Adenocarcinoma

Subsequent studies help explain who was benefiting from the drug. Non-smokers with BAC or adenocarcinoma had significant responses, in many cases over 35%. This group was tested and found to have had genetic damage in the tyrosine kinase portion of the EGFR. Iressa is a tyrosine kinase inhibitor. Harvard Genetics Lab performs testing to identify the tyrosine kinase mutations which predict response to Iressa. (See 15.7. Harvard Laboratories Gene Test). Since Iressa targets a specific cellular component rather than dividing cells, its side effects are substantially less than chemotherapy drugs. Beyond the non-smokers with adenocarcinoma, studies found Japanese citizens and women had better responses. Yet while the results seem impressive, studies have not clearly documented a substantial decrease in mortality. Today, Tarceva, a stronger EGFR inhibitor is being tested.

20.43 Squamous Cell Smokers

If the Iressa studies were promising for non-smokers with adenocarcinoma, they were unimpressive for other subgroups. Squamous cell patients had response rates less than 6%, and little improvement in survival. It appears Iressa can provide only a modest period of disease stabilization and symptom improvement. Since some of the early studies grouped various types together, it is difficult to see whether Iressa benefited everyone to some extent, or whether the perceived benefits were attributable to dramatic results in certain subgroups. Whether Tarceva can substantially benefit this group is being tested.

20.44 EGFR Alternatives

Iressa seems to work well on a small subgroup of patients with tyrosine kinase damage which can be address with Iressa, or perhaps Tarceva, other tyrosine kinase inhibitor. For those without this disease presentation, alternatives deserve consideration. While Iressa works on the tyrosine kinase portion of EGFR, other EGFR drugs attempt to prevent EGFR binding, a somewhat different mode of action. Drugs like Erbitux need to be tested on squamous cell smokers whose disease presentation does not seem to fit the mode of action of Iressa. If abnormal EGFR binding is an important part of this subgroup's lung cancer, the drug may be more effective than Iressa.

Herceptin has been used with breast cancer and attacked Erb2, part of the Erb family of receptors. The precise significance of ERb 2 and its relationship to EGFR remain unclear. Patients may want to consider major research facilities and monitor research online through Medline (see chapter 42) and check presentations at annual presentations of the American Society of Clinical Oncology (ASCO).

20.5 ANTI-ANGIOGENIC THERAPY

For the small group adenocarcinoma patients who are nonsmokers or former light smokers, EGFR drugs Tarceva and Iressa hold promise. These patients tumors appear to be driven at least in part by a malfunctioning EGFR tyrosine kinase which can be identified in a recent EGFR test. (See 15.7. Harvard Laboratories Gene Test). For the large group of smokers with lung cancer, it has not been shown that tyrosine kinase damage at the EGFR is a large part of their cancer. Iressa and Tarceva may provide modest benefit, though even that remains unclear particularly with Iressa.

Anti-angiogenic drugs like Avastin are showing promise. Cox-2 inhibitors like Celebrex are being evaluated. Finally, tissue testing is being evaluated, with the cells from removed tissue tested to see which drugs are likely to provide a response. While the method holds promise, it has not yet been refined to provide sufficient reliability to obtain mainstream approval.

20.6 SITES OF METASTASIS FOR LUNG CANCER

20.61 The Variability of Metastatic Behavior in Lung Cancer

Exactly where and when a tumor will metastasize is difficult to determine:

"It has been known that the biological behavior of NSCLC is heterogeneous; for example, distant metastasises occur early in most patients, but late in others, and there are also significant differences in responsiveness to irradiation or chemotherapy, even in patients with the same histological type." Fu, (5).

The frequent sites for distant metastasises were the bone, brain, liver and adrenal glands. Hanigiri, (6).

20.62 Brain

Approximately 10% of non-small cell patients will have some type of brain metastasis at time of presentation and by time of death, some 30% of patients will display some evidence of cranial metastasis. Pass (6) at 1011, (Quantin, (7), Rodriqus(8). Family members need to be alert to significant changes in personality or functioning. Single metastasises account for 30-50% of metastases. Pass (6) at 1011.

Radiation is the primary treatment though surgery may also be utilized. Some have advocated stereotactic radiosurgery, the use of computerized techniques to identify targets and focus large single doses of radiation on specific areas, while attempting to minimize exposure to adjoining tissues. Chemotherapy is used to generally combat metastatic cancer, while radiation and surgery are directed to specific areas.

20.63 Bone

A study found that 13% of non-small cell patients had bone metastasis. Hanigiri, (7). Bone scanning is a sensitive examination to detect bone metastases. A standard x-ray is also possible but,

"Fifty per cent of bone material content must be lost before changes are apparent on plain radiographs . . . . [Thus] plain radiograph is an insensitive method of investigating localized bone pain. Radiopharmaceutical bone scans are, in contrast, highly sensitive though non-specific. Bone scanning is thus only indicated in those patients who have bone pain, elevated alkaline phosphatase levels, or recent exacerbation of bone pain . . . MRI may be useful to assess localized areas of persistent bone pain which appear normal on bone scan and plain radiographs." Carney (10) at 65-66.

20.7 PSYCHOLOGICAL ISSUES AND THE PHYSICIAN

20.71 Performance Status as the Best Indicator of Survival

While stage and extent of metastasis are important, performance status continues to be the critical factor in determining the patient's status. Performance status is a medical term which evaluates a patient's mobility and status. An ambulatory patient conducting his usual activities has a high performance status, a bed-ridden fatigued patient would have a low performance status.

> "Three studies that have included large numbers of patients with cancer at all stages found that functional or performance status was the accurate predictor of survival. Decline in activities of daily living including bathing, continence, dressing and transfer, were very strongly associated with decreased survival." (Devita 6). and enjoying some reasonable quality of life in the process.

Contrariwise, an ability to perform most of the activities of life generally shows no immediate danger.

20.72 Selection of a physician

Results vary for stage 4 patients. While many will pass away within a year, some will survive longer. The diversity of this group with different areas of metastases, subtypes, age, and performance status makes prediction difficult. Many patients and their families will want to be fighters, searching for the best treatment, and maintaining a positive approach in the face of adversity. Support groups encourage this group providing inspiring stories of patients surviving 2, 3 and even 5 years after diagnosis,

Not every physician will have this approach. Some doctors worry that if they predict or suggest success, they will be blamed for failure, the patient reasoning that the doctor's lack of skill or knowledge was the cause. Others believe the patient is owed a stark candor. For various reasons, many some doctors will present a pessimistic approach. It is therefore important to carefully select a physician and, if need be, make a change. Family members may have to push some doctors to be aggressive. Advanced age may periodically play a role, and older patients and family may need to search for an aggressive physician if they believe that is the best course.

So beware of the negativity which may be present in some circumstances. Where a particular drug does not appear to be working, the aggressive patient will ask to have its impact evaluated and be willing to test another drug regimen. He may not accept side effects as the result of the disease, but consider changes, since many drugs have roughly equivalent efficacy.

REFERENCES

1. Wu, *Post-operative staging and survival based on the revised TNM staging system for non-small cell lung cancer*, Zhonghua Zhong Liu Za Zhi 1999 Sep;21(5):363-5.

2. Naruke, *Implications of staging in lung cancer*, Chest 1997 Oct;112(4 Suppl):242S-248S.

3. Devita, *Principles and Practice of Oncolology* (6th Ed. 2001).

4. Bianco, *Gemcitabine as single agent chemotherapy in elderly patients with stages III-IV non-small cell lung cancer (NSCLC): a phase II study*. Anticancer Res 2002 Sep-Oct;22(5):3053-6.

5. Guarino, *A dose-escalation study of weekly topotecan, cisplatin, and gemcitabine front-line therapy in patients with inoperable non-small cell lung cancer*, Oncologist 2002;7(6):509-15.

6. Devita, Cancer *Principles and Practice of Oncology 3078* (Lippincott 2001).

CHAPTER 21

SMALL CELL LUNG CANCER

21.0 OVERVIEW

Small cell is a quick-moving cancer, rapidly spreading to lymph nodes and other organs. Characterized by rapid cell division, SCLC long-term survival can be low because many patients have widespread disease at the time of diagnosis. "The biologic nature of small cell lung cancer causes dissemination to regional lymph nodes and/or distant metastatic sites in {most} patients at the time of initial presentation." NCI (1). This is particularly true in the U.S. where no program of screening or early detection of lung cancer exists. Metastases can be in the bone, liver, brain, or pleura.

Chemotherapy is the standard treatment for small cell lung cancer. In more than half of the cases, small cell initially responds well to chemotherapy which reduces the tumor by half or completely eliminates any evidence of tumor on x-ray. Sadly, the tumors frequently return, and the phenomenon of multi-drug resistance (MDR) means the tumor system develops ways to resist the chemotherapy.

Radiation may be used to target specific areas of the tumor in the lung or areas of metastasises. Surgery remains controversial, and is used more frequently outside the United States. Some studies indicate a favorable prognosis for surgically treated patients with limited disease at the time of diagnosis. New forms of gene therapy have shown good results on non-small cell patients and are being evaluated with small cell.

21.1 SMALL CELL STAGING

21.11 The Limited Extensive Demarcation

Exactly how small cell should be staged is somewhat controversial, with differing approaches to staging indicating different approaches to treatment. Recall that non-small cell cancer is divided into four stages (seven, if we count 1 A and 1 B, 2A . . .) based on the involvement of lymph nodes and other organs.

In contrast, most United States physicians divide small cell into but two categories: limited and extensive. Our National Cancer Institute explains,

"Because occult or overt metastatic disease is present at diagnosis in most patients, survival is usually not affected by small differences in the amount of locoregional tumor involvement. Therefore, the detailed TNM staging system developed for lung cancer by the American Joint Committee on Cancer (AJCC) is not commonly employed in patients with small cell carcinoma. A simple 2-stage system developed by the Veterans Administration Lung Cancer Study Group is more commonly used for staging small cell lung cancer patients." NCI (1).

Non small cell is divided into stages because the determination of whether to perform surgery depends upon stage. If surgery is not generally recommended for small cell patients, a four stage demarcation is unnecessary.

21.12 Countries Utilizing A Four Stage Categorization for Small Cell

In contrast, Japan employs the four step staging of non-small cell cancer to small cell and surgery is a more frequent option in Japan. Japan has an extensive system of screening for lung cancer which means that more early tumors are more frequently seen, allowing for surgery. Indeed, some physicians have admired and written about the Japanese approach. Sandler (12). Given the difficult prognosis of small cell patients, the use of surgery must be considered. One can argue the two step staging system contains an implicit bias against surgery, since surgical decisions need to utilize accurate information about tumor status that the simplified two stage analysis may not always provide.

21.13 How is Stage Determined?

The basic aim of staging procedures is to determine and measure the extent of metastasises to lymph nodes and other organs. Staging procedures commonly used to document distant metastasises include bone marrow examination, computed topographic or magnetic resonance imaging scans of the brain, computerized topographic scans of the chest and the abdomen, and radio nuclide bone scans.

21.14 Limited Stage

Limited stage small cell lung cancer means tumor confined to the hemothorax, mediastinum, and supraclavicular nodes, and which can be encompassed within a radiation therapy port. There is no universally accepted definition of the term limited stage, and patients with pleural effusion, large tumors, and positive contralateral supraclavicular nodes have been both included within and excluded from limited stage categorization.

21.15 Extensive Stage

Extensive stage small cell lung cancer means tumor that is too widespread to be included within the definition of limited stage disease above. Patients with distant metastasises (M1) are always considered to have extensive stage disease. [1,2].

21.16 Cellular Classification

The current classification of subtypes of small cell lung cancer are:

1. small cell carcinoma,
2. mixed small cell/large cell carcinoma, and
3. combined small cell carcinoma (small cell lung cancer combined with neoplastic squamous and/or glandular components).

Since the treatment of small cell is different from non-small cell, identifying the correct type is important and generally done through pathology, examination of tissue.

21.2 CHEMOTHERAPY AS THE PRIMARY FORM OF TREATMENT

In the United States, chemotherapy is the primary form of treatment for small cell lung cancer. Initial results are usually promising but the cancer frequently returns.

> "(Chemotherapy) regimens will result in response rates of 85-95% in limited disease and 65-85% in extensive disease patients. Complete responses, prerequisite for potential cure, can be achieved in about 50% limited disease patients and in about a quarter of extensive disease patients. Depending on the addition of radiotherapy, in limited disease patients about a third will have disease-free survival in excess of 2 years." Carney (1) at 157. Simon (14).

21.21 Recurrence and Drug Resistance

While the initial success of chemotherapy for small cell cancer is indeed promising, the propensity for recurrence and difficulties combating that are troubling. "Chemotherapy is the main treatment modality for small cell lung cancer. The disease is highly chemoresponsive and around 50% of patients receive complete response. In the great majority of these, however, the disease recurs within a few months and is progressively chemoresistant." "A primary cause of treatment failure in SCLC (Small Cell Lung Cancer) is the emergence of drug-resistant cell clones during chemotherapy." Carney, (1) at 158.

21.22 Second-Line Chemotherapy

Second-line chemotherapy (after the initial administration has failed) has been debated. A proponent explains,

> "Numerous clinical trials demonstrate that some patients benefit from treatment, achieving prolonged survival, symptom

palliation, improved quality of life, and the opportunity, albeit rare, for durable remission. Additionally, several novel chemotherapeutics are available that alone or in combination help patients lead an improved quality of life. Finally, alternative routes and schedules—oral formulations, weekly administration, and prolonged treatment vacations—have been developed to deliver chemotherapy to patients with poor performance status or multiple comorbidities." Eckhardt (12).

21.3 TREATMENT FOR LIMITED STAGE SMALL CELL LUNG CANCER

21.31 Surgery and the Stage 1 or Limited Stage Patient

Even if we assume that at least 90% of small cell patients have advanced disease, that leaves a critical 10% with timely diagnosed tumors confined to part of a single lung. That subgroup has a excellent prognosis perhaps almost equivalent to stage 1 *non-small cell* patients. One text states,

"Shields analysis of patients with small cell carcinomas in the VASOG trials also demonstrated the importance of TNM (tumor, node, metastasis) staging for tumors of this cell type. Sixty percent of patients with T1, No, Mo tumors were alive at 5 years, whereas there were almost no 5-year survivors among the patients who presented either with T2-3 tumors or with mediastinal lymph node involvement. Patients with T1 tumors with only hilar or bronchopulmonary nodes involved had an intermediate survival of approximately 30%. In fact, these survival results are similar to those of patients who have undergone complete surgical resection for non-small cell lung cancer of equivalent stage." Aisner (11).

21.32 Impressive Japanese Results with Surgery and Stage 1 and 2 Small Cell Patients

A Japanese study found good results with surgery for small cell patients. "The 4 year survival rate of the patients in stage I was 50%, and that of those in stage II and IIIA was 50% and 37.5%." The authors boldly conclude, "Surgical resection for limited SCLC should be recommended in patients with stage I, II and T3NoMo or T3N1Mo disease." Ohkubo, (5).

Aisner concludes, "Although there was general acceptance by the 1970's that surgical resection was inappropriate for the majority of patients with small cell lung cancer, the observations of Shields and his colleagues suggested that there might be a subpopulation of patients with small cell cancers for whom a surgical approach could be considered." Id. at 441. The notion that small cell treatment is comparable to non-small cell treatment would be rejected by most American physicians and investigators. However, at least at early stage 1, there are significant similarities and the same favorable prognosis. In many areas surgery is not performed upon small cell patients, even in earlier stages. The small cell patient will want to carefully review his options and review his options. If surgery is a realistic option, this highlights the need for early detection. As I discuss later in the book, neither the American Cancer Society nor the National Cancer Institute recommend screening as a means to assure timely diagnosis and improved long term survival.

Thus, even if we consider surgery, there are certain limitations. Patients with poor performance status, limited breathing capacity or other health problems may not be candidates for surgery.

21.33 Chemotherapy and Radiation for Limited Stage Patients

A combination of chemotherapy and radiation is standard treatment for even limited stage patients in the United States. Radiation is used to reduce the size of the tumor while chemotherapy is designed to address the areas of metastasis as well as the tumor itself.

"It is useful to identify patients with limited-stage disease as several randomized controlled trials employing combined modality therapy (chemotherapy and thoracic irradiation) in this group have demonstrated survival advantage over treatment with chemotherapy alone." Richardson & in Carney (3), at 114. NCI states,

> "In patients with small cell lung cancer, combination chemotherapy produces results that are clearly superior to single-agent treatment, and moderately intensive doses of drugs

are superior to doses that produce only minimal or mild hematologic toxicity. Current programs yield overall objective response rates of 65%-90% and complete response rates of 45%-75%. Because of the frequent presence of occult metastatic disease, chemotherapy is the cornerstone of treatment of limited stage small cell lung cancer. Combinations containing two or more drugs are needed for maximal effect."

"Mature results of prospective randomized trials suggest that combined modality therapy produces a modest but significant improvement in survival compared with chemotherapy alone. Two meta-analyses showed an improvement in 3-year survival rates of about 5% for those receiving chemotherapy and radiation therapy compared to those receiving chemotherapy alone. Most of the benefit occurred in patients less than 65 years of age. Combined modality treatment is associated with increased morbidity and, in some trials, increased treatment-related mortality from pulmonary and hematologic toxic effects; proper administration requires close collaboration between medical and radiation oncologist." NCI (1). Another study combining radiation with two chemotherapy drugs showed 5 year survival rates of at least 15% of limited stage patients. (12)

21.34 Particular Chemotherapy Drugs Used

As with non-small cell, defining combinations of drugs, maximum doses, and other variables is a continuing process with sometimes conflicting results. "Clinical trials have failed to show superiority of one chemotherapeutic regimen over another." Reddy (4). Cisplatin/etopiside is a frequently used combination, though physicians continue to examine Carboplatin instead of Cisplatin because of its lesser tendency towards nausea. Cyclophosphamide, Iritocecan and Ifosfamide are also used, and physicians are now looking at Taxol and other drugs used for non-small cell tumors.

21.35 Chemotherapy and Radiation

Many believe combining chemotherapy with radiation improves results:

"Combined modality therapy appears to result in improved complete response rates, but with increased toxicity. There is a benefit associated with the addition of radiation therapy to multiagent chemotherapy, compared with chemotherapy alone. Recent Intergroup data published in the *New England Journal of Medicine* reported improved overall survival with the use of concurrent twice-daily fractionated radiotherapy and cisplatin/etopiside. Patients with limited-stage SCLC (N = 417) were randomized to once-daily (45 Gy/25 fractions/5 weeks) or twice-daily (45 Gy/30 fractions/3 weeks) radiotherapy given concurrently with cycle 1 of cisplatin/etopiside. The median survival for all patients was 20 months, with a 40% 2-year survival rate. Overall survival was significantly better in the twice-daily arm compared with the standard fractionation arm (26% vs 16%, respectively). An increase in transient grade-3 esophagitis was seen in the twice-daily arm." Reddy, (4) at 1.

21.36 Gene Therapies

Most of the clinical trials with gene therapies have dealt with non-small cell lung cancer. However, many of the same rationales for treatment apply to small cell, and we can expect gene therapies like Iressa to be tested on small cell patients, alone and in conjunction with chemotherapy and radiation.

21.4 EXTENSIVE STAGE SMALL CELL LUNG CANCER

NCI states, (1) "As in limited stage small cell carcinoma, chemotherapy should be given as multiple agents in doses associated with at least moderate toxicity in order to produce the best results in extensive stage disease. Doses and schedules used in current programs yield overall response rates of 70%-85% and complete response rates of 20%-30% in extensive stage disease." Since overt disseminated disease is present, combination chemotherapy is the cornerstone of treatment of this stage of small cell lung cancer. Combinations containing two or more drugs are needed for maximal benefit.

The relative effectiveness of many 2- to 4- drug combination programs appears similar, and there are a large number of potential combinations. Optimal duration of chemotherapy is not clearly defined, but there is no obvious improvement in survival when the duration of drug administration exceeds 6 months.

Combination chemotherapy plus chest irradiation does not appear to improve survival compared with chemotherapy alone in extensive stage small cell lung cancer. However, radiation therapy plays an extremely important role in palliation of symptoms of the primary tumor and of metastatic disease, particularly brain, epidural, and bone metastasises . . .

Patients with small cell lung cancer treated with chemotherapy with or without chest irradiation who have achieved a complete remission can be considered for administration of prophylactic cranial irradiation (PCI). Patients whose cancer can be controlled outside the brain have a 60% actuarial risk of developing central nervous system metastasises within 2-3 years after starting treatment.

Retrospective studies have shown that long-term survivors of small cell lung cancer (>2 years from the start of treatment) have a high incidence of central nervous system impairment. However, prospective studies have shown that patients treated with PCI do not have detectably different neuropsychological function than patients not treated. Therefore, additional neuropsychologic testing of patients beyond 2 years from the start of treatment will be needed before concluding that PCI does not contribute to the decline in intellectual function.

Many more patients with extensive stage small cell carcinoma have greatly impaired performance status at the time of diagnosis when compared to patients with limited stage disease. Such patients have a poor prognosis and tolerate aggressive chemotherapy or combined modality therapy poorly. Single-agent intravenous, oral, and low-dose bi-weekly regimens have been developed for these patients. However, prospective randomized studies have shown that patients with a poor prognosis who are treated with conventional regimens live longer than those treated with the single-agent or low-dose regimens.

Chemotherapy drugs include Etopiside, Cisplatin or Carboplatin, Doxorubicin and Vincristine, with a number of combinations used for SCLC.

21.41 The Controversy Over Prophylactic Cranial Radiation

One of the sad sequalae of small cell cancer are metastasises to the head. Given their frequency, would it make sense to irradiate the patient before the tumor metastasises are seen on x-ray. Radiation may stem a metastasises while arguably causing only limited discomfort to the patient. At least this is what some scientists have suggested, with prophylactic cranial radiation an important and controversial topic in current treatment of small cell lung cancer. Many patients and their families would reject the notion of applying a potentially toxic substance to the brain where disease was not even identified in that area. Here is a discussion of PCI from the New England Journal of Medicine:

> "A major cause of morbidity and mortality in patients with small-cell lung cancer is brain metastasis, which in most patients results in multiple tumors. At the time of initial diagnosis, brain metastasises can be detected in up to 10 percent of patients, and 1 to 2 percent of these patients have metastasises only in the brain. However, among patients who complete chemotherapy, an additional 30 to 70 percent subsequently have clinically apparent brain metastasises, and even more have such metastasises at autopsy . . ."
>
> "For many years, prophylactic cranial irradiation has been used in patients with small-cell lung cancer in the belief that the treatment of microscopic or subclinical metastasises would prevent or delay the onset of symptomatic brain metastasises, but its efficacy for this purpose has been uncertain. Those who advocate prophylactic cranial irradiation point out that it is a safe way to reduce the overall incidence of brain metastasises, even if only a small number of patients benefit . . . . Others argue against routine prophylactic cranial irradiation. They point out that the brain is rarely the sole site of recurrence, that radiation can be neurotoxic, and that radiation therapy does not prolong survival. In this issue of the Journal, Auperin et al. report the results of a detailed meta-analysis of the efficacy of prophylactic cranial irradiation in 987 patients (847 patients with limited disease and 140 patients with extensive disease) who took part in seven trials and who had complete remission with chemotherapy, with or without thoracic irradiation. Prophylactic cranial irradiation was associated with an absolute decrease of 25.3 percent in the cumulative incidence of brain metastasis at three years, from 58.6 percent in the control group to 33.3 percent in the treatment group. More important,

prophylactic cranial irradiation was also associated with an absolute increase in overall survival of 5.4 percent at three years, from 15.3 percent in the control group to 20.7 percent in the treatment group. Prophylactic cranial irradiation was beneficial in patients with either limited or extensive disease . . . ."

"We still do not know how best to integrate prophylactic cranial irradiation with chemotherapy in patients with small-cell lung cancer. The optimal dose of radiation, volume of tissue to be irradiated, and duration and timing of prophylactic cranial irradiation have not been determined. Also, questions remain regarding the safety and long-term neuropsychological consequences of prophylactic cranial irradiation. The study found a significant survival benefit, but it should be noted that four of the trials included in the meta-analysis had fewer than 100 patients, which suggests that there may have been some selection bias."

There are ongoing studies and we cannot expect this question to be quickly or conclusively resolved.

21.5 SMALL CELL LUNG CANCER AND GENE THERAPY

21.51 Overview

Scientists have also looked to gene therapy for both patients with limited and extensive disease. Given the apparent success of drugs like Iressa in prolonging the lives of non-small patients with even metastatic disease, scientists are looking for comparable treatments for the small cell patient. "Recent clinical trials of gene therapy for patients with thoracic cancers have shown that these treatments were well tolerated with minimal side effects and that we need to further enhance specificity as well as efficiency of gene transfer to target cancer cells." (9). Gene therapy is a broad category encompassing drugs which seeks to frustrate the cancer process in many different ways.

While some laboratory studies have documented favorable response on cells, there have been few clinical trials showing favorable results for small cell, though this may have changed at the time of publication.

21.52 The Role of P-53

One method is to restore the body's natural tumor suppressor genes which may have been damaged during the carcinogenic process. One of the most important tumor-suppressor genes is P-53, the subject of a separate chapter.

"The protein is recognized as an important cell regulatory element that arrests the growth of cells containing damaged DNA. A reversible arrest in the G1 phase of the cell cycle allows DNA repair before DNA synthesis. When optimal repair is impossible, p53 expression may trigger apoptosis, an irreversible process culminating in cell death. Thus, loss of wild type p53 function may result in relative resistance to treatment as a consequence of abrogation of p53-dependent apoptosis . . . ."

"Reports show the frequency of p53 mutations in SCLC cell lines and tumors (about 70-100% in different series). The alterations in the p53 gene are common and perhaps critical events in lung carcinogenesis, but probably they are not the first, although these alterations are essential for the maintenance of malignant phenotypes in the progression of SCLC on the relationship between p53 status and clinical outcome. The available data in the literature results are controversial. Iggo et al.performed immunohistochemical p53 study and p53 gene secuentiation in 47 lung tumors, and found p53 altered expression in all SCLC: nine samples. In all of these cases it was correlated with missense mutations in p53 gene (G toT transversions). Finally they suggest that the presence of p53 mutations in SCLC implies a poor prognosis while D'Amico analyzed p53 mutations in 16 cell lines and in 20 tumors, and found p53 gene abnormalities in 100% cell lines and in 80% tumors, but they did not find correlation between location or type of mutations and clinical characteristics, stage, response to therapy or survival." Salas (7).

21.53 2 Herpes Simplex Viral Treatment

A Japanese group is investigating treatments designed to attack the myc oncogene implicated in small cell cancer:

"We previously reported that myc-overexpressing SCLC cell lines became selectively sensitive to ganciclovir (GCV) by transducing the herpes simplex virus thymidine kinase (HSV-TK) gene under the control of the Myc-Max response elements (a core nucleotide sequence, CACGTG) and that this construct (MycTK) could be utilized to develop a novel treatment against chemo-radio-resistant SCLC . . ."

"In vitro infection with AdMycTK selectively rendered myc-overexpressing SCLC cell lines 63- to 307-fold more sensitive to GCV. In vivo injections with AdMycTK followed by GCV administration markedly suppressed the growth of myc-overexpressing tumors established in the subcutis or in the peritoneal cavity of athymic mice. On the other hand, infection with AdMycTK did not significantly affect either in vitro GCV sensitivity of the cells expressing very low levels of the myc genes or the growth of their subcutaneous tumors. Moreover, we observed no apparent side effects of this treatment including body weight loss or biochemical abnormalities in contrast to the treatment with AdCATK that conferred strong but nonspecific expression of the HSV-TK gene. These results suggested that AdMycTK/ GCV therapy is effective on SCLC patients whose tumors overexpress myc family oncogenes." Nusino (9).

Results have been mixed. Another researcher states,

"Replication-incompetent adenoviruses (Ad) carrying the herpes simplex thymidine kinase (HSVtk) gene have been used in a number of human cancer gene therapy trials, however transduction has generally been limited to a small minority of tumor cells . . . . Our results indicate that addition of HSVtk to a replicating Ad virus will not likely be useful in augmenting antitumor effects." (10).

21.6 ADDRESSING MULTI-DRUG RESISTANCE

The development of MDR frustrating chemotherapy and allowing the cancer to grow is the primary problem with SCLC. We have the recurrent theme of normal functions corrupted with cancer. "Many enzymes (names omitted) are involved in DNA repair. An efficient DNA repair mechanism may thus be responsible for cytotoxic drug resistance. Reduced DNA damage and increased DNA repair in cisplatin, . . . resistant cell lines have been reported." Gupta (15). Sadly, the body's own repair mechanisms help rebuild DNA damaged in cancer cells, frustrating chemotherapy.

21.61 P-glycoprotein

21.611 Its Function in Normal Tissue

P-glycoprotein (p-gp) is one of the major causes of MDR. P-gp is encoded by the MDR1 gene and belongs to the ATP binding family. Other members of this family are associated with MDR. In normal tissue, P-gp helps regulate cell differentiation, apoptosis, and cell reproduction. It is found in liver bile ducts, the kidney, and the colon and appears to also detoxify certain organs. Lavie (17). Tumors arising from cells that have high expression of P-gp are generally resistant to chemotherapy. Lavie (17).

21.62 Verapanil

This is a calcium-channel blocker, and was used to treat hypertension. The drug also inhibits P-gp as well as other mediators of MDR. Some call it a chemo-sensitizer, since it is designed to make cells more receptive to chemotherapy. Its effectiveness remains debatable.

> "Drugs such as verapamil, diltiazem and quinidine have been found to overcome multidrug resistance in cell culture and in some animal experiments. For example, verapamil has been used to reverse adriamycin resistance in human ovarian cancer cells. Verapamil has been used clinically in an attempt to reverse multidrug resistance (though) a Phase I-II study failed to demonstrate a potentiation of doxorubicin therapy with verapamil in eight drug-resistant ovarian cancer patients." Principles (17).

However, a 1990 clinical trial found a 34% partial response rate from a combination of verapamil and tamoxifen for SCLC, though the lack of clear controls in this phase I study make it difficult to interpret. (18). "First generation MDR drugs were not specifically developed for inhibiting MDR. They often had other pharmacological activities, as well as a relatively low affinity for MDR transporters." (18).

MDR represents a failure of apoptosis (gene death). P-53 helps arrange gene repair and apoptosis, and clinical trials are investigating the insertion of P-53 genes.

REFERENCES

1. NCI.net. The NCI publishes its analysis and recommended protocols from which these excerpts have been taken. Since the NCI frequently revises its materials and excerpts have been taken from the Internet, precise quotations may be missing or changed in the latest version.

2. Twentyman, *Mechanism of Drug Resistance in Lung Cancer Cells*, in Carney, Lung Cancer (Arnold Publ. Co. 1995).

3. Carney *Chemotherapy of Small Cell Lung Cancer*, 157, in, Lung Cancer (Arnold Publ Co. 1995).

4. Reddy, *Small Cell Lung Cancer: Improving Outcomes,*Presentation, American Society for Therapeutic Radiology and Oncology 42nd Annual Meeting, excerpted on medscape.

5. Ohkubo, (4) *Surgical Analysis for Small Cell Lung Cancer of the Lung*, Kyobu Geka 1999 Dec; 52 (13) 1061-6.

7. Salas, *Correlation of p53 oncoprotein expression with chemotherapy response in small cell lung cancer*, Lung Cancer, Vol. 34 (1) (2001) pp. 67-74.

8. Carney, *Prophylactic Cranial Irradiation and Small-Cell Lung Cancer*, The New England Journal of Medicine Vol. 341, No. 7 (August 12, 1999).

9. Nushino, *Adenovirus-mediated gene therapy specific for small cell lung cancer cells using a Myc-Max binding motif,*. Int J Cancer 2001 Mar 15;91(6):851-6.

10. Lambright, *Inclusion of the herpes simplex thymidine kinase gene in a replicating adenovirus does not augment antitumor efficacy*, Gene Ther 2001 Jun;8(12):946-53.

11. Aisner, et. al., *Comprehensive Textbook of Thoracic Oncology* 441 (Williams & Wilkins 1996).

12. Eckhardt, *Second-line treatment of small-cell lung cancer. The case for systemic chemotherapy.*Oncology (Huntingt) 2003 Feb;17(2):181-8, 191; discussion 191-2.
13. Sandler, *Extending Survival in SCLC with Irinotecan: Building on the Japanese Experience,* http://www.medscape.com/viewarticle/429347_7.
14. Simon, *Small Cell Lung Cancer, Chest.* 2003;123:259S-271S.
15. Gupta, *Multi Drug Resistance in Human Lung Cancer and its Pharmacological Reversal, www.indianchestsociety.org/journal/apr-june/ra_multi_drug.htm.*
16. Lavie, *Cancer Multidrug Resistance: A Review of Recent Drug Discovery Research,* Idrugs 2002 5(4) www.weizmann.ac.il/home/lhliscov/IDrugs_2002.pdf.
17. *Principles of Clinical Cancer Chemotherapy and Drug Resistance,* http://ocw.mit.edu . . .
18. *Addition of verapamil and tamoxifen to the initial chemotherapy of small cell lung cancer. A phase I/II study,* Cancer. 1990 May 1;65(9):1895-902, Cancer. 1990 May 1;65(9):1895-902.

CHAPTER 22

TREATING METASTASES

22.1 ORGANIZATION

In the foregoing chapters, we discussed treatment by stage or type. We learned that different forms of chemotherapy were prescribed depending on type. Beyond chemotherapy, there are some specific issues and treatments with certain areas of metastases. Frequently, the treatments will be the same or similar even if the tumor type can vary. Therefore, this chapter is divided by organ.

22.2 METASTASIS TO BONE

Bone is an unfortunately common source for metastasis. "Bone metastases occur in 20% to 40% of patients with lung cancer." Pass (3) at 1012. While the most common presentation for lung cancer is progressive chest pain and discomfort, for some, the first symptom may be bone difficulty. A patient may be first diagnosed with lung cancer following a fall.

22.21 Where are the Metastases Located

Lung cancer metastasis most commonly affects the spine, ribs, pelvis, and proximal long bones. A unique feature of this lesion is its ability to spread to the bones of the hands and feet. Half of all mets to the hand bones are from lung, as well as 15% of lesions in the feet. This is thought to be due to the ability of a tumor in the lung to shed malignant cells directly into the arterial blood flow, from where they can be seeded far and wide. Other tumors shed cells into the veins, from which they go first to the lung or liver, which may act as filters and trap metastatic cells.

Lung cancer metastases normally appear purely lytic, with poor margination, no matrix and cortical destruction. Bone Tumor.org (1). Brain metastasises are an unfortunate but somewhat common consequence of advanced non-small cell (and small cell) lung cancer. There is much misinformation on the Internet about the effectiveness of various treatments. Generally, effectiveness can only be measured by assessing clinical trial results.

22.22 Diagnostic Tools

X-ray, MRI, Ct Scan, Petscan, and bone scan are diagnostic tools to detect bone metastasis. X-rays are the least sensitive tool, but the least costly and easiest to give. One writer estimates that "80% of patients (with metastases) will show abnormalities on plain spinal radiography." Pass (3).

22.23 Speed to Diagnosis and Treatment

Pass' treatise recommends prompt diagnosis and treatment:

"The evaluation of the patient with SCC (spinal cord compression) must be speedy and decisive. Delay may allow the development of irreversible neurologic deficit." Pass (3), at 1014.

Treatment can incorporate a number of different approaches:

"Currently, the treatment of bone pain remains palliative . . . with systemic therapy (analgesics, hormones, chemotherapy, steroids, and bisphosphonates) as well as local treatments (such as surgery, nerve blocks, and external beam radiation)."

"Ninety percent of patients with symptomatic bone

metastases obtain some pain relief with a low-dose, brief course of palliative radiation therapy." Kvale (6).

22.24 Steroids

Steroids can reduce pain and limit neurologic progression prior to definitive therapy. The presumed mechanism is reduction of edema (swelling)." Pass (3).

22.25 Surgical Treatment—Vertebroplasty

Some advocate vertebroplasty, a procedure to decrease pain by injecting cement in the tumor area on the bone:

> "Percutaneous vertebroplasty (PV) is an interventional radiological procedure for the treatment of pain in patients with vertebral compressions caused by osteoporosis, metastases or hemangioma . . . . It consists of percutaneous injection of bone cement (polymethylmethacrylate) into the vertebral body under fluoroscopy guidance. PV has proved to be effective and safe . . . . The complication rate is low, less than 3% for patients with osteoporosis and up to 10% in patients with metastases. We report on the first 17 patients (11 with osteoporosis, 3 with metastases and 3 with hemangiomas) treated in Sweden at the Department of Interventional Neuroradiology, Sahlgrenska Hospital, Goteborg University. We obtained complete pain relief in 71% and partial pain relief in 17% of cases. The majority of the patients improved in mobility and quality of life."

See also, Hierholzer, (4) ("Percutaneous vertebroplasty proved to be a highly effective, minimal invasive interventional procedure to treat severely painful bone lesions of benign and malignant origin.").

These were foreign studies. Certainly one should not minimize the risks of delicate spinal surgery, in a patient with compromised pulmonary reserve. The studies did not deal with and therefore did not discuss any special problems associated with lung cancer patients with bone metastases. Nonetheless, where a patient has significant pain, given the difficult prognosis for stage 4 patients today, this type of surgical procedure will be considered by some. A U.S. study also advocated the procedure but not some risks:

> "Based on experience, published data, and published series, the authors recommend the use of vertebroplasty for painful destructive vertebral lesions. In the authors' opinion, the greatest difficulty lies in denying the treatment to patients with advanced metastatic disease, where other surgical or medical treatments may have greater morbidity and mortality. The few complications reported have been related to excessive PMMA injection, underlining the need for excellent imaging conditions to control the cement injection."

22.26 Bisphosponate Drugs Zomata

Zomata is used to stabilize the area, prevent fractures, and maintain the patient's mobility and quality of life.

22.3 CRANIAL AND BRAIN METASTASES

22.31 Stereotactic Radiosurgery.

Chemotherapy designed to address all metastasises and radiation directed to particular areas of metastasises are standard treatment. Some doctors are investigating stereotactic radiosurgery. It appears to remain experimental though some physicians report improved results.

22.32 Decadron

One site discusses a patient's experience with Decadron, a treatment for brain metastasises. While the drug initially worked surprisingly well, a family member noticed a change and new assertiveness in the patient's personality which was gradually eliminated with a change in dose. Fetto (2). For many patients, going to support groups and speaking with others experiencing similar side effects can be very helpful. While one should certainly speak with the oncologist, in a managed care world, there may be limited time for sympathy, empathy, or extensive discussion.

REFERENCES

1. Bonetumor.org.
2. Rodriquez, *Percutaneous vertebroplastyBa new method for alleviation of back pain,* Lakartidningen 2002 Feb 28;99(9): 882-90.
3. Pass, *Lung Cancer: Principles and Practice* (Lippincott, 2000).
4. Serafini, *Therapy of metastatic bone pain,* Nucl Med 2001 Jun;42(6):895-906.
5. Fetto, *The Drug, A Steroid's Tale,* 5 www.cancerlynx.com/ decadron.html.
6. Kvale, *Palliative Care, Chest.* 2003;123:284S-311S.

CHAPTER 23

LONG AND SHORT-TERM SURVIVAL

23.0 SURVIVAL AND THE SIGNIFICANCE OF METASTASIS

Cancer overall is a serious disease, with lung cancer particularly serious. Why? First, the existence of cancer in the lung itself is usually not a cause of death. Instead, it is the tendency of cancer to metastasize, going through lymph nodes or blood vessels to other organs which generally causes death. The seriousness of a cancer is directly related to its propensity to metastasize. Thus, prostate cancer usually has a good survival rate because the cancer does not easily move from the prostate; whereas, pancreatic cancer has a high mortality because the pancreas secretes hormones which are spread throughout the body. Likewise, lung cancer, with a network of lymph nodes and blood vessels going to and from the lung does have an unfortunate tendency to metastasize.

Survival with lung cancer is linked to stage which is connected with the tendency to metastasize. A stage one patient with a surgically resected tumor will generally do well, and we have five year survival rates ranging from 55% to 75%. One Japanese study found survival rates approaching 80% for stage one and stage 0 lung cancers (microscopic tumors only visible on cellular examination). Ideally, when a stage one cancer is surgically resected, there is no more cancer, and nothing to metastasize. Many of the 30-40% of stage 1 patients who have future problems were not really stage 1 patients at all; that is, there were cancer cells within the lymph nodes which could not be seen though available diagnostic tools.

As the cancer progresses, the chance of metastasis increases and the probability of long-term survival decreases. There is a direct relationship between stage and long term survival. Let us look at excerpts from American Cancer Society research with all cancers:

TYPE OF CANCER	ALL STAGES	LOCAL	REGIONAL	DISTANT
Breast	84%	97%	76%	21%
Cervix	69	91	49	9
Lung	14	49	18	2
Pancreas	4	15	5	2
Prostrate	89	100	94	31

This chart is based on cases diagnosed from 1986-1993. American Cancer Society (2). Survival rates today are higher, because these statistics are based on cases 7-14 years old. While the absolute numbers will be higher, the basic trend will remain constant. Where we have a stage 4 patient whose cancer has already reached another organ, the prognosis is dim, but not hopeless. With a stage 4 patient, the cancer has already spread, and the physician has the task of preventing further spread and arresting the cancer through chemotherapy, as well as treating the symptoms in the lung and the other organ.

23.1 WHAT TYPES OF SURVIVAL ASSESSMENTS PHYSICIANS CUSTOMARILY MAKE

Estimations of survival time generally represent a statistical assessment, not an assessment of a particular patient. We know on an aggregate basis that because stage 3 and 4 patients with non-small cell cancer have a greater tendency to metastasis that their probability of survival is decreased. However, in most cases, the doctor cannot venture an entirely accurate prediction as to a particular patient. Thus, if there is a 5 year survival rate for stage 3 patients, the oncologist usually cannot tell whether our patient will be the lucky one for whom chemotherapy will work successfully.

23.11 Performance Status as the Best Indication of Survival

While stage can provide a general estimate of survival time, performance status, how the patient is functioning during everyday activities, remains the best predictor. "Functional or performance status was the accurate predictor of survival. Decline in activities of daily living including bathing, continence, dressing and transfer, were very strongly associated with decreased survival." (Devita 10) There are various grades or assessments given for performance status.

23.2 PREDICTIONS ARE ACCURATE ON AN AGGREGATE, NOT INDIVIDUAL BASIS

Within a statistical group are people who live longer and shorter, and the doctor usually has no accurate way of determining the patient's precise period of survival. People with advanced stage 4 cancer do have remissions, albeit a small number. The term six months, frequently used, is a somewhat arbitrary number, accurately taking into account the uncertainty of prediction. Some doctors do not like to provide predictions, believing that they could in some way frustrate recovery by decreasing a patient's will to live, and that the patient may misinterpret an opinion as fact. When a doctor interprets a pathology slide as squamous cell carcinoma, that is a fact, or something very close to it, when he ventures an estimates on survival time, that is really an opinion, albeit an educated opinion.

23.21 The Misleading Nature of Statistics

There are some misleading aspects of published aspects. Most assessments are from clinical trials, yet the trials usually comprise people with advanced cancer who no longer benefit from conventional treatment and are therefore trying another approach. Thus the trials assemble survival data from the patient group with the dimmest prognosis. A recent Mayo Clinic study found a 5 year survival rate of 4% for stage 4 patients which exceeds many other estimates. That assessment was apparently based upon statistics for all patients rather than those restricted to clinical trials.

The five year statistic is dim but not without hope as it indicated a meaningful number surviving five years. The figure accords with many stories of hope on support groups.

23.3 STAGE

The primary factor in assessing survival is cancer stage. Many questions relating to treatment and status of particular cancers are discussed in chapter 4 (nonsmall cell) and chapter 5, small cell. The *Lung Cancer Manual* provides five year survival estimates as follows:

1. stage IA 60% to 67% (that is, 60 to 67% of people diagnosed stage 1A NSCLC are alive five years after being diagnosed,
2. stage 1B 36% to 71%,
3. stage 2A 34% to 55%,
4. stage 2B 24% to 39%,
5. stage 3A 13% to 23%,
6. stage 3B about 5%, and
7. stage 4 about 1%, Lung Cancer Manual 6.2 (1).

With respect to small-cell cancer, the median survival time for patients with limited SCLC is 14 to 30 months. From 10% to 25% of people diagnosed with limited stage SCLC live five years. With treatment, the median survival time for patients with extensive disease is 8 to 14 months. Only 1% to 5% of people diagnosed with extensive-stage SCLC live five years or more." Lung Cancer Manual (1).

An informative website on lung cancer presents these survival statistics based upon patients eligible for surgery:

Stage	TNM (Tumor Node Metastasis Staging)	5 Year Survival
1a	T1N0Mo	67%
1b	T2N0Mo	57%
2a	T1N1Mo	55%
2B	T2N1Mo;, T3NoMo	39%
3a	T3N1Mo;T1-3N2Mo	23%
3b	any T,N3, MO; T4,any N, Mo	<5%,
4 (Surgery not performed)	any T, any N, M1,	<5%,

Adapted from www.cancer.about.com.

23.31 Since Survival is Directly Related to Stage at Diagnosis, We Need to Create Early Detection Programs

The fact that survival is so directly related to stage is a strong argument for early detection programs. Such programs would increase the number of patients diagnosed with early stage cancers and thereby increase survival. As noted, there is no established program for early detection of lung cancer in the United States. The American Cancer Society and the National Cancer Institute have only recommended against smoking; they have failed to establish programs to enable smokers to have their disease diagnosed in early and treatable stages. In contrast, the lesser-known lung cancer advocacy group Alcase, authors of the Manual cited above, have strongly urged the creation of early detection systems.

23.32 Limits to Predicting Survival Based on Stage

The information above is helpful is assessing long-term survival, but there are a number of variables not noted. For example, performance status, the type of lung cancer and overall health of the patient, is an important factor. As noted, we cannot provide an accurate prediction in individual cases. We look at survival issues at stage 1 and 4 below.

23.33 Stage 1 Tumors

Stage 1 tumors have five year survival rates of 50% to 70%. The Stage 1 survival rate is improved when the tumor can be surgically removed. Stage 0, or tumors known by cellular analysis but which cannot be seen on an x-ray or bronchoscope, have an even better prognosis of 70 to 80%. Thus anyone with a stage 0 or 1 tumor which has been surgically removed has an excellent prognosis. Indeed, as a society, we need to work harder to diagnose lung cancer at earlier stages. One treatise reports on the favorable experience of stage 1 patients:

"Results were reported recently with surgical treatment of 598 patients with stage 1 tumors. The male to female ratio was 1.9 to 1 and the median age was 62 years. The primary tumor was located in the upper lobe in 67% of the patients, in the middle or lower lobes in 30%, and in the main bronchus in 3%. The histology was squamous carcinoma in 233 patients and nonsquamous carcinoma in 365 (adenocarcinoma, 253; Bronchoalveolar in 98; large cell carcinoma, 14). The overall 5- and 10 year survival rates (Kaplan-Meier) were 75% and 67%, respectively (Fig 14.2). Patients with T1 tumors fared better than those with T2 tumors. Survival in patients in T1 tumors was 82% at 5 years and 74% at 10 years, compared with 68% at 5 years and 60% at 10 years for those with T2 tumors." Martini (3).

23.34 Stage 3 Tumors

Stage 3 patients are frequently studied in clinical trials. One study "calculated three year survival rates at 35% for stage 3A patients and 26% for stage 3B patients." Impact (4).

23.35 Stage 4 Tumors

Stage 4 tumors, tumors involving metastasis to other organs have a dim prognosis. There are periodic reports of cures and long-term survival. Statistically, we seem unable to develop adequate chemotherapy and radiation regimens to attack and permanently cure metastatic cancer. For many stage 4 lung cancer victims, treatment is palliative, designed to reduce pain, extend life for a period, or limit the spread of the tumor. Within stage 4, it appears prognosis is most adverse where there are metastasis to the bone marrow, liver or brain, whereas the prognostic impact of spread to pleura, skin or peripheral nodes, or the presence of an abnormal bone can have less impact on mortality.

Many of the clinical studies involve stage 4 patients. There we know that there is an approximate rate of response to chemotherapy of 25%, with some recent reports indicating higher success rates, and success defined as a partial or complete response. Thus, at least one in 4 patients overall will enjoy some favorable response with chemotherapy. However, the cancer cells develop some immunity or tolerance to the chemotherapy and second line or second round chemotherapy is usually less successful than the first. In short, a complete cure is possible, and can be hoped with current modes of treatment, which have the capacity to eradicate cancer and have done so in a few cases. Statistically, chemotherapy with stage 4 patients usually does not effect an overall cure, though it does improve the patient's condition.

23.4 OTHER PROGNOSTIC FACTORS

23.41 Performance Status

Physicians use the term performance status to assess a patient's functioning. One performance standard measure rates activity on a scale of 0 (normal) to 4 (bedridden). Survival levels have been correlated with a patient's performance status. For specific articles, and recent developments, go to Medline, the world medical database, at www.healthgate.com.

23.42 Predictive Measures

One study examined medical history in patients with good survival with advanced cancer, "6 independent prognostic factors were: good performance status (ECOG 0), no appetite loss, previous surgical resection, number of metastatic sites (<4), no metastases in liver or subcutaneous tissue".

23.5 EARLY MEASUREMENTS OF METASTASIS

23.51 Micro-Vessel Density

Tumor growth and progression depends partly upon angiogenesis, the development of new sources of blood supply for the tumor. One method of measuring angiogenesis is micro-vessel count. In various cancers, there is a significant correlation between density of micro vessels and the status of the cancer itself. Thus, density of microvessels is a good predictor of future metastasises and perhaps revealing present ones not easily observed. Here are excerpts from studies showing the prognostic importance of micro-vessel density:

- "In our study, we demonstrated that the risk of relapse for patients affected by NSCLC, who have had radical surgical treatment, is directly correlated with the intratumoral microvessel density, namely with tumor angiogenesis." Dazzi (5).

- "Macchiarini et. al demonstrated a statistically significant correlation between the incidence of metastasises and the density of microvessels in 87 Stage 1 NSCLC patients." Machirini (6).
- In a study of 101 non-small cell patients, tumor micro-vessel count found to be the most important prognostic factor. Matsuyama (7).

23.52 The Significance of Micro-Vessel Density

In one sense, these results are predictable—we know that survival is related to stage and stage, in turn, relates to the nature and extent of metastasis. These studies only tell us that microvessel density is a means of assessing present and future metastasis. Nonetheless, we can identify several areas of research and investigation from these findings. These studies identify a subgroup of patients with a likely poorer prognosis. Thus, we may wish to assess stage one patients for micro-vessel density and consider chemotherapy, radiation, and other therapies for those with high levels.

23.6 GENE MEASUREMENTS

23.61 Apoptosis Measurements

Apoptosis is cell death and scientists have devised a way of assessing the percentage of cells that are dying. Not surprisingly, where the percentage of cancer cells dying is high, the patient can do relatively well since the disease has essentially stabilized. "The group with the highest apoptotic index (greater than 25/1.00) revealed the most favorable prognosis because apoptotic cell death overcame cell proliferation." Put negatively in another study, the group with lower levels of cell death had a poorer prognosis. Junker (8) Apoptosis (9).

23.62 Apoptosis and Chemotherapy

One way P-53, a tumor-suppressor gene, works is by prompting cells with defects to undergo apoptosis. Not surprisingly, some studies have found that low levels of P-53 are a negative sign for patients, indicating that programmed cell death is not occurring and that instead the tumor cells are allowed to proliferate. Some forms of chemotherapy work by causing apoptosis or cell death. One study examined whether patients do better with chemotherapy after surgery, and divided the patients in a number of groups. The study found that, "For patients with higher apoptotic index 5-year survival rate of the UFT group (83.3%) was significantly higher than that of the Control group (67.6%, P = 0.039)". Chemotherapy seemed to particularly help those patients with already high indexes perhaps enabling those with less serious tumors to prevent proliferation and spread.

REFERENCES

1. Alcase, *The Lung Cancer Manual* 7.2 (1999).
2. www.bioscience.org, American Cancer Society Surveillance Research, 1998.
3. Martini, Treatment of Stage 1 and 2 Disease, 340 in Aisner, *Comprehensive Textbook of Thoracic Oncology* (Williams & Wilkins 1996).
4. *Impact of Preoperative Biomodality Induction including twice-daily radiation on tumor regression and survival in stage III non-small-cell lung cancer*." J. Clin Oncol 1999 Apr, 17 (4) 1185.
5. Dazzi, et. al., *Prognostic and Predictive Value of intratumoral Microvessels Density in Operable Non-Small-Cell Lung Cancer*, Lung Cancer, Vol. 24 (2) (1999), pp. 81-88.
6. Macchiarini, *Relation of Neovascularization to Metastasises of Non Small Cell Lung Cancer*, Lancet 340 (1992) 145-46.
7. Matsuyama, *Tumor Angiogenesis as a Prognostic Marker, in Inoperable nonsmall cell lung cancer*, Ann Thorac Surg 65 (1998) 1405.
8. Junker, *Prognostic Factors in Stage 1/I Non-Small Cell Lung Cancer*, Lung Cancer, Vol 33 (1001) (2001) p S17-S24.
9. *Apoptosis and Bcl-2 expression as Predictors of Survival in radiation-treated Non-small-cell Lung Cancer*. Int J Radiat Oncol Biol Phys 2001 May 1;50(1):13.
10. Devita. *Cancer Principles and Practice of Oncology* (Lippincott 2001).
11. Hoang, *A clinical model to predict survival in chemonaive patients with advanced non-small cell lung cancer (NSCLC)*, Proc Am Soc Clin Oncol 22: page 624, 2003 (abstr 2508).

CHAPTER 24

CLINICAL TRIALS

24.1 WHAT IS A CLINICAL TRIAL?

How do we know if a particular form of treatment works? Self-reporting by doctors, hospitals or pharmaceutical companies could be subject to exaggeration or at least inaccuracy. Instead, what is needed is a scientific method of assessing the reliability of certain treatments and comparing them with what is used today. Clinical trials are designed to test new drugs, compare them with existing treatments, and determine if they provide better results, fewer side effects, or other benefits. Before a drug can be approved for use by the FDA, clinical trials must show it has some type of demonstrable positive effect.

24.2 DIFFERENT STAGES OF A CLINICAL TRIAL

There are three stages in clinical trials. The stages are progressive, stage one, being a basic test to see if a drug has some effect and to establish the maximum amount which can be given without substantial side effects, stage two, to evaluate the drug and assess its success, usually based upon the maximum allowable does established in stage one, and stage 3, measuring the drug against conventional treatments being used, to see if it provides better or at least comparable benefits.

24.3 STAGE ONE TESTS

Stage one is the first step to see if a particular drug or other form of therapy works, and to define a maximum allowable dosage assuming it does. For example, if interleukin has been successful with some forms of cancer, a phase one trial could be used to see if it works by reducing the size of lung tumors. Individuals entering the study would be prescribed interleukin, measurements would be made, and the study authors would attempt to ascertain whether the drug positively impacts patients.

In addition to seeing if the drug has some impact, in stage one, the study authors try to define a maximum dose, that is, what amount of the drug can be prescribed without significant side effects. Using Interleukin, we may administer the drug in various doses to see what is the maximum amount which can be tolerated without substantial side effects. Note that a clinical trial can be stopped or modified if a clear pattern emerges. For example, if people given large amounts of Interleukin suffer severe effects, we may decide to reduce the amount to prevent injury. Likewise, if it becomes clear that certain doses of the drug are providing clearly beneficial results, we may change the design so that all patients receive the benefit from the drug. Typically, however, the results are not clear, and conclusions about the drug are made after a phase of the study is completed. Here is how the American Cancer Society describes stage one:

> "During a phase I trial-the initial investigation of a treatment's safety and effectiveness in humans—a promising new therapy is tested to learn if it is worthy of further investigation. In the case of a new drug, this is when researchers learn about its effects by gradually increasing the dosage in a step-wise fashion and carefully analyzing the response among the participants. These are preliminary trials in which the researchers learn, for example, how well the drug is absorbed by the body, how much of it reaches the blood stream, and how it is metabolized and eliminated from the body." American Cancer Society, *Informed Decisions* 230 (1997).

24.31 Stage One is Not Designed to Assess the Success of a Drug

While we want to see if a drug works in stage one, defining the extent of tumor reduction is not really our purpose. A phase 1 trial might administer a drug in different dosages with response rates depending on the dosage. We would not measure the success or failure at stage one. If we have five different dosages used at stage 1, it is difficult to tell whether the drug works. If we have 18 participants in a stage 1 trial given three different doses of a new drug and in the group given the maximum there are two persons with partial responses, it is somewhat misleading to conclude that the drug has a 33% response rate at its maximum dose. Most scientists would instead call the results in phase 1 "promising" and proceed to realistically assess the drug at phase 2.

24.32 A Stage One Protocol

Here is an example of a description of a phase 1 clinical trial:

Phase I Study of Irinotecan and Gemcitabine in Patients
With Unresectable or Metastatic Solid Tumors

Objectives

1. Determine the *maximum tolerated dose* (MTD) and the principal toxicities of irinotecan and gemcitabine in patients with surgically unresectable or metastatic solid tumors.

2. Determine if the principal toxicities and MTD of this combination regimen are affected by drug sequencing in this patient population.

3. Determine the potential for gemcitabine to alter the pharmacokinetic characteristics when administered with irinotecan in these patients.

4. Describe the influence effected by varying the

administration sequence of this combination regimen in this patient population.

Protocol Entry Criteria

Disease Characteristics

Histologically confirmed metastatic or surgically unresectable solid tumor, having received the following maximum number of prior therapies for advanced disease:

> Breast cancer—no more than 2 prior therapies . . .
> Lung cancer—no more than 1 prior therapy
> (*this clinical trial deals with different forms of cancer, others may be restricted to lung cancer, or even to a particular stage and type of lung cancer*) . . .
> No prior irinotecan, topotecan, or gemcitabine. Prior adjuvant chemotherapy allowed, if at least 1 year between last dose of adjuvant chemotherapy and recurrence of cancer.

The study seeks to test two chemotherapy drugs which have shown some prior success in reducing the size of tumors and what is experimental is apparently a unique combination of the two being tested. The study involves a number of different cancers and patients with some but not extensive chemotherapy are permitted.

24.33 Participation in Phase 1 Tests

Some scientists would say that it is overly simplistic to say that phase 3 tests are the safest, phase 2 second, and phase 1 the least safe. What we can say is that by phase 3, a drug has been initially tested for maximum allowable dose, shown some promise in stage 2 in reducing tumors without creating significant side effects, and is now measured against standard treatment in stage 3. No such track record is present for drugs used in phase 1 and they are at least to some extent, an unknown quantity. We are probably unsure of the drug's efficacy, at the least we do not know the appropriate dose that should be administered.

Thus, most physicians would advise caution before entering a phase I trial. While it may be initially appealing to participate in a trial involving an innovative new treatment, the practical reality is that too much remains to be done at stage 1. Only those patients with a poor prognosis who have been told that conventional treatment is unlikely to do any good and who are ineligible for stage 2 and 3 trials would want to participate in a stage 1 assessment. One can note that in a stage 1 trial, the patient will frequently get excellent care and attention from physicians intimately acquainted with the particular disease.

24.4 STAGE 2 TESTS

Stage two clinical trials test treatments shown to have promise in stage 1. With hopefully a decent sample size, we now administer the maximum dose and see how the drug performs. In particular with lung cancer, we will assess partial response rate, usually defined as reduction of tumor size by one half, complete response, elimination of the tumor on x-ray or Ct Scan, and survival rate. For example, let us assume that for a drug to be used to treat non-small cell cancer, it should show at least a 20% response rate, that is, at least 20% of the patients' tumors show at least a partial response, without significant side effects, at least as compared with other forms of chemotherapy.

The American Cancer Society describes stage two trials this way,

"Once researchers confirm the possible value of a drug (or other treatment) and determine the safe dosage and other specifics of administering it, they focus on how effective it is in people with one (a particular form of) cancer . . . . to gather information about how well people are responding, researchers may measure the size of tumors for shrinkage . . . . The study may also involve monitoring the patient's blood for substances called tumor markers that often indicate whether their cancers are growing or shrinking." (ACS) (1).

If good results are shown in stage 2, we are now ready for stage 3.

We will compare the new drug with the standard treatment used, with patients randomly assigned to either group. Thus, if Interleukin works at stages one and two, we compare its success in a phase 3 trial against, for example, a cisplatin based chemotherapy. Obviously if it is no better than existing treatments, there is no reason for its usage. For example, Gemcitabine may not show significantly better response rates than Cisplatin, but its diminished side effects merit its FDA approval.

The stages are progressive, stage one, being a basic test to see if a drug has some effect and to establish the maximum dosage, if it does appear to work, stage two is designed to refine the dose and assess side-effects, and finally, stage three, measuring the drug against conventional treatments being used. Once a drug shows positive results in stage 3 it is generally ready to be marketed. Here is a description of a phase 2 clinical trial:

> "In a prior Cancer and Leukemia Group B (CALGB) Phase II trial of patients with advanced, previously untreated mesothelioma, diyhdro-5-azactidine (DHAC) demonstrated a 17% response rate, including 1 complete response, with only mild myelosuppression. This Phase II study (CALGB 9031) was conducted to determine the effectiveness of and toxicities that would result from adding cisplatin to DHAC administered to the same patient population. Overall, 5 objective responses were observed in 29 evaluated patients (objective response rate, 17% . . . . The major toxicity noted was significant chest/ pericardial pain, . . . (s)significant leukopenia was observed in 29% of the patients. The addition of cisplatin to DHAC did not increase the response rate over that observed with DHAC alone in patients with mesothelioma; however, it did increase toxicity, especially leukopenia. This combination is not recommended for further studies involving mesothelioma patients." Samuels, et. al, *Di-hydro-5-azacytidine and Cisplatin in the Treatment of Malignant Mesothelioma: a phase II study by the Cancer and Leukemia Group B*, Cancer, 1998 Apr, 82:9, 1578-84.

Let us review the results from this trial:

1. We can infer that there was a phase I clinical trial involving DHAC where the drug was shown to diminish

tumor size (partial response) without unwarranted side effects. A phase II trial followed which showed a modest 17% response rate for use of DHAC, and in the trial various doses of DHAC were likely tried.

2. Most physicians use multi-modal chemotherapy, administering various types of anti-cancer drugs to attack the disease in different ways. Cisplatin is a well-known chemotherapy drug which has been shown to have demonstrated ability to reduce tumor size in many trials involving non-small cell lung cancer. Its efficacy in attacking mesothelioma, a rare type of lung cancer, is not known. In this phase II trial, Cisplatin was combined with DHAC, in the hope of improving response rates without creating additional side effects. If the study were successful, a phase III trial would occur, comparing DHAC and Cisplatin against the standard treatment being used, with patients randomly assigned to either group.

3. This Phase 2 trial was not successful. The response rate did not improve upon existing forms of treatment while the rate of side effects did, and the authors concluded that this combination did not warrant further investigation.

4. This appears to be part of an on-going study. The study authors will now have to determine whether the 17% response rate using DHAC alone merits a phase III trial. If other chemotherapy drugs show a response rate of more than 17%, then the drug would presumably not be FDA approved. The study authors may decide to combine DHAC with another drug, or take other action to improve the response rate. These changes would be evaluated in additional phase I or II trials and if successful, compared against the prevailing form of treatment in phase III.

24.5 STAGE THREE

Assume that interleukin showed promise in stage 1 with a maximum dosage being determined, in stage 2 there were good results with that dosage, the drug is now ready for stage 3 comparison testing. In stage 3, the drug will be compared with conventional methods of treatment.

24.51 Patients are Divided by Type of Cancer and Stage

To accurately assess a form of treatment, the participants must be restricted to those with a particular form of disease at a particular stage. Thus non-small cell and small cell trials would almost always be done separately, and usually trials would be restricted to stage. Thus our hypothetical trial could be called, *Assessment of the Effect of Interleukin with Chemotherapy versus Chemotherapy Alone in Stage 3 B non-small cell lung cancer patients*. Since the study authors, (sometimes with a pharmaceutical company's assistance) are interested in demonstrating a positive result, they will frequently restrict participation to those in otherwise good health. Thus, a clinical protocol, the summary of how and what will be done, may restrict the trial, and prohibit those with other health problems from participating.

If the stage 3 trial shows a positive result, then other trials might be conducted to confirm the results and meet FDA requirements before allowing the product to be marketed to the public. Sometimes clinical trials will display inconsistent or contradictory results, which is why a series of trials is more reliable than one. For example, an increase in survival in a 20 person clinical trial might be due to one patient doing very well for reasons which could be unrelated to the particular drug tested. A meta-analysis is combining the results of many tests to reach particular conclusions.

24.6 TERMINOLOGY AND PARTICIPATION

24.61 Protocol and Control Group

Protocol is the written outline of a clinical trial. The patient receives an informed consent document which will provide an abbreviated description, but you can request and obtain the protocol itself. Standard treatment refers to the therapy that is accepted by the medical community and has FDA approval. For example, the forms of treatment set forth in chapters four and five are generally the standard treatments. Placebo is a harmless substance given to members of the control group when the study is attempting to evaluate the benefit of adding a new drug to current treatment. American Cancer Society (1).

Control group refers to the people in a clinical trial receiving the standard treatment, and not the experimental treatment. Randomization means the participants are randomly assigned to either an experimental or a control group. In a double-blind study, neither the physicians nor the participant's know which treatments are administered to whom until the study is completed. This is done to prevent some types of conscious or unconscious bias. In a blind study, the patients are not told whether they are receiving the experimental treatment, but the doctors are informed.

24.62 Limited Use of Placebos

Cancer clinical trials typically do not use placebos unlike other trials for the following reason. These clinical trials typically test a new cancer drug or formulation in phases one and two and measure it against standard treatment in stage 3. The primary measuring point is likely to be tumor reduction and there is usually no place in this framework for the absence of treatment, i.e., a placebo.

24.63 Lists of Clinical Trials

To learn about pending clinical trials, go on the Internet to the National Cancer Institute (NCI) site: http://CancerTrials.nci.nih.gov. Prominent hospitals such as M.D Anderson and Sloan Kettering also provide lists of clinical trials.

For general information, call the National Cancer Institute's Cancer Information Service and ask for the booklet What Are Clinical Trials All About, or view the videotape "Patient to Patient: Cancer Clinical Trials and You." The Cancer Information Service can be reached by dialing 1-800-4-CANCER (1-800-422-6237). An excellent book is Finn, Cancer Clinical Trials (OReilly 1999).

24.64 Considerations in Entering Clinical Trials

Where there is effective available conventional treatment, it makes sense for the patient to get it, rather than be randomly assigned a form of treatment which may or not be effective. That is why participants in clinical trials are generally limited to those for whom conventional treatment has not been proven effective. Thus, stage 3B and stage 4 lung cancer patients are eligible for clinical trials, because conventional treatment is not usually curative.

Occasionally, you will see clinical trials for patients for whom conventional treatment works. There is one clinical trial attempting to assess the efficacy of sampling some lymph nodes versus all lymph nodes in surgical resection. Participation in such clinical trials seems to make little sense from the patient's perspective. Instead, a clinical trial makes sense when available treatment appears may not to be sufficient. Here are some of the advantages and disadvantages of clinical trials:

ADVANTAGES

1. Potentially useful for advanced stage patients for whom conventional treatment does not appear effective,
2. Treatment is usually provided in fine medical institutions by specialists who are among the best in their field, and
3. A feeling of helping others and the medical profession towards a cure for lung cancer.

DISADVANTAGES

1. Treatment can be guided by considerations in the clinical protocol,
2. Historically, only a small portion of clinical trials in non-small cell lung cancer have had significant results, and
3. Treatment can sometimes occur in a distant medical center, rather than a local hospital.

For advanced stage patients, clinical trials are clearly an option, but must be discussed with the treating oncologist.

24.65 Eligibility and Conflicts

The creators of the clinical trial seek first and foremost to establish that their drug works which is determined by looking at statistics of how the drug performs during the trial. For example, if existing chemotherapy drugs have a 25% partial response, a successful trial would show a 30% reduction. Thus, it is in the interest of the study creators to pick those patients who are most likely to fare well. If we know that those patients have severe existing health problems or are generally less likely to respond to new drugs, then the study creators may want to exclude them from the trial. (Note that in a stage 3 trial at least theoretically that would not matter, because we are selecting two equivalent groups.) Many trials exclude patients with prior unsuccessful chemotherapy, and those with severe health problems. It is conceivable that some of these people could benefit or at least might want to participate.

24.66 Limitation and Patient Selection

Generally patients with severe or advanced disease are selected for clinical trials. The great majority of lung cancer trials deal with stage 4 and 3B cancers, the ones which are generally most resistant to newer forms of treatment. Thus it is possible that some new forms of treatment which could have had some benefit on earlier stage patients have been abandoned. Traditionally, clinical trials are offered to patients who will no longer benefit from conventional treatments.

However, stage 1 and 2 patients could benefit from timely intervention. Approximately 65% of timely diagnosed stage 1 patients do not have recurrences but the 35% remaining is a disturbing percentage. It makes sense to attempt to identify tumor markers and other features which may indicate recurrence and test methods of treatment and identification through clinical trials.

REFERENCES

1. American Cancer Society, *Informed Decisions* 230 (1997).
2. Oyama, *Molecular genetic tumor markers in non-small cell lung cancer,* Anticancer Res. 2005 Mar-Apr;25(2B):1193-6.
3. Borczuk, *Molecular signatures in biopsy specimens of lung cancer,* Am J Respir Crit Care Med. 2004 Jul 15;170(2):167-74

CHAPTER 25

MESOTHELIOMA

25.1 OVERVIEW

25.11 How Mesothelioma was Named

Most cancers are named after the part of the body where the cancer originates. Mesothelioma begins in the tissue that surrounds different organs inside the body. This tissue, called mesothelium, protects organs by making a special fluid that allows the organs to move. Mesothelium surrounds the lungs, stomach, and heart, and tumors can begin in any of these areas. Three quarters of mesothelial tumors begin in the pleura of the lungs, with the remainder in the peritoneum (stomach), and a small number in the heart.

25.12 Differences from Other Lung Cancers

For many patients with other forms of lung cancer, this chapter may be better ignored since many statements about mesothelioma will not apply to other forms of lung cancer. The presentation of mesothelioma as well as its treatment varies from non-small cell or small lung cancer.

25.13 Why a Rare Cancer Has Been So Intensively Studied

Mesothelioma is a rare cancer which has attracted much attention. First, it is perhaps the only cancer with a clear environmental component.

Mesothelioma is directly related to exposure to asbestos with about 80% of mesotheliomas tied to asbestos exposure. The disease is studied to understand how a cancer develops in relation to a specific causative agent.

25.14 Why Surgery is Difficult

The ideal treatment for lung cancer is surgical resection of the tumor which can eliminate the prospect of metastasis (transfer of the cancerous cells to other organs) and removes the tumor from the lung. Five year survival rates of between 50% and 80% have been reported in early stage one patients with other forms of lung cancer. Surgery has been difficult to perform with mesothelioma because it is really a group of tumors.

25.15 Diffuse Malignant Mesothelioma

Unlike other cancers where a single tumor develops in the large or small breathing pathways, with mesothelioma, a group of tumors develops in the pleura. A more accurate term for mesothelioma is diffuse malignant mesothelioma. The disease is described in a textbook (17) at page 757 of the Comprehensive Textbook of Thoracic Oncology:

> "Mesothelioma of the pleura is characterized by local growth and invasion of contiguous structures and by relatively late spread to distant organs. Recent studies provide evidence that pleural mesothelioma begins in the parietal layer and subsequently spreads to involve the visceral pleura. Pleural effusion (fluid in the pleura of the lung) usually is present . . . . Proliferation of mesothelioma cells and accompanying stromal elements form firm, gray nodules that subsequently coalesce [and] the pleura gradually thickens."

The nature of the disease unfortunately makes it difficult to treat. When tumors can be surgically removed, the patient enjoys a good prognosis. With mesothelioma, since there is usually a group of tumors spread throughout the pleura, surgery can be difficult to perform, though there is literature discussing it as an option.

25.16 Smoking Not A Cause

While most lung cancer is associated with smoking, that appears to play little or no role in mesothelioma. Studies do not indicate a clear increased risk with smoking and the tumors do not develop in the breathing areas of the lung.

25.17 Long Latency

When questioned, some patients may not recall recent exposure to asbestos. However, mesothelioma has a long latency period, (period to develop) and heavy asbestos exposure has been traced 20 and 30 years before the patient developed the disease. A heavy exposure, sometimes y of short duration, may create the conditions for the disease. It is a cancer which develops and spreads slowly. Here is a summary of the differences and similarities with non-small cell cancer and mesothelioma.

CONDITION OR FEATURE	MESOTHELIOMA	NON-SMALL CELL LUNG CANCER
Typical Presentation	A group of nodules in the pleura part of the lung	Single nodule
Primary Danger	Loss of breathing capacity and serious problems in the lungs themselves	Metastasis to lymph nodes, and other organs
Role of Asbestos	Primary Cause	Limited role, may combine with smoking to play causative role
Chemotherapy	By injection or sometimes applied to the area itself.	Given by injection to disseminate throughout the body.
Smoking	Apparently little if any role.	Primary cause
Epidermal Growth Factor Inhibitors and Iressa	Clinical trials continuing with some studies discussing a role.	Helpful in non-smokers, efficacy in others unclear.
P-53 Tumor Suppressor Gene	Debatable impact, and P-53 genetic damages is not seen in many studies. Regulation of apoptosis is a problem.	Significant role in cell repair and apoptosis. P-53 abnormalities significant in non-small lung cancer as well as other cancers.
Surgery	Complex procedure on the pleura, performed at only a few specialized facilities, with used other treatment modalities.	Removal of the nodule. a common procedure. Post-surgical chemotherapy or radiation for stage 1 patients remains experimental.

SIMILARITIES

Chemotherapy	Platinum-based chemotherapy such as Cisplatin or Carboplatin is the main form. Extends life but does not provide an overall cure.	Same
Radiation	Effective at local control of tumor and relieving symptoms. Long-term survival benefit is uncertain	Same
Surgery	Used only for early stage disease	Same

25.2 DIAGNOSTIC TOOLS AND STAGING

A physician will look inside the chest cavity with an instrument called a thorocoscope. This test, called thororcopy, is usually performed at a hospital. Before the test, a local anesthetic is given. The physician may also look inside the abdomen (peritoneoscopy) with a special tool called a peritoneoscope. Biopsies (taking and analysis of tissue) are usually done during the thorocoscope or peritoneoscopy.

25.21 Staging

Mesothelioma uses a different staging system called the Butchert system using stages one through four to designate the extent of spread of mesothelioma:

Localized Mesothelioma

Stage I: The cancer is found in the lining of the chest cavity near the lung and heart or in the diaphragm or the lung.

Advanced mesothelioma

Stage II: The cancer has spread beyond the lining of the chest to lymph nodes in the chest.

Stage III: Cancer has spread into the chest wall, center of the chest, heart, through the diaphragm, or abdominal lining, and in some cases into nearby lymph nodes.

Stage IV: Cancer has spread to distant organs or tissues.

25.23 Types of Mesothelioma and Distinguishing Mesothelioma from Adenocarcinoma

There are three tissue types of mesothelioma. 50-70% of mesothelioma are of the epithelioid type. Less common are mixed byphasic and sarcomatoid. In some cases, mesothelioma is not easily distinguished from adenocarcinoma, a type of non-small cell lung cancer discussed in chapter 2. This has both medical and legal implications; substantial sums can be awarded for mesothelioma while the association between adenocarcinoma and asbestos is disputed. Medically, adenocarcinoma would be placed in the non-small cell category while mesothelioma is treated as a separate disease. Some mesothelioma tumors have a tubulopappilary growth pattern that presents like adenocarcinoma, and a Canadian panel disagreed on the diagnosis of mesothelioma in 30% of the cases. Immunohistochemistry and other tests can help distinguish the two diseases and provide better information for treatment or compensation.

25.24 Treatment Overview

If the mesothelioma is confined to a limited area, surgery may be tried. Unlike non-small cell lung cancer, a single tumor cannot be removed, and the surgery for mesothelioma is more complex. A three part program of surgery, radiation, and chemotherapy has been studied. For advanced mesothelioma, various forms of chemotherapy are used, though with limited success. Interestingly, with mesothelioma, chemotherapy may be applied directly into the tumor area, as opposed to injection into the bloodstream as with most forms of cancer.

25.3 CONTRIBUTING GROWTH FACTORS AND GENES

25.31 Apoptosis and Mesothelioma

Apoptosis, or cell death, is the body's way of getting rid of diseased or damaged cells. "Apoptosis is the carefully regulated process of programmed cell death that is critical for maintaining normal cell and tissue homeostasis. Dysregulation of cell death pathways often results in tumor initiation, progression, and drug resistance in many human cancers." Xia (15). In many forms of cancer, the process goes awry, with genetically damaged cells permitted to multiply. Some suggest failure of the apoptotic system o plays a critical role in mesothelioma. One study "found that three mesothelioma cell lines (1 with wild-type p53) were highly resistant to apoptosis induced by oxidant stimuli (asbestos, H_2O_2) or nonoxidant stimuli (calcium ionophore) compared with primary cultured mesothelial cells."

25.32 Survivin

The body is a complex system. Just as there are apoptosis proteins to signal cell death, there are anti-apoptosis proteins which impact the normal process of cell death. Such proteins can be elevated in various forms of cancer. Survivin is an apoptosis inhibitor that has been detected in many cancers. "Survivin a member of the IAP gene family, is . . . up-regulated in cancer cells and completely down-regulated and undetectable in normal adult tissues." Xia (15).

A recent study indicates its particular importance in mesothelioma, "Survivin was overexpressed in 7 of 8 (87.5%) mesothelioma cell lines assayed and in all (12 of 12; 100%) freshly resected mesothelioma tissues analyzed." Xia (15). Survivin is a reasonable target for gene therapy. "Survivin, an inhibitor of apoptosis protein, deserves attention as a selective target for cancer therapy because it lacks expression in differentiated adult tissues but is expressed in a variety of human tumors." Olie (16).

25.33 Platelet Derived Growth Factor

PDGF has also been associated with response to asbestos and development of mesothelioma:

"One early response to asbestos observed in rat inhalation models is the rapid induction both platelet-derived growth factor (PDGF) A and B chains in the bronchiolar-alveolar epithelium and underlying mesenchymal cells, which is sustained for at least 2 wk after exposure. Interestingly, the (PDGFR) receptor but not (PDGFR) is also elevated in asbestos-exposed rat lung suggesting a possible role for autocrine stimulation in the early stages of asbestos-associated lung damage." Metheny (6).

"Overexpression of PDGF-A is sufficient to cause tumorigenic conversion of T antigen—immortalized human mesothelial cells." That is, where the cells have already been altered, the addition of Platelet-derived growth factor can transform them in mesothelioma cancer cells. Thus, one reasonable hypothesis is that PDGF plays a role in many mesotheliomas as a partial cause. Identifying persons with elevated levels of PDGF through tissue sample could help early diagnosis. Developing a drug which inhibited the development of PDGF is also a possibility.

25.34 Vascular Endothelial Growth Factor and Mesothelioma

Vascular Endothelial Growth Factor (VEGF) is associated with the spread of tumors or angiogenesis. Scientists are investigating its role in mesothelioma and whether the new anti-VEGF agents being tested on NSCLC would work on mesothelioma.

25.35 Apoptosis and Mesothelioma

The failure of the body's normal system of programmed cell death or apoptosis appears to play an important role in mesothelioma.

"The unresponsiveness of this tumor to most conventional agents may in part be explained by a resistance to the induction of programmed cell death or apoptosis. Although the discrete mechanism of action varies, many conventional treatments depend on an ability to engender apoptosis as a final common pathway. Histone (20).

As with other cancers, the targets are two-fold, restore apoptosis and the work done by tumor-suppresor genes, and attack the growth factors which stimulate reproduction of cells. Histone found BCL-XL protein played a vital role and could be limited in a laboratory setting. "We also show that a reduction in BCL-XL protein expression is associated with cell death and apoptosis induced by NaB." Histone (20).

25.4 RELATIONSHIP TO ASBESTOS EXPOSURE

25.41 Asbestos is the Primary Cause of Mesothelioma

There is extensive and overwhelming evidence that mesothelioma primarily comes from exposure to asbestos. (Note, the author of this book is an attorney who represents mesothelioma plaintiffs in claims against asbestos companies.) Although the risks of asbestos exposure were known throughout the last 40 years, asbestos of widely used with few if any warnings. Insulators and pipefitters were exposed to substantial quantities of airborne asbestos on a regular basis. The notorious Sumner-Simpson documents explained how two major asbestos manufacturers concealed the dangers of asbestos.

Asbestos manufacturers failed to warn about known hazards or utilize other precautions to make their product safe, such as encapsulating the asbestos so it would not become airborne. Today in the United States, asbestos is essentially banned, though it continues to be used in some other countries. Sadly people around the world will continue to contract asbestos disease from their work in various occupations:

> Based on knowledge of past and current exposures to asbestos in industry, we can predict a future occurrence of clinical asbestos-related diseases-pleural changes, pulmonary fibrosis, bronchogenic carcinoma, and diffuse malignant mesothelioma. These cases of asbestos related disease are expected to occur in asbestos exposed workers from mining, milling, and manufacturing as well as in those with secondary exposures to asbestos-containing materials, including construction and maintenance workers, users of asbestos-containing consumer products, and the occupants of asbestos-containing buildings. (Dave 21)

25.42 Compensation for Mesothelioma Patients

Because the products were dangerous, not properly labeled and caused serious injuries, many victims of asbestos diseases, particularly mesothelioma have obtained substantial compensation. The largest producer/manufacturer of asbestos, Johns Manville developed a claims facility which has provided over billions of dollars in compensation to the victims of their asbestos products. While direct claims against manufacturers were filed in the 1980's and 90's, today's claims include distributors and others involved in the process. In addition to compensatory damages, some courts have awarded punitive damages, because of the disregard of known risks by the manufacturers.

25.43 Worker-Compensation Claims

In addition to claims against manufacturers, victims of mesothelioma may have claims for medical bills, temporary and permanent disability against their employers. In such cases, the worker would not only need to show his workplace exposure causes his illness, he would not need to identify the specific products used.

25.44 Jobs Where Asbestos Was Used

Unfortunately even brief exposure to asbestos may cause mesothelioma. These jobs have customarily involved the use of asbestos:

1. Insulators and pipefitters,
2. Brake mechanics, and
3. Janitors and roofers.
4. Construction, plumbers, electricians.

This is only a brief list since asbestos was widely used for insulation, heat prevention and other purposes.

25.45 Statute of Limitations Issues

Mesothelioma typically develops from 20-30 years after the date of first exposure. Obviously if the statute of limitations were two years from the date of exposure, virtually every claim would be time-barred. Most states use a discovery rule, finding that the statute of limitations begins two years or some other period after the date the patient knew or had reason to know of a claim. In some cases, the court will conclude that period begins when the patient is first diagnosed with the disease. Most patients with mesothelioma will be entitled to some form of compensation, frequently a significant amount. Anyone interested in filing a claim should promptly consult an attorney.

25.46 Claims for Those Outside the United States

The Johns Manville Claims Facility allows claimants from other countries to submit claims for asbestos-related mesothelioma. If an American company made an asbestos product which caused a disease overseas, frequently a claim can be presented in the United States.

25.47 Causation

The plaintiff would have the burden of identifying the products which caused his exposure. Frequently this is done circumstantially, by showing that co-workers were exposed to a particular product, or by demonstrating that a product was shipped to a particular site. While asbestos's causative role in mesothelioma is clear, precisely which type of fibers cause the disease continues to be investigated. (22)

25.48 Bankruptcies of Asbestos Manufacturers

A number of manufacturers have declared bankruptcy but established a claims facility to provide compensation to mesothelioma victims and their families. Indeed, because of the dangers their products presented, there are probably more asbestos companies in bankruptcy than not. Some argue that limited funds that should have been devoted to mesothelioma have instead been used to compensate those with less serious disease.

25.49 Asbestos Legislation

Legislation has been introduced to limit claims. In some ways, that would benefit mesothelioma patients by assuring that limited funds would be devoted to those whose illness was clearly causes by asbestos. While manufacturers have been assertive in limiting liability, less attention has been paid to funding research to develop cures. Since mesothelioma is a relatively rare disease, drugs companies have not devoted significant attention to it.

REFERENCES

1. Antman, *Asbestos-Related Malignancy*(Grune & Stratton 1989).
2. National Cancer Institute website, *Malignant Mesothelioma*.
3. Sugarbaker, et. al., (3) *Resection Margins, extra pleural nodal status, and cell type determine postoperative long term survival in trimodality therapy of malignant pleural mesothelioma: results in 183 cases.* J. Thoracic Cardiovascular Surgery 1999, Jan, 117:1, 54,65.
4. Faux, *EGFR Induced Activation of NF-kB in Mesothelial Cells by Asbestos Is Important in Cell Survival,*"Proceedings of the American Association for Cancer Res earch, AACR, Vol. 42, March 2001.
5. Caminschi, *Cytokine gene therapy of mesothelioma. Immune and antitumor effects of transfected interleukin-12.* Am J Respir Cell Mol Biol, 1999 Sep, 21:3, 347-56.
6. OReilly, *A phase II trial of Interferon Alpha-2a and Carboplatin in patients with Advanced Malignant Mesothelioma.* Cancer Invest, 1999, 17:3, 195-200.
7. Astoul, *Intrapleural administration of interleukin-2 for the treatment of patients with malignant pleural mesothelioma: a Phase II study* Cancer 1098 Nov, 83:10, 2099-104.
8. Amodio, *Gemcitabine in peritoneal mesothelioma: a case report]* Clin Ter, 1998 Nov, 149:6, 447-51.
9. Nakano, *Cisplatin in combination with irinotecan in the treatment of patients with malignant pleural mesothelioma: a pilot phase II clinical trial and pharmacokinetic profile.* Cancer, 1999, Jun, 85:11, 2375-84.
10. Porohit, *Weekly systemic Combination of Cisplatin and Interferon Alpha 2a in Diffuse Malignant Pleural Mesothelioma,* Lung Cancer, 1998, Nov. 22.:2, 119-25.
11. Ryan & Vogelzang, *A Review of Chemotherapy trials for Malignant Mesothelioma,* Chest, 1998, Jan. 113:1, Supp. 66s-73s."
12. Ardizzoni, *Systemic Drug Therapy of Malignant Pleural Mesothelioma,* Monaldi Arch Chest Dis, 1998 Apr, 53:2, 236-40.
13. Astra-Zeneca, www.egfr-info.com, publishers of Signal, a medical journal devoted to epidermal growth factor research.
14. Metitinas, *Cisplatin, Mitomycin, and Interferon-alpha2a combination chemoimmunotherapy in the treatment of diffuse malignant pleural mesothelioma.* Chest, 1999 Aug, 116:2, 391-8.

15. Xia, *Induction of Apoptosis in Mesothelioma Cells by Antisurvivin Oligonucleotides, Vol. 1, 687-694, July 2002* Molecular Cancer Therapeutics.

16. Olie, *A Novel Antisense Oligonucleotide Targeting Survivin Expression Induces Apoptosis and Sensitizes Lung Cancer Cells to Chemotherapy, Cancer Research* 60, 2805-2809, June 1, 2000.

17. Apoptosis, *A Target for Cancer Therapy*, Cancer Research Vol. 8, 2024-2034, July 2002.

The author explains the term's history and the mechanism of apoptosis.

"In 1972, Kerr described a distinct morphology of dying cells and called it apoptosis. The term was coined based on the fact that the release of apoptotic bodies by dying cells resembled the picture of falling leaves from deciduous trees, called in Greek "apoptosis." This type of cell death has also been called programmed or physiological cell death, and is characterized by a genetic controlled autodigestion of the cell through the activation of endogenous proteases. This process results in cytoskeletal disruption, cell shrinkage, membrane blebbing, nuclear condensation, and internucleosomal DNA fragmentation."

18. Narasimhan, *Resistance of pleural mesothelioma cell lines to apoptosis: relation to expression of Bcl-2 and Bax*, Am J Physiol Lung Cell Mol Physiol 275: L165-L171, 1998.

19. Zanella, *Asbestos-induced phosphorylation of epidermal growth factor receptor is linked to c-fos and apoptosis*, Am J Physiol Lung Cell Mol Physiol 277: L684-L693, 1999.

20. Histone, *Deacetylase Inhibitor Downregulation of bcl-xl Gene Expression Leads to Apoptotic Cell Death in Mesothelioma*, Am. J.Respir. Cell Mol. Biol., Volume 25, Number 5, November 2001 562-568.

21. Dave, *Occupational asbestos exposure and predictable asbestos-related diseases in India*, Am J Ind Med. 2005 Jul 19;48(2): 137-143

22. Suzuki, Short, thin asbestos fibers contribute to the development of human malignant mesothelioma: pathological evidence, Int J Hyg Environ Health. 2005;208(3):201-10.

CHAPTER 26

SURGERY AND RADIATION FOR MESOTHELIOMA

26.0 SURGERY IN TREATING MESOTHELIOMA

26.01 Overview

In early stage non-small lung cancer patients, the tumor is removed leading in some cases to a complete cure. That type of surgery is rarely an option in mesothelioma. "Because the tumor is either broadly extensive on the pleural surface or multi-focal at the time of detection, it does not lend itself to localized surgical excision." Butchart (1). Instead, a more complicated procedure called pleuropneumonectomy is used.

26.02 Surgery Combined with Chemotherapy and Radiation

Where surgery is recommended, it is generally combined with chemotherapy and radiation. This three-pronged approach was pioneered by Dr. David Sugarbaker at Boston's Langham and Woman's Hospital where they operated on a number of mesothelioma patients and generated at least four medical articles assessing longevity patterns. See, Butchert (1). Their conclusions as to when surgery is recommended have been adopted by many throughout the world, with the combination of surgery, radiation, and chemotherapy the starting point, though scientists continue to try to define the optimal mix, and investigate less intrusive gene therapies.

Given the complexity of this surgery, it is generally recommended only for patients with a certain type of early disease though scientists have not precisely defined when it should be performed. The originator of this treatment plan explains, "Cytoreductive surgery (pleuropneumonectomy) followed by sequential chemotherapy and radiotherapy have demonstrated improved survival, especially for patients with epithelial histology, negative resection margins, and no metastases to extrapleural lymph nodes." Jaklitsch (13).

26.1 PLEUROPNEUMONECTOMY

The primary surgery for mesothelioma is a pleuropneuemonectomy. "All of the ipsilateral pleura, lung and pericardium are removed, and because diaphragmatic pleura cannot be separated from the diaphramatic muscle . . . it is necessary to remove (that also)." Butchart (1). "The goal of pleuropneumonectomy is radical resection of the tumor, which often requires combined resection of adjacent structures."

26.11 Eligibility for Surgery

26.111 Performance Status

This is major and complicated surgery suitable for fit patients with normal cardiopulmonary function." Butchart (1).

"Patients were considered surgical candidates if they had a Karnofsky performance status of greater than 70%, a creatinine level within normal limits, liver function test results within the norm. (Exclusive criteria included lower readings on various pulmonary function tests.)" Sugarbaker (2).

26.12 Mortality Rates

Mortality levels from this surgery are not low, and one Japanese study estimated 6% mortality rate from the surgery. Takagi (6). A Scottish hospital reported 9% mortality during the course of its study, Aziz (3), while another English hospital reported 30 day mortality of 7.8% Martin (8). Sugarbaker's post-operative mortality of 4% is one of the lowest but is still substantial. Sugarbaker (3). Given the surgery risk and complexity, choosing a hospital and physician with substantial experience in the procedure should be a prerequisite.

26.13 Type

Studies have study found that patients with the epithelial type benefited most from the surgery. Sugarbaker states, "Univariate analysis found epithelial cell type associated with improved survival in the study, (52% 2 year survival, 21% 5 year survival, 26 month median survival)." Sugarbaker (2). In comparison,

> "The patients with non-epithelial cell type (sarcomatoid and mixed cell type) have a significantly worse survival, with only 16% living for 2 years after the operation. This suggests that our current trimodality treatment plan is having a small impact within this group with unfavorable histologic features, and new strategies for local control are needed."

Based on Sugarbaker's data, those within the non-epithelial group should consider alternatives such as chemotherapy and gene therapy. While his results are persuasive, Sugarbaker is less successful in explaining why cell type should be so important and what it is about epithelial type that improves prognosis. Or conversely, what do the other types do that diminishes one's chances for recovery? Another study found that cell type did not impact survival. Aziz (3). "Survival was, surprisingly, not affected by lymph node involvement (P=0.08) or pathological type of MPM." Aziz (3). However, an Italian study also found that epithelial type improved survival. Serisoli (7).

26.14 Stage

Not surprisingly, patients with limited disease received the most benefit from this surgery.

"Negative resection margins and lack of extrapleural lymph nodal involvement were significant prognostic factors associated with prolonged survival . . . The 66 patients with negative resection margins had a 2 year survival of 44% and a 5 year survival of 25% compared with the 110 patients with positive resection margins, who had a 2 year survival of 33% and a five year survival of 9%. The 136 patients with negative extrapleural nodal status had a 2 year survival of 42% and a 5 year survival of 17%; the 40 patients with extrapleural nodal status had a 2 year survival of 23% and none survived 4 years." Sugarbaker (2).

Similar findings were reported in an Italian study. Serisoli (7). This is consistent with results with non-small cell lung cancer and even small cell, with surgery recommended for those with early disease.

26.141 Stage 1 Patients

The impressive results of the tri-modal surgery make it a promising alternative for stage 1 patients. A later study reported "survival has improved to a mean of 35 months for patients treated by radical surgery followed by systemic post-operative chemotherapy . . . . In selected patients with MPM, complete surgical resection by EPP represents an important initial step in their management. Systemic chemotherapy improves survival in surgically treated patients." Aziz (3). Again, patients would have to be in otherwise good medical condition. As to stage 1 with epithelial type, Sugarbaker explains that. "thirty one patients with 3 positive variables had the best survival", 68% 2 year survival, 46% 5 year survival, median 51 months. Sugarbaker (2).

26.142 Stage 2 Patients

Perhaps the most difficult determinations are to be made in this group. For patients with early disease, the combined regimen makes sense, for those with advanced disease, the risks are clearly too great and the benefits too limited. Where there is or may be limited spread, intelligent minds can disagree. Even with positive resection margins, the 2 year survival of 33% and 5 year of 9% reported by Sugarbaker still exceeds most other treatments. If the results in this group exceed other treatments, it may make sense. Indeed, these results include epithelial and non-epithelial mesothelioma; if we include only epithelial type, the two and five year survival figures would be higher in Sugarbaker's study. But see Butchart, ("It would appear that patients with sarcomatous histology or involved intrathoracic nodes will derive little benefit from the trimodality therapy according to the protocols used by Sugarbaker and collagues." Butchart (1).

26.143 Quality of Life Issues

Difficult judgments must be made. Assessing quality of life in a demanding tri-modal regimen is difficult. Is 12 months of easier treatment better than 20 months enduring complex surgery, chemotherapy, and radiation? How does one evaluate the increased possibility of five year long term survival when it is still only in the area of 10%?

Sloan Kettering reported median survival of 33.8 months for stage 1 and II grouped together. This study used surgery and radiation without chemotherapy. Rusch (9).

26.15 Nodal Status

Sugarbaker did not report his results based on stage, but on nodes and other factors. Sugarbaker writes, "the 136 patients with negative extrapleural nodal status had a 2 year survival of 42% and a 5 year survival of 17%; the 40 patients with positive extrapleural nodal status had a 2 year survival of 23%, and none survived 5 years." Sugarbaker (2). Thus, the existence of positive nodes essentially precluded long-term survival in this tri-modal regimen. Positive nodes may not always be identified pre-operatively, indeed, it may be those with identifiable cancerous nodes would not have been eligible for the Sugarbaker trial surgery. However, one can conclude that positive nodal status would preclude this regimen.

In the future, more sophisticated techniques may identify positive nodes. Pet Scans were not extensively used in the mid-90's when the surgeries in the Sugarbaker study were conducted. Today, Pet-Scans, and other diagnostic tests may reveal positive nodal status.

Given the impact of positive nodes and positive resection margins, most physicians would not recommend the arduous tri-modal plan for patients with advanced mesothelioma. Sugarbaker found that positive lymph nodes essentially precluded long-term survival. Instead, less demanding chemotherapy and gene therapy regimens would be recommended because of the risks of surgery and to improve quality of life.

26.16 Specialized Facilities

Since mesothelioma is a relatively rare disease and pleuropneumonectomy is a difficult and unusual surgery, it should probably be done at a facility specializing in mesothelioma by a physician experienced in this surgery. "The attendant morbidity and potential mortality from extrapleural pneumonectomy stresses the importance of performing the procedure at specialized institutions." Sugarbaker (2). Indeed, with various types of surgery, experience not unexpectedly tends to reduce mortality rates.

26.2 PLEURECTOMY

A more modest surgery is called pleurectomy. Butchart distinguishes a pleurectomy as living diaphragmatic pleura in place which he suggest will usually result in some amount of tumor remaining. While pleurectomy is lesser surgery, its benefits are not clear.

26.3 OMITTED

26.4 RADIATION FOR MESOTHELIOMA

26.41 Its Curative Role

Radiation is used both to relieve symptoms of disease and increase survival. It is clear radiation is not a complete cure, and not even its proponents suggest it can eradicate the disease. Whether radiation increases survival alone or in combination with other treatments continues to be disputed. "External beam radiation therapy, like chemotherapy, has been ineffective in prolonging survival in mesothelioma patients, although several studies have demonstrated some degree of regression of gross disease."

Another author writes, "The effectiveness of primary radiation therapy remains controversial. Even very high doses of radiation cannot control tumor growth. It remains unclear whether radiation therapy may palliate tumor associated symptoms." There have been only a limited number of clinical trials testing radiation making it difficult to pinpoint its efficacy.

26.43 Hyperfractionation

Radiotherapy works by destroying the cancer cells in the treated area. The treatment is normally divided into several sessions (called fractions). An increase in the number of fractions is called hyperfractionated radiotherapy. One study with radiation found a higher than expected 5 year survival rate of 9%. Though the researchers experimented with 6 different fractionation schedules, "the pattern of progression was similar in each treatment group".

26.431 Dose Limitations

Higher doses could arguably improve radiation, however, "delivery of optimal radiation schedules, which may involve large fractions as well as large total doses, is limited by the presence of nearby dose-limiting structures". Ho (9).

26.44 Photodynamic Therapy

Photodynamic therapy is also being evaluated with or without surgery:

> "ALocal failure in particular is a large part of the natural history of mesothelioma, especially after surgery alone. Therefore, one of the major considerations in the development of new treatments is the inclusion of aggressive local therapies. Photodynamic therapy (PDT), a local treatment modality, is being evaluated as an adjuvant therapy to surgical resection."

REFERENCES

1. Butchart, Contemporary Management of Malignant Pleural Mesothelioma, Oncologist, Vol 4, No 6, 488-500, December 1999.

2. Sugarbaker, Resection Margins, extra pleural nodal status, and cell type determine postoperative long term survival in trimodality therapy of Malignant Pleural Mesothelioma: results in 183 cases. J. Thoracic Cardiovascular Surgery 1999, Jan, 117:1, 54,65.

3. Aziz, The management of malignant pleural mesothelioma; single centre experience in 10 years, Eur. J. Cardiothorac Surg 2002 Aug;22(2):298-305.

3. Melluni, Treatment of malignant pleural mesothelioma, Minerva Chir 2001 Jun;56(3):243-50.

4. Jaklitchs, Treatment of Malignant Mesothelioma, World J Surg 25:210-217 (2001).

5. Takahashi, Extrapleural pneumonectomy for diffuse malignant pleural mesothelioma. A treatment option in selected cases? Jpn J Thorac Cardiovasc Surg 2001 Feb;49(2):89-93.

6. Takagi, Surgical approach to pleural diffuse mesothelioma in Japan, Lung Cancer 2001 Jan;31(1):57-65.

7. Serrisoli, Therapeutic outcome according to histologic subtype in 121 patients with malignant pleural mesothelioma, Lung Cancer 2001 Nov;34(2):279-87.

8. Martin, Palliative surgical debulking in malignant mesothelioma. Predictors of survival and symptom control, Eur J Cardiothorac Surg 2001 Dec;20(6):1117-21.

9. Rusch, A phase II trial of surgical resection and adjuvant high-dose hemithoracic radiation for malignant pleural mesothelioma, J Thorac Cardiovasc Surg 2001 Oct;122(4):788-95.

10. Ho, Malignant pleural Mesothelioma.Cancer Treat Res 2001;105:327-73

11. Neumesister, Prognosis, staging and therapy of malignant pleural mesothelioma, Med Klin 2002 Aug 15;97(8):459-71.

12. Hahn, Photodynamic therapy for mesothelioma, Treat Curr Treat Options Oncol 2001 Oct;2(5):375-83.

13. Jaklitsch & Sugarbaker, Treatment of malignant mesothelioma, World J Surg 2001 Feb;25(2):210-7.

Leading Hospitals and Surgeons for Mesothelioma

Given that mesothelioma is a rare disease and the surgery is complicated, one would want to select a physician and hospital with considerable experience. I have listed some of the physicians and institutions which have done work specifically with mesothelioma and in some cases, journal articles where the institution is cited.

United States Hospitals

Brigham is probably the leading hospital for mesothelioma and is where the tri-modal treatment plan was pioneered.

Dr. David Sugarbaker, Department of Surgery, Division of Thoracic Surgery, *Brigham and Women's Hospital*, 75 Francis Street, Boston, Massachusetts 02115, USA.

Other U.S. Hospitals with specialized experience are:

M.D. Anderson Cancer Center, Houston, Texas

Sloan Kettering Cancer Center, New York, Rusch, A phase II trial of surgical resection and adjuvant high-dose hemithoracic radiation for malignant pleural mesothelioma. J Thorac Cardiovasc Surg 2001 Oct;122(4):788-95

Australia

University of New South Wales Department of Surgery, *St George Hospital*, Kogarah, New South Wales, Australia.

France

Institut Gustave-Roussy, Departement de Medecine, 39, rue Camille Desmoulins, F94805 Villejuif.

Italy

Department of Radiochemotherapy, *San Raffaele H Scientific Institute*, Via Olgettina 60, 20132 Milan, Italy. ceresoli.giovanni@hsr.it

Japan

Division of Thoracic Surgery, *National Cancer Center Hospital East*, Kashiwa, Japan.

Netherlands

Department of Thoracic Oncology, *The Netherlands Cancer Institute*, Amsterdam, the Netherlands.

United Kingdom

Dr. Eric Butchart, *University Hospital*, Cardiff, CF 4, 4XW, Wales UK.

Department of Thoracic Surgery, *Glenfield Hospital*, Groby Road, Leicester LE3 9QP, UK.

CHAPTER 27

CHEMOTHERAPY FOR MESOTHELIOMA

27.0 CHEMOTHERAPY OVERVIEW

Tri-modal therapy, surgery, chemotherapy, and radiation is recommended for patients with early epithelial mesothelioma. For others, chemotherapy will be an important option.

The results are similar to non-small cell lung cancer, with platinum-based chemotherapy probably the norm, and now used with the drug Taxol. A new drug, Alimta was recently FDA approved. Chemotherapy can extend life and reduce disease-related symptoms, though it usually does not provide a cure.

The percentage of partial responses with chemotherapy in clinical trials ranges from 20-35%, with a few studies above and below that range. A review from 1998 noted that various drugs are tested:

> "To our knowledge, no chemotherapeutic regimen has emerged as a standard of care. A review of the literature reveals that small activity against this disease has been shown by the anthracyclines, platinum compounds, and alkyllating agents, whereas higher activity has been reported with the antimetabolites. Dose-escalated chemotherapeutics regimens may offer an advantage, whereas combination chemotherapy has not shown any benefit over single-agent therapy. Favorable responses have

been reported with the administration of intrapleural biological response modifiers. Further trials and the investigation of new agents in the treatment of this disease are necessary."

"The role of chemotherapy in the management of pleural mesothelioma still remains uncertain. The available data indicate that although 10-20% of patients are known to achieve an objective response to a number of chemotherapeutic agents, the impact on survival appears limited and improvement in the quality of life remains uncertain." Ardizonni, (1).

Some studies have shown an increase in survival with chemotherapy:

"The influence of treatment on clinical outcome in pleural mesothelioma (PM) is uncertain. We studied 83 patients with PM treated at our institution to evaluate the impact of treatment modality on survival, Methods. Medical records of 83 patients with PM treated between 1978 and 1994 were reviewed. The following data were tabulated for each patient; age, sex, date of diagnosis, history of asbestos exposure, smoking history, method of diagnosis, histologic subtype, type of treatment and survival from diagnosis. Four treatment groups were analyzed; chemotherapy (C), surgery (S), combined modality (CM i.e. S + C with or without radiation therapy) and supportive care alone (SC). Survival curves were calculated and adjustment made for age . . . . Seventy-one males and 12 females with a mean age of 67 years were analyzed. Seventy-five percent were smokers and 74% reported definite or probable asbestos exposure. Treatment groups did not vary according to smoking or asbestos history. The CM group and SC groups contained similar proportions of patients with epithelial tumors (54% v 56%). Median survival for patients in the CM (combined modality) group was 23.9 months versus 4.5 months among those receiving SC (supportive care) (p < 0.01)." Huncharak (2).

While an impact of chemotherapy is seen, some have interpreted the study as supporting combined modalities, surgery and chemotherapy, and not chemotherapy alone. Another study we look at showed chemotherapy and immunotherapy lengthening survival in some patients.

27.1 PLATINUM-BASED CHEMOTHERAPY COMBINATIONS

Cisplatin is a widely used chemotherapy drug which has demonstrated effectiveness with non-small cell lung cancer, and other types of cancer. Cisplatin combinations have shown consistent responses, though Cisplatin is associated with nausea and stomach discomfort. Use of newer drugs to relieve stomach discomfort, and substitution of Carboplatin, a similar platinum drug with fewer side effects but similar effectiveness, may reduce the problems associated with the drug. Precisely what should be used with Cisplatin remains unclear, as other chemotherapy drugs, immunotherapy, and newer forms of gene therapy are all being tried.

27.11 Side Effects

Unfortunately Cisplatin's strength is also its weakness; its capacity to stop the division of cells may also create problems in some areas of the body where such division is a part of normal functioning. Cells in the stomach frequently divide as part of digestion, and Cisplatin has been associated with nausea and even episodic vomiting. However, one third of the patients had an episode of nausea or vomiting. Many patients will want to risk such side effects for the chance to extend life, but some may not, and side effects with Cisplatin combinations must be discussed with your oncologist.

Many of the combination therapies limit Cisplatin because of its potency. In the future, Carboplatin, a similar drug with few side effects, may be substituted, as it is with other forms of lung cancer.

27.12 Cisplatin and Irinotecan

A Japanese clinical trial combined Cisplatin with Irinotecan. The abstract states:

> "The purpose of this study was to assess the efficacy and toxicity of a combination of cisplatin and irinotecan (CPT-11) in the treatment of patients with malignant pleural mesothelioma . . . . METHODS: Fifteen previously untreated

patients with malignant pleural mesothelioma were treated with cisplatin (60 mg/m2 on Day 1) and CPT-11 (60 mg/m2 on Days 1, 8, and 15) administered intravenously and followed by a 1-week rest period . . . RESULTS: All patients were valuable for response and toxicity. Four partial responses (response rate of 26.7%) with a median response duration of 25.9 weeks and 2 regressions of valuable disease (overall response rate of 40%) were observed." Nakano. (Note the term response rate usually is defined as reduction in tumor size by at least 50%.)

27.13 Cisplatin and Interferon

Immunotherapy and gene therapy are frequently used to fight mesothelioma. In a phase 1 study of 13 patients with mesothelioma, four patients had a partial response, and one a complete response. A phase 1 trial is designed to determine tolerable doses as well as assess response. Some anemia and renal or kidney problems were noted from the therapy, but overall the study showed promise with phase 2 trials expected. Porohit (10).

27.14 Cisplatin, Etopiside and 5 Fluourouracil

A recent French study examined Cisplatin, Etopiside and 5-Fluourouracil, a combination previously used with other forms of lung cancer:

"The authors conducted a Phase II trial in which two drugs (etopiside and 5-fluorouracil) were added to the Cancer and Leukemia Group B cisplatin-mitomycin regimen in an effort to define a more effective chemotherapy. METHODS: Forty-five patients with confirmed Stage II malignant pleural mesothelioma were prospectively enrolled in the study. Thirty-one patients received cisplatin 60 mg/m2 on Day 1, 5-fluorouracil 600 mg on Days 1-4, folinic acid 100 mg/m2 on Days 1-4, mitomycin C 10 mg/m2 on Day 3, and etopiside 100 mg/m2 i.v. on Days 1-3, with prophylactic hematopoietic growth factors . . . . Histology included epithelial (in 33 cases), sarcomatous (in 6), mixed (in 3), and unspecified type (in 3). RESULTS: Two hundred eleven cycles were administered. Treatment was well tolerated and the major toxicity was hematologic: anemia in 30% of cases, neutropenia in 24%, and 2 probable cases of mitomycin-induced pneumonitis. The objective response rate was 38% (17 of 45 were partial responses), and the median response duration was 12 months. The median survival time was 16 months. There were no differences in response or survival between the 31 patients treated with growth factors and the 14 patients treated without them. Survival was slightly better for responders than for nonresponders who had stable disease or progression (20 vs. 10 months, P < 0.05). CONCLUSIONS: This four-drug combination was effective, with a notably high response rate, acceptable toxicity, and good adherence to protocol doses. The impact on survival was limited."

27.15 Cisplatin and Gemcitibine

Gemcitabine is a newer chemotherapy drug used to treat lung cancer. Its side effects are generally limited. Gemcitabine has been tried alone:

"Gemcitabine is broadly active in a variety of solid tumors, including malignant mesothelioma. In vitro, gemcitabine demonstrates activity against mesothelioma cell lines. The role of single-agent gemcitabine in patients with mesothelioma is unclear, since three phase II trials treated a total of 60 patients and achieved response rates of 0%, 7%, and 31%." Kindler (10).

Another study reported an unusually high partial response rate of 47% using Cisplatin and Gemcitabine. (Byrne 5). However, one third of the patients had an episode of nausea or vomiting. Another study reported more modest results with 4 of 25 patients having partial responses. The average time for the disease to progress was 6 months with median survival measured at 9.6 months, perhaps only a modest increase over nonintervention and non-chemotherapy based treatment. Finally, a new Japanese study found impressive rates of survival using a three drug combination. (Mariyuma 21)

27.2 NEW CHEMOTHERAPY DRUGS

27.21 Pemetrexed (Alimta)

A phase I study of pemetrexed in combination with cisplatin showed impressive response and survival rates. "Tumors shrank in 41 percent of patients on pemetrexed in combination with a more commonly used chemotherapy agent called Cisplatin." Additionally, patients with the combination survived 25% longer. Pemetrexed is a new antifolate which inhibits many reactions that are essential for cell proliferation. Another writer suggests that anti-metabolites combined with either Cisplatin or Carboplatin will be the preferred treatment:

> "Antifolates such as methotrexate are among the most active compounds in mesothelioma, albeit based only on phase II data. Recently two antifolate-based combinations with apparently higher efficacy than older regimens have emerged: the pemetrexed/cisplatin regimen and the raltitrexed/oxaliplatin regimen. In two phase I trials with pemetrexed combined with either cisplatin or carboplatin responses occurred in five of 11 and nine of 29 patients, respectively. In a phase I trial of raltitrexed/oxaliplatin, six of 17 patients (35%) with mesothelioma achieved a partial response. In a phase II trial of raltitrexed/oxaliplatin, 14 objective responses were confirmed in 72 patients (25%) with malignant pleural mesothelioma."

Precisely why these drugs are particularly effective remains to be established.

27.211 Side Effects

Some side effects are seen with this drug. A study of non-small cell cancer showed grade 3 or 4 neutropenia was seen in 25 patients (42%).

> "The early studies of pemetrexed showed that the important dose-limiting toxicities were myelosuppression, mucositis, and diarrhea, all of which are common with any antimetabolite.

Subsequent studies described in this article will show that these toxicities can be significantly reduced by the use of vitamin supplementation with folate and B(12), and that pemetrexed has considerable activity in non-small cell lung cancer and mesothelioma." Clark (8).

In February, 2004, Alimata was FDA approved. It is recommended with Cisplatin.

27.22 Oxaliplatin and Raltitraxed

"In a phase I study, the combination of oxaliplatin and raltitrexed was shown to be active against malignant pleural mesothelioma. Four partial responses, 1 regression of disease (objective response rate, 45%; 95% CI, 15.6-74.4%), 4 stable diseases and 2 progressions of disease were observed. An improvement in disease-related symptoms was recorded in all responders and in 2 patients with stable disease. Toxicity was mild, with no toxic-related death and only 1 episode of grade 4 neurotoxicity. CONCLUSIONS: We consider the combination promising and worthy of further studies." Maisano (5).

27.23 Intrapleural Administration of Chemotherapy

For most tumors including non-small cell, the drug is given either orally or intravenously. However, a new form of treatment where the drug is applied directly to the tumor has been utilized with mesothelioma with some success. Several investigators have studied direct intrapleural delivery of chemotherapy with the rationale of achieving high local drug concentrations while minimizing systemic toxicity. Intrapleural delivery requires the presence of a patent pleural space, which limits the candidate pool to those with earlier stages of disease, because the pleural space is often obliterated in advanced mesothelioma.

REFERENCES

1. Ardizzoni, *Systemic Drug Therapy of Malignant Pleural Mesothelioma*, Monaldi Arch Chest Dis, 1998 Apr, 53:2, 236-40.

2. Huncharak, *Treatment and survival in diffuse malignant pleural mesothelioma; a study of 83 cases from the Massachusetts General Hospital*, Anticancer Res 1996 May-Jun;16(3A):1265-8.

3. www.Cancer.gov. *Largest-Yet Mesothelioma Study Shows Survival Benefit with New Drug.*

4. Ho, *Malignant pleural Mesothelioma.Cancer* Treat Res 2001;105:327-73.

5. Maisano, *Oxaliplatin and raltitrexed in the treatment of inoperable malignant pleural mesothelioma: results of a pilot study*, Tumori 2001 Nov-Dec;87(6):391-3.

6. Clark, Phase II trial of pemetrexed disodium (ALIMTA, LY231514) in chemotherapy-naive patients with advanced non-small-cell lung cancer, Ann Oncol 2002 May;13(5):737-41.

7. Rusch, *A phase II trial of surgical resection and adjuvant high-dose hemithoracic radiation for malignant pleural mesothelioma*, J Thorac Cardiovasc Surg 2001 Oct;122(4):788-95.

8. Holsti, *Altered fractionation of hemithorax irradiation for pleural mesothelioma and failure patterns after treatment.* Acta Oncol 1997;36(4):397-405.

9. Stenman, Advances in the Treatment of Malignant Pleural Mesothelioma, Chest. 1999;116:504-520).

10. Kindler, *The role of gemcitabine in the treatment of malignant mesothelioma*, Semin Oncol 2002 Feb;29(1):70-6.

11. Magnegold *Pemetrexed for diffuse malignant pleural mesothelioma* Semin Oncol 2002 Apr;29(2 Suppl 5):30-5.

12. Byrne, *Cisplatin and gemcitabine treatment for malignant mesothelioma: a phase II study*, J Clin Oncol 1999 Jan;17(1): 25-30.

13. Fisazzi, *The emerging role of antifolates in the treatment of malignant pleural mesothelioma*, Semin Oncol 2002 Feb;29(1):77-81.

14. Bunn, *Incorporation of pemetrexed (Alimta) into the treatment of non-small cell lung cancer (thoracic tumors)*, Semin Oncol 2002 Jun;29(3 Suppl 9):17-22.

15 Butchart, *Contemporary Management of Malignant Pleural Mesothelioma*, Oncologist, Vol 4, No 6, 488-500, December 1999.

16. Sugarbaker, *Resection Margins, extra pleural nodal status, and cell type determine postoperative long term survival in trimodality therapy of malignant pleural mesothelioma: results in 183 cases.* J. Thoracic Cardiovascular Surgery 1999, Jan, 117:1, 54,65.

17. Aziz, *The management of malignant pleural mesothelioma; single centre experience in 10 years*, Eur. J. Cardiothorac Surg 2002 Aug;22(2):298-305.

16. Melluni, *Treatment of malignant pleural mesothelioma*, Minerva Chir 2001 Jun;56(3):243-50.

18. Jaklitchs, *Treatment of Malignant Mesothelioma*, World J Surg 25:210-217 (2001).

19. Takahashi, *Extrapleural pneumonectomy for diffuse malignant pleural mesothelioma. A treatment option in selected cases?* Jpn J Thorac Cardiovasc Surg 2001 Feb;49(2):89-93.

20. Takagi, *Surgical approach to pleural diffuse mesothelioma in Japan*, Lung Cancer 2001 Jan;31(1):57-65.

21. Maruyama, *Triplet Chemotherapy with Cisplatin, Gemcitabine and Vinorelbine for Malignant Pleural Mesothelioma*, Jpn J Clin Oncol. 2005 Jul 8A.

CHAPTER 28

IMMUNOTHERAPY AND GENE THERAPY FOR MESOTHELIOMA

28.1 IMMUNOTHERAPY

Immunotherapy and gene therapy are important investigational drugs to fight mesothelioma.

> "The rationale for immunotherapy is the existence of immune abnormalities in patients with MPM. Moreover, some human mesothelioma cell lines are sensitive to cytokines like interferon—,—IFN, and interleukin 2, and to some immune cells, which suggests that immunointervention would be beneficial. Intrapleural administration of interleukin 2 has resulted in objective responses in 19 to 55% of the cases in two trials including low numbers of patients in the early stages of disease."
> Monnert (1).

28.11 Interferons

Interferons are proteins secreted by immune cells that "interfere" with a virus's ability to reproduce and proliferate. Interferon has had some significant beneficial effect in treating mesothelioma though significant side effects have been associated generally with Interferon. In the laboratory, low concentrations of Interferon help boost the power of natural killer T cells. With some tumors, interferons can help inhibit the development of the blood vessels that tumors need to metastasize and grow, a process called angiogenesis. There are three main types and 17 subtypes of interferon.

28.12 Studies with Interferon and Mesothelioma

One study reported an impressive response rate for patients with stage 1 disease:

> "Eighty-nine patients were included over 46 months. Eight histologically confirmed complete responses and nine partial responses with at least a 50% reduction in tumor size were obtained. The overall response rate was 20%. Most responses were achieved in patients with early stage disease. The response rate for patients with Stage I disease was 45%. Tolerance of interferon was good. Treatment was performed on an outpatient basis. The main side effects were hyperthermia, liver toxicity, neutropenia, and catheter-related infection. CONCLUSIONS: Gamma-interferon is effective mainly in Stage I mesothelioma, especially if the tumor is confined to the parietal or diaphragmatic pleura (Stage IA)." Boutin (4)

Unfortunately, the abstract does not report median survival figures. The favorable results for stage 1 can be interpreted as indicating the effectiveness of Interferon with this subgroup or that most therapies will be more successful on patients with limited disease.

28.13 Why Interferon Works

A recent study explains how Interleukin works on laboratory animals.

> "Malignant mesothelioma appears to be sensitive to immunotherapeutic approaches, and one of the most powerful immunomodulatory cytokines with antitumor effects is interleukin (IL)-12. We have previously shown in a murine model of MM that systemic administration of recombinant IL-12 induces a potent anti-MM immune response. The nature and accessibility of MM

tumors means that they are suitable candidates for direct cytokine and gene-transfer therapeutic approaches. In mixing experiments, paracrine IL-12 production inhibited growth of untransfected MM cells provided that cells producing IL-12 represented more than 50-80% of the inoculum . . . . This study shows that paracrine secretion of IL-12, generated by gene transfer, can induce immunity against MM that can act locally and also at a distant site. In addition, there was no evidence of toxicity, which has been associated with the systemic administration of IL-12, indicating that this cytokine is a good candidate for experimental gene therapy in MM." Caminschi (5).

However, a study at New York's renowned Sloan Kettering reported,

"The combination of low-dose interferon alpha-2a and carboplatin did not result in greater antitumor activity than that reported for single-agent carboplatin in advanced malignant mesothelioma. Although toxicity was mild, carboplatin and low-dose interferon, given at this dose and schedule, cannot be recommended for this patient group." O'Reilly (6).

28.14 Complimentary Effects of Inferon and Chemotherapy

Perhaps the lesson is that low doses of Interferon are unlikely to effect favorable results, and the dosage must be compared with the more favorable studies. Significant side effects have been reported with Interferon so defining the maximum tolerable dose is no easy task. The median survival is somewhat higher than with other treatments as is the progression to more serious disease. Initially, the results of a 2002 study of interpleural administration of Interferon are modest. "Among the 14 evaluable patients, 2 patients (patients 4 and 11) had a partial response. The overall response rate of patients actually treated was 14%." Monnert (1). The author explains,

"After completion of the cellular therapy, 10 patients were treated by chemotherapy as their diseases progressed. Two patients (patients 13 and 15) achieved a stabilization of their disease. The disease in patient 13 again progressed after 26 months, and this patient died at 45 months. Patient 15 was still alive in December 2000, with a follow-up of 47 months. The median survival of patients actually treated, including those who received chemotherapy after AM treatment, was 29.2 months. At last follow-up (December 2000), 4 of the 17 patients were alive. Patient 4 had completed chemotherapy and had a very slow-progressing disease. The disease in patients 15 and 3 was progressive at 47+ and 41+ months, respectively; patient 1 was still disease-free at 69+ months." Monnert (1).

The median survival rate of 29.2 months and the results of several patients surviving at or close to four years is impressive. Yet the partial response rate of 14% is unimpressive. This indicates to me that the most potent impact of the Interferon was its later favorable impact upon chemotherapy for several patients. A Turkish study found moderately favorable results, a response rate of 24% combining Interferon with Cisplatin. Metintas (14).

"OBJECTIVE: To investigate the therapeutic activity and toxicity of combination chemoimmunotherapy with cisplatin, mitomycin, and interferon (IF)-alpha2a, by comparing the responses in a group of patients with diffuse malignant pleural mesothelioma (DMPM) to the responses in a control group of DMPM patients given supportive care alone . . . . Forty-three patients with DMPM received chemoimmunotherapy until the end of the survey; 19 patients were given supportive therapy alone after refusing chemoimmunotherapy. INTERVENTIONS: Drugs were administered according to the following schedule: IV cisplatin, 30 mg/m2 qd on days 1 and 2; IV mitomycin, 8 mg/m2 on day 1; and subcutaneous IFN-alpha2a, 4.5 million IU twice weekly . . . . A total of 10 objective responses (ORs) in 43 patients (23%) were assessed, including 2 complete responses (5%), 4 partial responses, and 4 regressions. Seventeen patients had stable disease, and 16 patients had progression. The median survival time was 11.5 months for the 43 patients who received chemoimmunotherapy and 7.0 months for the 19 patients who received supportive therapy alone. The difference in survival times between the chemoimmunotherapy and supportive therapy groups was not significant. However, the median survival time for the patients who had OR was 21.3 months, which is significantly longer than that of the patients who received supportive care alone and that of patients with progressive disease (6 months). The toxicities associated with the treatment schedule of this study were, for the most part, tolerable. CONCLUSIONS: The drug combination used in this study is moderately effective and well tolerated in patients with DMPM, especially in those who responded to the treatment."

28.15 Cellular Studies of Interferon and Chemotherapy

Some cell studies support the hypothesis that Interferon can improve the efficacy of chemotherapy. One study reported, "A combination of IF-alpha and IF-gamma consistently augmented the response of the cell lines to methotrexate, by as much as 75% for one cell line, although the response to the individual IFNs was variable." Hand (3).

28.2 INTERLEUKIN

28.21 Interleukin

A 1995 study of Interleukin reported modest results:

"Partial response (PR) occurred in 4 of 21 evaluable patients (19%; 95% confidence interval 5-42%) with a median time to progression of 12 months (range 5-37). Stable disease (SD) occurred in seven patients with a median time to progression of 5 months (range 2-7). There were no complete responses (CRs). The median overall survival was 15.6 months (range 3.0-43). No relationship between the dose of IL-2 and response rate was observed. We conclude that IL-2 given intrapleurally is accompanied with acceptable toxicity and has anti-tumour activity against mesothelioma."

In a phase 1 study of 13 patients with mesothelioma, four patients had a partial response, and one a complete response. A phase 1 trial is designed to determine tolerable doses as well as assess response. Some anemia and renal or kidney problems were noted from the therapy, but overall the study showed promise with phase 2 trials expected. Porohit (10). In a French phase II study, over 50% of the participants showed some tumor reduction from Interleukin-2:

> "Several clinical studies have demonstrated objective antitumoral responses to intrapleural interleukin-2 (IL-2) administration in the treatment of malignant pleurisy . . . . Based on these results, a Phase II study was conducted, in which intrapleural IL-2 (21 x 10(6) IU/m2/day for 5 days) was given to patients with MPM (malignant pleural mesothelioma) . . . . Twenty-two patients entered this study. Of the 22 cases of MPM, 19 were epithelial, 2 were mixed, and 1 was fibrosarcomatous. Three patients had Stage IA disease, 1 had Stage IB, 16 had Stage II, 1 had Stage III, and 1 had Stage IV (Butchart classification) . . . . There were 11 partial responses and 1 complete response. Stable disease occurred in 3 patients and disease progression in 7 patients. The overall median survival time was 18 months; the median survival time of responders differed significantly from that of nonresponders (28 months vs. 8 months, $P < 0.01$). The 24- and 36-month survival rates for responders were 58% and 41%, respectively. CONCLUSIONS: These results confirm that intrapleural administration of IL-2 is well tolerated and has antitumor activity in patients with MPM. Astroul (7).

28.3 EPIDERMAL GROWTH FACTOR INHIBITORS AND MESOTHELIOMA

28.31 Overview

Given the limited success of surgery and chemotherapy, scientists are evaluating other forms of treatment for mesothelioma. The development and spread of cancers are prompted by growth factors, signals from one cell to another.

A prominent growth factor is the epidermal growth factor. The epidermal growth factor (EGF) is associated with the creation and spread of lung cancer as well as other types of cancer. Connecting with its receptor, EGFR, this sets in motion various carcinogenic events. Use of epidermal growth factor inhibitors have stabilized disease in some lung cancer patients, though the rates of complete cure or even partial response (reduction of tumor volume by one half) have been low. Since the EGFI's do not affect all cells, but target a specific receptor, they have much fewer. The most common side effect is skin irritation since the epidermal growth factor is connected with skin (dermal) regeneration.

Rather than disrupting the immune system as with Interferon, or performing risky surgery, this treatment is minimally intrusive. Drugs which inhibit this growth factor are beginning to play an important role in treatment of patients with advanced non-small cell cancer, and may play an equal role in treating mesothelioma. Our chapter on EGF and Iressa discusses these drugs and recent studies, and here we look at such drugs specifically in relation to treatment for mesothelioma.

> "Govindan and colleagues have investigated EGFR receptor expression in mesothelioma tissue, using Zymed™ antibodies. They found that nearly 60% of samples overexpressed EGFR, while none overexpressed HER-2, suggesting that it is worth considering anti-EGFR therapy in patients with mesothelioma." (13 egfrinfo.com).

A recent presentation found that asbestos prompted production of the epidermal growth factor and this could be duplicated in the laboratory:

> "Over-expression of the epidermal growth factor receptor (EGFR) is a common finding in many solid tumors, including lung, breast and mesothelioma, and has been shown to correlate with both a poor prognosis and resistance to radiation and chemotherapy . . . . Recent evidence suggests that up-regulation and activation of EGFR may play a critical role in early carcinogenic events . . . . carcinogenic asbestos fibers upregulate the expression of the EGFR. Exposure of MET 5A cells to asbestos leads to the activation of nuclear factor-kB (NF-kB), a transcription factor important in the regulation of a

number of genes intrinsic to inflammation, proliferation and lung defences. This study set out to examine the relationship between EGFR and NF-kB in MET 5A cells exposed to asbestos fibers . . . The selective EGFR tyrosine kinase inhibitor, PKI166 (Novartis), inhibited the DNA binding of NF-kB mediated by crocidolite asbestos fibers . . . . Modulation of the asbestos-mediated EGFR/NF-kB signaling pathway may be important in the development of novel therapeutic strategies for both the chemoprevention and treatment of malignant mesothelioma." Faux (4).

28.32 Mesothelioma Cell Studies

A recent cell study concludes, "The EGFR mediates both asbestos-induced proto-oncogene expression and epithelial cell proliferation, providing a rationale for modification of its phosphorylation in preventive and therapeutic approaches to lung cancers and mesothelioma." Manning (15). Iressa is the most well-known EGFR.

28.33 Human Studies

Investigation is continuing with clinical trials, though I have not located published reports.

28.34 Iressa Use with Mesothlioma

Iressa is an FDA approved drug for non-small cell lung cancer. Since it is FDA approved, doctors can prescribe it for other uses, so-called off-label. While the drug has not been approved or found effective for mesothelioma, some patients could seek its use, particularly if other alternatives were not available for various reasons. A doctor would then have to determine whether the drug should be used off-label.

28.35 Recent Studies on Iressa and Testing

Non-smokers with adenocarcinoma showed significant response to Iressa. Interestingly, mesothelioma is a type of cancer which non-smokers contract and has limited association with smoking. The non-smokers benefiting from Iressa had damage to the tyrosine kinase portion of the epidermal growth factor receptor, causing the receptor to malfunction. Iressa is a tyrosine kinase inhibitor.

The Harvard Genetics Laboratory recently developed a test to detect this type of tyrosine kinase damage. Mesothelioma patients may wish to be tested for this abnormality. At this point we do not know whether this abnormality is present in mesothelioma and whether mesothelioma patients can benefit from Iressa.

Iressa impacts the tyrosine kinase preventing autophosphylation. Tarceva is a similar drug which some believe is stronger than Iressa. Erbitux is another drug which prevents binding at the EGFR level, a somewhat different mode of action.

Patients will want to review recent studies on Medline (www.ncbi.nlm.nih.gov) to see if new studies or clinical trials are showing progress with EGFR inhibitors and mesothelioma. Leading hospitals may have greater access to clinical trials.

28.4 COX-2 INHIBITORS AND MESOTHELIOMA

28.41 Overview

Cox-2 is produced in response to inflammatory process. As our section on cox-2 inhibitors discusses (16.4) Cox-2 is associated with various carcinogenic processes. "Cyclooxygenase-2 (COX-2) plays an important role in solid tumor growth, invasiveness, and angiogenesis." Edwards (17).

Cox-2 inhibitors like Celebrex present the possibility of inhibiting some cancer processes.

2004 saw several studies linking long-term use of cox-2 inhibitors with an increased risk of heart attack. These studies cast doubt on the routine use of products like Celebrex and Vioxx for normal aches and pains and even arthritis. Nonetheless, the long-term hazards of cox-2 inhibitors for mesothelioma patients may be less than with standard forms of chemotherapy like Cisplatin. Chemotherapy impacts a wide number of dividing cells while Celebrex's impact is primarily seen with cox-2. Given the limited success of other treatments, Celebrex remains an alternative for mesothelioma, or at least an area where clinical trials and further research is merited.

28.42 Cox2's role in Mesothelioma

Cox-2 appears to play a role in the development and spread of mesothelioma. Edwards (17) "The data presented here demonstrates that cells in mesothelioma tissue, as opposed to normal mesothelial linings, express detectable levels of the inducible enzymes, NOS2 and COX2." Manning (16). "Human mesothelioma tumors have been shown to overexpress COX-2 and high levels of COX-2 protein have been demonstrated to be a prognostic factor, indicating poor outcome in this tumor."

28.43 Cell Studies of Cox-2 Inhibitors

A recent study looked at Celebrex and mesothelioma. "We determined that inhibition of COX-2 by oral administration of Rofecoxib significantly slowed but did not cure the growth of small tumors in mesothelioma-bearing mice." (Delong 19).

Celebrex and other cox-2 inhibitors should be tested on mesothelioma, probably in conjunction with other established therapies.

28.5 OTHER DRUGS

28.51 Lovastatin

A 1998 study reported that concentrations of Lovastatin, induced apoptosis (cell death) in human malignant mesothelioma cell lines. Mesothelioma cell viability was decreased in a dose-dependent manner by Lovastatin. Rubins (18). The reasons why more research has not been performed on Lovastatin for mesothelioma are unclear and are likely to be more economic than medical. Here, too, the prospect of developing a cure for a rare disease, may not provide sufficient incentive for expensive clinical trials and product development, which may not be successful.

28.52 Need for More Research Funds

Manning's found a substance called NS 398 inhibited mesothelioma in a laboratory. It would make sense to have the substance developed into a drug and tested in clinical trials. Because of mesothelioma's relative rarity, pharmaceutical companies have not moved quickly to develop drugs to attack the disease, and more money for research is needed. Generally, the companies have developed drugs for more prevalent diseases

28.6 SV 40 AND MESOTHELIOMA

28.61 What is SV 40?

Simian virus 40 (SV40), is a virus associated with monkeys which has been recently associated with the development of mesothelioma. Some suggest that SV 40 can come into contact with humans through contaminated polio vaccines. Polio vaccine was grown on the kidneys of rhesus monkeys. Brierly, (12).

SV 40 has been found in mesothelioma cells, animal studies and human cell biopsies. Foddis found that "SV40, a DNA tumor virus was present in approximately 50% of mesothelioma biopsies in the USA." (4). Klein states, "In 1994, PCR and protein studies suggested that SV40 DNA sequences and proteins were present in 29/48 (60%) USA human mesothelioma samples." McLaren found SV 40 in Australian mesothelioma tissue:

> "We examined five human mesothelioma cell lines that were established in our laboratories. In addition, we examined several tumour biopsies from seven different patients. SV40 like sequences were present in all the cell lines and in at least one sample from each of the patients examined. CONCLUSIONS: The large T antigen of SV40 or an SV40 like virus is expressed in Australian mesotheliomas and therefore could be aetiologically-associated with tumourigenesis."

Results have not been uniform—"a study in 1996 and a presentation made at the International Mesothelioma Interest Group, IMIG in 1997 failed to detect SV40 in mesotheliomas." Klein (5). This has prompted some discussion of the pathological techniques to ascertain the presence of SV40.

We studied tissue sections from 18 paraffin embedded mesothelioma specimens diagnosed by the Pathology Department of S. Chiara Hospital of Pisa. Using PCR analysis and Southern blot hybridization we examined the specimens for the DNA regulatory region of the virus. 10/18 (55.5%) of the samples tested contained SV40 DNA regulatory sequences, and of these positive samples, 80% were found to contain Tag sequences by PCR and Southern Blot hybridization. These results confirm that SV40 can be amplified and detected in paraffin embedded mesothelioma samples.

28.62 Relationship to Prognosis

McLaren found that levels of SV 40 were a negative factor in length of survival of mesothelioma patients indicating that the drug played a role in the pathogenesis of the disease.

28.63 SV 40 and Tumor Suppressor Genes

At its simplest level, cancer arises from the triggering of a growth factor and the inactivation of a tumor suppressor gene which would normally act as a brake. P53 is the most well-known tumor suppressor gene with its absence or mutation playing a role in many cancers. P53 may trigger apoptosis or cell death of genes with abnormalities, and otherwise inhibit or stop the abnormal reproduction which is cancer. In this delicate and complex system, SV 40 triggers Tag which, in turn, may frustrate the normal functioning of tumor suppressor genes.

"The simian virus 40 (SV40) oncoprotein large T antigen (Tag) plays a crucial role in the transformation of human cells and causes cell-cycle derangement of human mesothelial cells (HMC). The effects of Tag are caused by its ability to bind the tumor suppressor gene products p53 and retinoblastoma family (Rb)proteins." Thus SV 40 is an anti-tumor suppressor gene.

28.64 Significance of P 53 and Rb in Mesothelioma Continues to be Debated

P53 and RB are genes commonly associated with the development of various cancers including non-small cell lung cancer. Boccheta writes, "p53 plays an important role in down-regulating the replication of SV40 genomes in infected HM and in preventing HM lysis." (1). However, some suggest that the significance of P53 and RB are unclear in mesothelioma. See Waheed 12. ("These neoplasms are unique in that they rarely if ever exhibit Rb and p53 mutations, which frequently disrupt G_1 restriction point control in thoracic malignancies; these observations suggest that growth constraints mediated by these tumor suppressor genes are circumvented by mechanisms more subtle than those typically observed in solid tumors.")

28.641 Animal Studies of SV 40

Bocchetta writes, "SV40 is highly oncogenic in rodents. We found that intracardial injection of SV40 induced MM (malignant mesothelioma) in 60% of hamsters, whereas intrapleural injection caused 100% incidence of MM in 3-7 months." Bocchetta (1). "Rat pleural mesothelioma cells expressing SV40 T exhibit disrupted cell cycle progression, abnormal mitoses, and aneuploidy." Waheed.

28.65 SV 40 and Growth Factors

28.651 Vascular Endothelial Growth Factor

Vascular Endothelial Growth Factor or VEGF is associated with the spread of lung and other cancers. Recent studies have identified a connection between VEGF and SV 40.

"Vascular endothelial growth factor (VEGF), an important angiogenic factor, regulates cell proliferation, differentiation, and apoptosis (programmend cell death) through activation of its tyrosine-kinase receptors, such as Flt-1 and Flk-1/Kdr. Human malignant mesothelioma cells (HMC), which have wild-type p53, express VEGF and exhibit cell growth increased by VEGF. Here, we demonstrate that early transforming proteins of simian virus (SV) 40, large tumor antigen (Tag) and small tumor antigen (tag), which have been associated with mesotheliomas, enhanced HMC proliferation by inducing VEGF expression. SV40-Tag expression potently increased VEGF protein and mRNA levels in several HMC lines." Catalano (2).

28.652 Hepatocyte Growth Factor

While the association between VEGF and cancer metastasis is well-known and documented, recent research discovered a connection with a lesser known growth factor.

> "Recent studies suggested that simian virus 40 (SV40) may cause malignant mesothelioma, although the pathogenic mechanism is unclear. We found that in SV40-positive malignant mesothelioma cells, the hepatocyte growth factor (HGF) receptor (Met) was activated."

28.66 Teleromerase

Imagine cutting one inch off a 10 inch stick, ultimately the stick would disappear. Each cell has a predetermined number of divisions and a certain size so that divisions must end. Something called teleromerase allows the cells to evade these predetermined restrictions and is associated with cancer. One study found SV-40 A induced telomerase activity in primary human mesothelial cells. Foddis (4).

28.67 Asbestos and SV 40

Asbestos is the chief cause of mesothelioma. What is the connection between asbestos and SV 40? One hypothesis, "Asbestos appears to increase SV40-mediated transformation of human mesothelial cells in vitro, suggesting that asbestos and SV40 may be cocarcinogens." Carbone (3). The cocarcinogen hypothesis is consistent with the long latency of mesothelioma, making it likely that multiple carcinogens are needed for cancer transformation. Since only a portion of those exposed contract lung cancer, it makes sense that a genetic weakness is a contributing factor in the disease. "The role of asbestos in causing MM has been firmly established epidemiologically; however, it has been difficult to reconcile the epidemiological findings with the inability of asbestos to transform mesothelial cells in tissue culture." Bocchetto (1).

Here is a similar theory:

> "Mesothelioma, a malignancy associated with asbestos, has been recently linked to simian virus 40 (SV40). e found that

infection of human mesothelial cells by SV40 is very different from the semipermissive infection thought to be characteristic of human cells. Mesothelial cells are uniformly infected but not lysed by SV40, a mechanism related to p53, and undergo cell transformation at an extremely high rate. Exposure of mesothelial cells to asbestos complemented SV40 mutants in transformation. Our data provide a mechanistic explanation for the ability of SV40 to transform mesothelial cells preferentially and indicate that asbestos and SV40 may be cocarcinogens." Boccheto (1).

28.68 SV 40 Treatment Options

Determining that a particular gene, enzyme, or growth factor plays a role in the creation or spread of disease is only the first step in crafting a cure or remedy. One must determine if the damage can be corrected, create a delivery system for an anti-virus or other suppressant, and determine that the new drug carries no untoward side effects.

28.681 Vaccine

One possibility is a vaccine:

"The identification of SV40 as a possible cause of human cancer leads to the question of whether the unique properties of the virus can be exploited to treat patients with SV40-positive mesotheliomas, which are otherwise refractory to successful intervention. A modified SV40 T antigen, from which the transforming domains have been removed, has been cloned into a vaccinia virus vector and tested in animal tumor model systems. It has been shown to be effective against both subsequent tumor challenge and pre-existing tumors. Thus, the potential exists for use of such a vaccine in mesothelioma patients."

Another writer reports success in cell studies:

"An adenoviral vector expressing an antisense transcript to SV40 early region inhibited T antigen expression and mediated significant growth inhibition and apoptosis in T-antigen-positive mesothelioma cells and SV40-transformed COS-7 cells.

Abrogation of T/t antigen expression coincided with enhanced p21/WAF-1 expression, suggesting that restoration of p53-mediated pathways may have contributed to the growth inhibition and apoptosis induced by the antisense construct. These effects were not observed after similar treatment of mesothelioma or lung cancer cells containing no SV40 DNA sequences. Collectively, these data suggest that SV40 oncoproteins contribute to the malignant phenotype of pleural mesotheliomas and indicate that interventions designed to abrogate their expression may be efficacious in the treatment of individuals with these neoplasms."

28.682 Why Isn't More Money Spent Searching for a Cure for Mesothelioma?

The Waheed study was done in 1999; why aren't we close to a clinical trial of an SV40 anti-virus? While millions, indeed, billions have been spent on litigating asbestos mesothelioma cases, a far lesser amount has been spent on research on this disease. Given the relatively small number of people with mesothelioma, a drug which addressed the disease might not be as profitable as drugs which attacked more prevalent diseases. One hopes that additional public pressure will prompt needed research.

28.683 Assessing SV 40 Values and Treatment

Instinctively, one might ask if patients should be tested for SV 40 and those testing positive should receive targeted treatment. Some analogous issues are presented with the drug Iressa, which targets the epidermal growth factor, related to the development and spread of lung cancer. While the drug targets the epidermal growth factor receptor, treatments are not discriminating based on levels of that growth factor.

28.684 P16 Tumor Supressor Gene

P16ink4a is a lesser known tumor suppressor gene which seemingly plays a greater role in mesothelioma. "Examination of p16^{INK4a} was suggested by the frequent loss of the chromosome 9p region encoding p16^{INK4a} and p14^{ARF} in primary mesothelioma and in mesothelioma cell lines, as well as the association of p16^{INK4a} loss or methylation with extension of lifespan in culture."

SV 40 SECTION REFERENCES

1. Bocchetta, *Human mesothelial cells are unusually susceptible to simian virus 40-mediated transformation and asbestos cocarcinogenicity*, Proc Natl Acad Sci U S A 2000 Aug 29;97(18):10214-9.
2. Catalano, *Enhanced expression of vascular endothelial growth factor (VEGF) plays a critical role in the tumor progression potential induced by simian virus 40 large T antigen*, Oncogene 2002 Apr 25;21(18):2896-900.
3. Carbone, *The pathogenesis of mesothelioma*, Semin Oncol 2002 Feb;29(1):2-17.
4. Foddis, *SV40 infection induces telomerase activity in human mesothelial cells*, Oncogene 2002 Feb 21;21(9):1434-42.
5. Klein, *Association of SV40 with human tumors*, Oncogene 2002 Feb 14;21(8):1141-9.
6. Caccioti, *SV40 replication in human mesothelial cells induces HGF/Met receptor activation: a model for viral-related carcinogenesis of human malignant mesothelioma*, Proc Natl Acad Sci U S A 2001 Oct 9;98.
7. McLaren, *Simian virus (SV) 40 like sequences in cell lines and tumour biopsies from Australian malignant mesotheliomas*, Aust N Z J Med 2000 Aug;30(4):450-6.
8. Procopio, *Simian virus-40 sequences are a negative prognostic cofactor in patients with malignant pleural mesothelioma*, Genes Chromosomes Cancer 2000 Oct;29(2):173-9.
9. Stearly, The Forty Year Legacy of Tainted Polio Vaccine, www.ioa.com/~dragonfly/vaccine2.html.
10. Cristaudo, SV40 can be reproducibly detected in paraffin-embedded mesothelioma samples, Anticancer Res 2000 Mar-Apr;20(2A):895-8.
11. Imperiale, Prospects for an SV40 vaccine, Semin Cancer Biol 2001 Feb;11(1):81-5.
12. Waheed, Antisense to SV40 early gene region induces growth

arrest and apoptosis in T-antigen-positive human pleural mesothelioma cells, Cancer Res 1999 Dec 15;59(24):6068-73.

13. Lixin, Asbestos induction of extended lifespan in normal human mesothelial cells: interindividual susceptibility and SV40 T antigen, Carcinogenesis, Vol. 20, No. 5, 773-783, May 1999.

14. Cristaudo, *SV40 Enhances the Risk of Malignant Mesothelioma among People Exposed to Asbestos: A Molecular Epidemiologic Case-Control Study*, Cancer Res. 2005 Apr 15;65(8):3049-52

OTHER REFERENCES

1. Monnert, *Intrapleural Infusion of Activated Macrophages and— Interferon in Malignant Pleural Mesothelioma*, Chest. 2002;121:1921-1927.

2. Goey, *Intrapleural administration of interleukin 2 in pleural mesothelioma: a phase I-II study*, Br J Cancer 1995 Nov;72(5):1283-8.

3. Hand, *Interferon (IFN)-alpha and IFN-gamma in combination with methotrexate: in vitro sensitivity studies in four human mesothelioma cell lines*, Anticancer Drugs 1995 Feb;6(1):77-82

4. Boutin, *Intrapleural treatment with recombinant gamma-interferon in early stage malignant pleural mesothelioma.* Cancer 1994 Nov 1;74(9):2460-7.

6. OReilly, *A phase II trial of Interferon Alpha-2a and Carboplatin in patients with Advanced Malignant Mesothelioma.* Cancer Invest, 1999, 17:3, 195-200.

7. Astoul, *Intrapleural administration of interleukin-2 for the treatment of patients with malignant pleural mesothelioma: a Phase II study*, Cancer 1098 Nov, 83:10, 2099-104.

8. Amodio, *Gemcitabine in peritoneal mesothelioma: a case report*] Clin Ter, 1998 Nov, 149:6, 447-51.

9. Nakano, *Cisplatin in combination with irinotecan in the treatment of patients with malignant pleural mesothelioma: a pilot phase II clinical trial and pharmacokinetic profile.* Cancer, 1999, Jun, 85:11, 2375-84.

10. Porohit, *Weekly systemic Combination of Cisplatin and Interferon Alpha 2a in Diffuse Malignant Pleural Mesothelioma*, Lung Cancer, 1998, Nov. 22.:2, 119-25.

11. Ryan & Vogelzang, *A Review of Chemotherapy trials for Malignant Mesothelioma*, Chest, 1998, Jan. 113:1, Supp. 66s-73s."

12. Ardizzoni, *Systemic Drug Therapy of Malignant Pleural Mesothelioma*, Monaldi Arch Chest Dis, 1998 Apr, 53:2, 236-40.

13. Astra-Zeneca publishers of Signal, a medical journal devoted to epidermal growth factor research.

14. Metitinas, *Cisplatin, Mitomycin, and Interferon-alpha2a combination chemoimmunotherapy in the treatment of diffuse malignant pleural mesothelioma*. Chest, 19922.66.

15. Manning, *A Mutant Epidermal Growth Factor Receptor Targeted to Lung Epithelium Inhibits Asbestos-induced Proliferation and Proto-Oncogene Expression. Cancer Res*, 2002 Aug 1;62(15):4169-75.

16. Manning. *Human Mesothelioma Samples Overexpress Both Cyclooxygenase-2 (COX-2) and Inducible Nitric Oxide Synthase (NOS2): In Vitro Antiproliferative Effects of a COX-2 Inhibitor*, Cancer Research 60, 3696-3700, July 15, 2000.

17. Edwards, *Cyclooxygenase-2 Expression Is a Novel Prognostic Factor in Malignant Mesothelioma*, Clinical Cancer Research Vol. 8, 1857-1862, June 2002.

18. Rubins, Lovastatin Induces Apoptosis in Malignant Mesothelioma Cells, Am. J. Respir. Crit. Care Med., Volume 157, Number 5, May 1998, 1616-1622.

19. Delong, *Use of cyclooxygenase-2 inhibition to enhance the efficacy of immunotherapy*, Cancer Res. 2003 Nov 15;63(22):7845-52.

CHAPTER 29

NON-SMOKER'S LUNG CANCER

29.1 CHARACTERSTICS AND DISTINGUISHING FEATURES

While lung cancer is mostly associated with smoking, an estimated 10% of cancer patients have no smoking history. Recent studies have shown their disease may have some unusual characteristics, mandating some differences in treatment.

29.11 Areas of Genetic Damage

Initial research indicates many non-smokers with lung cancer have damage to the tyrosine kinase area of the epidermal growth factor receptor. Several studies have found this area of damage in non-smokers and very light former smokers while few smokers have this area of damage. Lynch (1). Non-smokers lung cancer may be characterized by fewer areas of genetic damages and be easier to treat. Rather than the multiple areas of damage to growth factors and tumor suppressor genes, we may have only a few areas which when accurately identified, can be treated.

29.12 Adenocarcinoma and Bronchioloalveolar Lung Cancer

These non-smokers generally have adenocarcinoma and bronchioloalveolar lung cancer (BAC), and Iressa is discussed in the separate chapter on epidermal growth factor inhibitors.

29.13 Iressa and Epidermal Growth Factor Inhibitors

Iressa suppresses chemical reactions leading to cancerous signaling at the tyrosine kinase part of the epidermal growth factor receptor. As such, it is a drug designed for the BAC or adenocarcinoma egfr tyrosine kinase driven lung cancer many non-smokers have. "Patients with nonBsmall-cell lung cancer who had striking responses to gefitinib had somatic mutations in the *EGFR* gene that would indicate the essential role of the EGFR signaling pathway in the tumor." Lynch (1). Many of the responders to Iressa are nonsmokers with BAC or adenocarcinoma.

29.14 Implications for Treatment

Smoking history should be a part of medical history and be considered in formulating treatment plans. We are at the point of contouring treatment plans depending upon the type of disease, smoking history, cell studies, and other factors.

29.15 Brain Metastases and Iressa

Some recent studies have suggested that Iressa alone can provide relief to nsclc patients with cranial metastases. Ishida (5). One study testing Iressa reported, AA disease control rate of 46% (objective response rate 8.7%) and 1-year survival of 29% were documented. Histology (adenocarcinoma) and a "never-smoking" history were predictive of response. A Iressa is being tested as first line treatment, with chemotherapy, or after chemotherapy for patients with cranial metastases.

REFERENCES

1. Lynch, *Activating Mutations in the Epidermal Growth Factor Receptor Underlying Responsiveness of NonBSmall-Cell Lung Cancer to Gefitinib*, Volume 350:2129-2139, May 20, 2004 (full text available online).
2. Miller, *Bronchioloalveolar pathologic subtype and smoking history predict sensitivity to gefitinib in advanced non-small-cell lung cancer*, J Clin Oncol. 2004 Mar 15;22(6):1103-9.

3. Chang, *Successful treatment of multifocal bronchioloalveolar cell carcinoma with ZD1839 (Iressa) in two patients*, J Formos Med Assoc. 2003 Jun;102(6):407-11.

4. Pao, *EGF receptor gene mutations are common in lung cancers from "never smokers" and are associated with sensitivity of tumors to gefitinib and erlotinib*, Proceeding National Academy of Science, NAS September 7, 2004, vol. 101, no. 36 13306-13311. www,pnas.org.

5. Ishida, *Gefitinib as a first line of therapy in non-small cell lung cancer with brain metastases*, Intern Med. 2004 Aug;43(8):718-20

6. Haringhuizen, *Gefitinib as a last treatment option for non-small-cell lung cancer: durable disease control in a subset of patients*, Ann Oncol. 2004 May;15(5):786-92.

CHAPTER 30

HEALTH INSURANCE ISSUES

30.1 A HEALTH INSURANCE POLICY IS A CONTRACT

Under American law, two parties can agree to pay for a service or enter into any other contract. Under extreme circumstance, an agreement can be said to be so unfair as to be unconscionable, or be unenforceable because it involves illegal conduct or conduct which offends public policy. However, in most contract cases including those involving health insurance, the court's task is to determine what was intended, first by looking at the written agreement. "It is the duty of the courts to enforce an insurance policy as it is written, and the courts are not at liberty to rewrite policies of insurance to provide coverage where no coverage was intended. Likewise, we are not at liberty to rewrite an insurance policy simply because we do not favor its terms or because its provisions produce harsh results. In the absence of fraud, overreaching or unconscionability, the courts must give effect to an insurance policy if its language is clear and its intent certain." Black v. Aetna Ins (1).

Thus, the first task for any patient or family member is to assemble the relevant papers and to review what the health care agreement and the plan itself provides. The chief areas of dispute are as follows:

1. Is the treatment medically necessary and therefore should the health care provider be required to pay for it?
2. May the patient choose a hospital or physician?

30.2 WHAT IS MEDICALLY NECESSARY?

The health care policy typically states that the provider will reimburse for what is medically necessary.

30.21 Consider and Evaluate What the HMO says, Though You Do Not Have to Accept It

In some cases, HMO's act unreasonably and for their own financial interests. Sometimes however, a patient may fail to understand medicine or the nature of the HMO. Initially, the HMO does not have to refer you to the physician or hospital that you would like or prefer. They do not have to provide the best care, only acceptable care with the standard of care of the particular specialty or area. The very nature of the HMO is to achieve cost savings through negotiation and centralization of certain tasks. Thus, if the HMO has retained qualified hospital A to provide certain treatment, you may not simply opt for hospital B because you like it better, even if there is evidence that B is a better hospital.

30.22 Change of Hospital

You do have a right to select a hospital, or more accurately participate in the selection process, if the particular physician or hospital is not as well-equipped to perform a task as your own. Thus you would need to demonstrate their selection's lack of, at least lesser qualification as compared with your choice.

30.23 Defining What is Medically Necessary

Let us look at three examples of HMO problems, noting that the approach to each will be different:

1. John Smith has stage 4 lung cancer. The doctor has prescribed an FDA approved medication to relieve pain which while

effective is very expensive. The HMO has delayed providing the appropriate approvals.

2. After being given a negative prognosis from the treating oncologist, the Smith family decides that the approach which has the best chance of cure is an innovative approach being taken by a physician located in Los Cacos, Mexico. There are reports on the Internet of exceptional results, though the procedure is not FDA approved.

3. United States physicians have experimented with a new drug in clinical trials though the FDA has not yet approved same.

The HMO's delay in 1 is wrong and a breach of its contract. Relief of pain is a legitimate medical objective, and the patient or his family should be assertive in vindicating the patient's rights. The HMO's refusal to approve 2 is correct and lawful. The treatment is unproven, and the HMO contract likely precludes experimental treatments. 3 is similar and there is usually no enforceable right to experimental treatment. In a few circumstances with support from the patient's physician, the patient can convince a court that the treatment is needed and medically appropriate.

30.3 BE ASSERTIVE BUT KNOW AND FOLLOW YOUR CONTRACT

Assuming the HMO is acting unreasonably, as a lawyer, one sees a somewhat strange phenomenon in how people approach the legal system. You may see a client send four letters and file a formal complaint over damage to a $121.00 dress. In a divorce, two combatants may spend hours arguing over the disposition of a piece of furniture or a lamp. Yet sometimes people with real concerns, and family members of those with cancer are strangely passive. Certainly, if you believe a particular type of treatment is necessary, you should be aggressive in demanding. Document your concerns in a letter.

30.31 Make Sure that Necessary Papers Have, In Fact, Been Submitted by Your Physician

In some cases HMO's delay things, but in others their requests for information or supporting documentation are ignored. Certainly it is irritating for a well-regarded oncologist to spend hours each week justifying a decision he made to a junior clerk at an HMO, but it must be done. In example 1 above, an expensive pain-reliever, an HMO auditor may ask why a less-expensive drug could not be substituted, and ask the doctor as a participating physician to provide information supporting his decision. Generally, the doctor must provide information reasonably requested and pertinent to the treatment decision. As a patient, you may need to check that your anger is properly directed towards the HMO, and not a doctor who neglected to supply information the HMO requested.

30.32 Your Contract and Appeal Procedures

Most HMO contracts provide for a specified appeal procedure. If you go to court, many judges will require you to first exhaust the contractual procedures before seeking the court's assistance. Get your contract, read it, understand your procedures, and follow them. If you believe you are right, continue to appeal.

30.4 ITEMS TO INCLUDE IN AN HMO LETTER

Assuming you believe the HMO is at fault, a letter to them should outline the following:

1. The treatment which is needed, and has been rejected,
2. The medical justification for the treatment, attaching your physician's letter of explanation, and any medical studies or other data you have located,
3. A statement that the plan member will suffer severe and irreparable physical injury as a result of the delay in treatment, and noting that such injury may have already occurred because of the HMO's delay, and
4. Noting that you are contacting an attorney to institute legal action as a result of the HMO's willful and deliberate disregard of the patient's health and well-being, and expect to institute legal action against the responsible individuals as well as the plan itself.

Consider placing particular responsibility upon the particular person who rejected the treatment. You should fight, and in most cases you will win. From an health insurer's point of view, they may want to limit certain types of health care costs, but will alter their position if the possibility of legal or other exposure exists. There have been several large verdicts against HMO's.

30.5 WHOM TO CONTACT WHEN YOU HAVE AN HMO PROBLEM

If an HMO fails to authorize treatment which you believe is medically justified, you could write to the following:

1. The HMO case manager,
2. His or her supervisor,
3. The state insurance commission who deals with health care issues,
4. The central office of the health insurer,
5. Members of the board of directors of the HMO,
6. Your local newspaper or radio station,
7. State assemblyman or representative, and/or
8. An Internet website dealing with this issue.

Generally form letters and copies receive less attention than the original. If you want action, address your correspondence to each of the above. Letters should be direct but brief. No letter should be longer than a page, but do include some brief documentation supporting your position.

30.6 LEGAL ACTION

If an HMO refuses to authorize necessary treatment, you can contact an attorney to file a lawsuit. A lawsuit or claim is usually initiated by filing a complaint with the court which identifies the litigants, what the defendant has done wrong and why, and how the plaintiff has or will be injured by that wrong. While it is preferable to have an attorney representing you, set forth below is a form of complaint designed for use by an individual representing himself.

ROBERT PATIENT

Plaintiff

SUPERIOR COURT OF NEW JERSEY
ESSEX COUNTY—LAW DIVISION

vs

Civil Action

INSURANCE COMPANY,

Defendant

COMPLAINT AND JURY DEMAND
Docket No.

COUNT ONE (BREACH OF CONTRACT)

1. Plaintiff resides at 43 Spring Street, Maplewood, New Jersey. Defendant is a health maintenance organization (HMO) licensed by the State of New Jersey, with offices at 40 Broad Street, Newark, New Jersey.

2. Under a contract with the Defendant, Plaintiff is entitled to medical and hospital treatment with the costs of such services to be paid by the HMO.

3. Plaintiff has lung cancer. On July 23, 1999, Plaintiff's physician recommended hospitalization to provide relief from pain associated with plaintiff's cancer. Such recommendation was reasonable and necessary for treatment of Plaintiff's condition.

4. Defendant HMO has failed to approve reimbursement to the appropriate medical and hospital providers for such treatment despite oral and written requests from Plaintiff and his physician.

5. As a result, Plaintiff has been denied medically necessary treatment. More particularly, as a result, Plaintiff has suffered substantial pain and his medical condition has deteriorated as a result of the defendant HMO'S willful and deliberate refusal to perform its contractual obligations.

6. Plaintiff believes and therefore alleges, that defendant has constructed procedures to deprive plaintiff and others of the medical treatment to which they are entitled for the purpose of reducing its costs. Furthermore, Defendant HMO has concealed and misstated its reasons for denying treatment to delay and

frustrate Plaintiff and his physicians from arranging for required medical services. The above conduct violates the terms of the Plaintiff's insurance contract, insurance statutes and other applicable law.

WHEREAS, Plaintiff demands judgment against Defendant for compensation damages, punitive damages, and injunction requiring Defendant to perform its contract and restraining it from further violating applicable insurance claims.

JURY DEMAND
Plaintiff requests a trial by jury.
Dated: July 5, 2003

_____

Robert Patient

30.61 Comment on the Form of Complaint

This is based on New Jersey practice; practices vary from state to state. Generally, what a complaint does is explain who the Plaintiff and Defendant are where they are located, what the Defendant did wrong, how the Plaintiff was injured by the Defendant's acts, and what Plaintiff is seeking.

File the complaint with the court with the necessary filing fee, get a docket number or a copy of the complaint marked "filed", and serve that complaint on the Defendant. You can ask a local process-server or subpoena service to serve or hand deliver the complaint to the HMO.

You may wish to send the accompanying Letter to the Defendant:

Enclosed please find a copy of the complaint which I have filed with the Superior Court. I confirm that as of this date, you have not authorized the treatment which I need. If this changes, please immediately call me and my physicians. If you have any questions regarding this Complaint, you may call me directly at 973-467-8040 though I may be retaining counsel shortly.

30.7 COURT DECISIONS

One federal court rejected a proposal for high-dose chemotherapy with stem cell transplants for a small cell lung cancer patient:

"The court finds that the evidence establishes that HDC/
PSCR [high-dose chemotherapy with peripheral stem cell rescue]
for small cell lung cancer is an experimental or investigational
rather than an accepted standard of practice. The protocol, the
consent form, the medical evidence received each described the
procedure in terms which emphasized its experimental or
investigational nature. The purpose for which the plaintiff is
being treated is to either cure or give him relief from his condition
or prolong his life, and in utilizing HDC/PSCR, there is no evidence
to this point that that will be accomplished."

"The court also found that the treatment was not medically
necessary as defined by the policy since the "efficacy of this
procedure is undetermined, and it is not possible to know
whether the procedure could be omitted without adversely
affecting plaintiff's condition or the quality of medical care."
Hendricks (2).

There is a tendency to paint the HMO as a heartless bureaucrat
denying patients needed therapy to save money. However, the therapy
that was proposed never became standard (chemotherapy with stem cell
rescue) and there was no medical basis for a court or an HMO to believe
that it would extend life. While on a humanitarian basis one would like
to give a patient and his physician the right to select the treatment they
deem best, that is not the HMO's role. Instead the HMO need only
provide reimbursement for treatments with demonstrable validity, leaving
the patient to pay for unusual and unverifiable experimental treatments
from his own pocket.

REFERENCES

1. Black v. Aetna Ins. Co., 909 S.W.2d 1, 3 (Tenn. App. 1995).
2. Hendricks v. Central Reserve Life Insurance Co., 39 F.3d 507, (4th Cir. 1994).

CHAPTER 31

SYMPTOMS AND DIAGNOSIS OF LUNG CANCER

31.1 SYMPTOMS OF LUNG CANCER

The primary symptoms of lung cancer are chest pain, dyspnea, loss of breath, fatigue, loss of weight. Lung cancer should be suspected in any smoker with new or worsening respiratory symptoms including hemoptysis (spitting up blood), or indication of systemic illness such as loss of energy, appetite, or weight. Here is an outline from Devita's leading text, Cancer, Principles and Practice Of Oncology:

Symptoms secondary to central or endobronchial growth of the primary tumor include:

1. Cough,
2. Hemoptysis (spitting up blood),
3. Wheeze and stridor,
4. Dyspnea (shortness of breath or difficulty breathing), and
5. Pneumonitis from obstruction (fever, productive cough).

Symptoms secondary to peripheral growth of the primary tumor include:

1. Pain from pleural or chest wall involvement,
2. Cough,
3. Dyspnea on a restrictive basis, and
4. Lung Abscess syndrome (1).

Small cell cancer has similar symptomology: "The main symptoms of SCLC are similar to those of other lung cancers and include cough, hemoptysis, chest pain, obstructive dyspnea, or signs secondary to pneumonitis. Uncommon but more specific to SCLC are the manifestations of paraneoplastic syndromes such as Cushing's or Eaton-Lambert or inappropriate secretion of antidiuretic hormone." (2) Textbook of Oncology.

Here is a similar summary:

"In later stages, lung cancer may give one or more of the following symptoms: **Cough**—people who smoke and already have a chronic smoker's cough often report a change in the nature of the cough. Bloody cough (hemoptysis) is a major warning sign and should never be ignored. **Wheezing**/Shortness of Breath—smokers may already have emphysema which may cause wheezing and shortness of breath. However, a tumor which causes blockage of a breathing passage may bring these symptoms on more acutely. Pneumonia Symptoms—such as fever with phlegm-producing couch which does not clear with antibiotic treatment may be an indication of a lung cancer. **Fatigue**—and loss of endurance with routine activities may be a consequence of lung cancer. **Pain**—in the chest may be caused by lung cancer which has spread into the lining of the lung or chest wall; pain in the back or ribs may be indicative of cancer which has spread to bones. Hoarseness—may be a sign of lung cancer which has affected the recurrent laryngeal nerve (the nerve which controls the movement of the vocal cords). **Weight Loss**—for reasons which are not well understood, lung cancer, especially in advanced stages, may cause a person to lose weight. Headache and Other Neurologic Signs—may be caused by cancer which has spread to the brain and nervous system." www.infolane.com/pamp/lungcncr/lungcncr.html, Care Sheet for Lung Cancer.

31.2 WHY LATE DIAGNOSIS IS SO COMMON

In between 60 and 80% cases, lung cancer is diagnosed at an advanced stage. Timely diagnosis is the exception. Why? We can identify several reasons.

31.21 Non-Specificity of Symptoms

The physician's job is not easy; virtually all of these syndromes are nonspecific, that is, they can indicate another disease, and many are already a part of the smoker's life. Shortness of breath, loss of breathing capacity, and perhaps periodic chest discomfort are the usual lot of the smoker.

A doctor may check lungs with a stethoscope or order routine blood work, neither of which will reveal a lung tumor. As we noted earlier, lung cancer screening for smokers is not standard practice. The difficulty of promptly diagnosing cancer based upon the patient's complaints alone, and the critical importance of that task, are again reasons for testing all smokers and aggressive use of available diagnostic tools.

31.22 Difficulties in Predicting in Seeing the Course of Disease

One would think the natural course of a tumor is to enlarge and spread. Yet, scientists have shown there may be necrosis, cell death, and the progress can vary. Thus, symptoms can be alleviated, patients can feel better, all of which may serve to confuse the physician and delay diagnosis. Some male patients may not return to a physicians, or their visits again may not correlate with what one would think to be the ordinary course of the disease. Sometimes symptoms specific to the lung manifest themselves at a late stage.

31.23 Late Arrival of Serious Symptoms

Pain in the lung area or breathing problems may be evident only after the tumor has spread.

31.3 SOLUTIONS TO THE DIAGNOSIS PROBLEM

31.31 Early Detection Tools like Ct Scan

All these problems indicate an aggressive approach is appropriate. We have already discussed screening, that is, the use of diagnostic tools for patients at high risk who do not display symptoms.

31.32 Aggressive Intervention

A closely related approach is using Ct Scan whenever some abnormality potentially indicative of cancer is shown. Today many physicians wait for the classical symptoms to display themselves. In contrast, an aggressive approach might be to utilize Ct Scan or other tools whenever smokers display even one symptom or sign such as fatigue, weight loss, chest pain, or persistent cough.

Cancer is a product of many genetic abnormalities and changes which occur over a period of years. The ideal approach would be to intervene before a tumor develops. Genetic screening which tells smokers that some abnormalities have developed may induce some smokers to quit.

REFERENCES

1. Devita, Cancer Principles and Practice of Oncology, 607 (3d Ed. 1989).
2. Aisner, Comprehensive Textbook of Thoracic Oncology 459 (Williams & Wilkins 1996).

CHAPTER 32

SCREENING AND EARLY DETECTION OF LUNG CANCER

32.1 WHY MOST LUNG CANCERS ARE DETECTED AT ADVANCED STAGES

The diffuse nature of lung cancer symptoms together with the pattern of delayed detection has made screening an important topic. Sadly, most lung cancers are diagnosed late, when the cancer has infiltrated significant organs and created pain, difficult breathing, and other symptoms. "Unfortunately, by the time a sign, symptom, or visible nodule appears, dissemination to regional or distant lymph nodes or distant extra nodal sites usually has occurred." Devita (1)

"In its early stages, lung cancer is asymptomatic. The lung parenchyma is not generously supplied with pain fibers, and primary lung cancers can reach considerable size without causing any symptoms. This lack of symptoms is particularly true for more peripheral lesions. Less than 5% of lung cancers are discovered in patients who have no symptoms of the disease." Pass (10).

32.11 There is No Program of Early Diagnosis of Lung Cancer in the United States

Given the attention paid to lung cancer, one would expect an impressive program of early detection. Lung cancer is the largest cause of cancer death in the United States and the second overall. In its earliest stages, lung cancer is treatable through surgery, with stage 1 patients having 5 year survival rates approximating 70%. One could assume early detection programs would compliment anti-smoking programs, reinforcing the potential hazards of the tobacco but providing timely early treatment for those at risk. That assumption would be wrong.

We do not in this country routinely check smokers for signs of lung cancer, nor is there any organized program to detect lung cancer in its earliest and most treatable stages. Thus well over 60% of lung cancers are diagnosed late, when the cancers are at advanced stages having spread to lymph nodes or other organs and medical science is least able to treat them.

32.12 Comparison with Early Diagnostic Programs for Other Cancers

One of nine women contract breast cancer, and yearly mammograms for women over 40 helps detect breast cancer in its earliest and treatable stages. PSA tests for prostate cancer help create an over 95% survival rate by insuring that prostate cancer is diagnosed in its earliest and most treatable stages. Pap smears for women are now part of exams for many women and also help provide timely detection of cervical cancer.

While approximately one in ten men and women who smoke will contract lung cancer there is no program of early diagnosis in the United States. With that said, why don't we institute a program for early diagnosis? Indeed, lung cancer kills more women each year than breast and cervical cancer combined, each of which have sensible early detection programs in place to improve survival and qualify of life. Preoccupied with telling smokers not to smoke, a laudable if difficult goal, we have ignored the equally important point of getting those at risk diagnosed at early and treatable stages.

32.2 WHY THERE IS NO PROGRAM OF EARLY DETECTION IN THE UNITED STATES

The explanations for a lack of early detection are, in my opinion, unpersuasive, though they merit examination. Basically the merit of any form of treatment must be established through testing. We learned in tenth grade biology that a hypothesis can be formed, but it must be confirmed through an actual experiment. In this case, the experiment is some type of examination of how two groups do, one with the treatment and the other without—in this case, with and without screening.

According to the National Cancer Institute, early detection programs have not established a significant improvement in patient survival; therefore it cannot be implemented as a reliable form of treatment. Here is a summary of two important studies:

"In the Johns Hopkins and Memorial Sloan Kettering Studies, patients in the screened group received chest radiographs annually and sputum cytology every 4 months, whereas the control group received only an annual chest radiograph. In the Mayo Clinic study, the screened group received a chest x-ray and sputum cytology every 4 months, where the control group received the standard Mayo advice of the time, consisting of an annual chest radiograph and annual sputum cytology, but without reminders to comply after the first visit . . . The conclusion from all three trials,; however, was that screening with chest radiography and sputum cytology was of no benefit in reducing lung cancer mortality. Despite lower stage at presentation, increased resectability, and an apparently higher 5 year survival rate in lung cancer patients in the screened group (35% in the screened group versus 15% for the control group), the cumulative lung cancer mortality and overall survival were the same for both screened and control populations in all three trials." Aisner (2).

Based on these studies, researchers conclude that screening does not save lives. Let us look at the errors in those findings.

32.21 The Critical Positive Findings of the Study Were Ignored

In the Mayo Clinic study, five year survival was higher in the intensively screened group. More importantly, both groups had appreciably *higher survival* rates than the general unscreened population. Both groups were essentially screened, one group receiving chest x-rays and sputum cytology, and the other instructions to see their physicians for an annual checkup and have a chest x-ray performed there. As one observer explains:

> "The Johns-Hopkins and Memorial Sloan Kettering randomized studies showed that addition of sputum cytology and more frequent chest films did not decrease mortality compared to annual chest films. The trials were not designed to evaluate chest films as such, and there was no control group that had no chest films. Charles Smart has pointed out that the 5-year survival rate for the men diagnosed in these studies was 35% in the study group and 25% in the "control" group, both far better than lung cancer patients not involved in a screening trial."

A reasonable interpretation of the study was that screening or annual chest-x-rays reduces mortality, with the only issue determining the optimum combination. Instead researchers concluded that screening did not save lives, a finding directly contrary to the study's findings regarding overall mortality in both groups.

32.22 The Difficulties of Performing a Clinical Trial with Healthy People

If we have two groups of cancer patients, both in poor health, we can ethically create a study to try one type of an experimental treatment on one group and compare it with the currently accepted mode of treatment. We cannot tell people at risk not to be seen by a doctor. That is one reason there was a small difference between the two groups, because the study authors could not create conditions which would deliberately endanger the control group.

32.221 An Example of the Same Type of Specious Reasoning

Pedestrian accidents for children is a serious problem. There is no study however showing that holding a child's arm while crossing the street saves lives or reduces injuries. A clinical trial is run at which one group holds the child's hand while crossing, and the other checks for cars and tells the child to be careful and look both ways. Results are the same with no accidents in either group. The study authors therefore conclude there is no clinical evidence that holding a child's hand while crossing reduces accidents or provides any ascertainable benefit, and cannot be recommended. The conclusion is obviously erroneous because precautions in both groups led to safety.

32.23 The Difference in Treatment Between Screened and Un-screened Was Not Tremendously Significant in the Mayo Clinic Study

In the Mayo Clinic study, one group received bi-annual screening with the other instructed to consult a physician each year, who might provide the same tests as the screened group. Not a significant difference. The problem is again to develop an effective, yet ethical clinical trial. We could have one group of heavy smokers given bi-yearly sputum cytology and chest x-rays while the other group is told not to undergo these tests for a five year period. Such a test would likely highlight differences in treatment but place the unscreened group at risk. Yet by not screening, we are essentially doing the same thing in overall treatment that we would hesitate to do in a test.

Thus, Japanese researchers have found some value in x-ray screening:

> "In Japan, a national mass program using chest x-rays was introduced for all residents over 40 years of age. Since the program was introduced, the 5-year survival rate has increased to 58%, as compared with 38% in the pre-screening period. The increase in 5 year survival rate was attributed to a 12% increase in the proportion of stage I cancers at diagnosis." Marshall (8).

32.24 Limits of X-Ray Screening

Even as we recognize that x-rays may extend lives by detecting lung cancer before it become symptomatic, we must also recognize its limitations. In one study chest x-rays were only able to detect 7 of 27 stage 1 tumors visible on Ct Scan. Henschke (3). Chest-x-rays are ineffective at detecting smaller, highly curable tumors. Thus, while it is clear that x-rays play some role in detecting lung cancer, its utility is limited, and its reliability in detecting small nodules questionable. Recent attention has focused on developed a more effective and sensitive method of detecting lung cancer.

32.3 CT SCREENING OF HEAVY SMOKERS

An important study screened present and former smokers using a special type of CT Scan. From the 1,000 asymptomatic participants, 27 tumors were seen, most small treatable stage 1 nodules. Hentscke (3). The results were excellent, with many lives saved by early detection of tumors and prompt surgery. Many including Alcase, the American cancer advocacy group, suggested Ct screening for heavy smokers and former smokers. With clinical proof, we hope that major cancer organizations like the American Cancer Society and the National Cancer Institute will recommend screening of those at risk.

32.31 Studies Finding CT Scan to be Effective in Diagnosing Lung Cancer

A Japanese study confirms the Cornell findings:

"From September 1993 to December 1998, 1669 individuals underwent a biannual screening program for lung carcinoma. The program included posteroanterior radiograph, sputum cytology, and low dose spiral CT . . . . A total of 9993 examinations were carried out . . . RESULTS: Peripheral lung carcinoma was detected in 31 of 9993 examinations (0.3%). Of the 31 cases, 24 tumors (77%) were detected by low dose spiral CT but were not visible on standard chest radiography. Twenty-two of the 24 tumors were Stage IA (T1N0M0, according to staging system revised in

1997). CONCLUSIONS: Low dose spiral CT shows promise for lung carcinoma screening." Computed tomography in Japan (5).

Another Japanese study concluded:

"Small peripheral lung cancers can be detected by spiral or helical computed tomography (CT). We applied mobile spiral CT as the first step in further examination (or secondary screening) for lung cancer. We detected 86 lung cancers per 100,000 persons without spiral CT, and 102 patients with spiral CT. Using the latter method, the resection rate and the rate of early-stage lung cancer increased significantly from 48.6% to 67.3% . . . Good results were obtained with mobile CT, especially in women. The mean tumor size of lung cancer detectable with CT was 7 mm smaller than that detected by the previous method . . . . Overall 787 lung cancers per 100,000 persons were detected using spiral CT for primary screening (1,039 lung cancers/100,000 in men)" Kusonoki (6).

32.32 The Interrelationship between CT Scans and Smoking Cessation

Many smokers unfortunately wait until a cancer is diagnosed to quit. A test which alerts them to the substantial dangers of smoking with respect to their own lungs may prompt many smokers to quit— "An unanticipated benefit of the screening was that many of the enrollees quit or decreased smoking after enrollment, and stated that the review of their CT images with the Elcap radiology, had prompted the change and provided the necessary focus for maintenance of their non-smoking behavior." Minnesota State Analysis (4).

32.4 OTHER TESTS

32.41 Sputum Cytology

Sputum cytology has been successful at detecting small centrally located squamous cell tumors, but less successful at detecting adenocarcinomas. Combining standard sputum cytology with sophisticated DNA testing for aberrations remains a possibility.

32.5 EARLY DETECTION AND HMO'S

When health maintenance organizations were created, there was a theory that would emphasize prevention as well as cure. That has not proven to be the case. Many HMO's resist early detection and screening, though they sometimes publicly say the opposite.

HMO's may reason that tests should be taken only where there is a demonstrated need. From the patient's perspective, all necessary tests should be taken where there is a possibility of this disease, since the consequence of delay may be a difference of life and death, or at least the time of survival. Doctors are caught in the middle. However, smokers and their families need to be far more vigilant in demanding follow up in situations where the disease is a possibility. Again, it is not smoking that causes lung cancer death; it is smoking combined with a delay in diagnosis.

32.6 WHAT YOU CAN DO

Consider the following:

1. **Create an effective anti-smoking program in your schools** which vividly explains the consequences of smoking. Have cancer patients come to schools to explain the consequences of their illness, and the pain they experience. Too many anti-smoking programs are boring recitals of numbers, figures, and medical terminology. Explain to students that the consequence of smoking can be pronounced suffering and even death at ages as young as 40, that about 1 in 10 smokers will contract lung cancer, and that we have no clear cure for advanced stage lung cancer, which is when most people are diagnosed.

2. **Write to the American Cancer Society** and the National Cancer Institute and suggest that they institute early detection program. Tell people about the recent study showing that CT Scans can detect cancer at early stages. Help save the lives of your friends and neighbors.

3. **Tell smokers** not only of the importance of quitting but **of the need for CT Scans**, chest-x-rays, sputum cytology and other diagnostic tools,

4. Ask your family physician and your HMO if they have early detection programs in place for high risk patients such as smokers, those exposed to heavy amounts of dust, and people with family histories of lung cancer.

5. Contact ALCASE, and other lung cancer advocacy groups to **lobby for more effective detection.**

33.61 Contacting the American Cancer Society

If you believe in early detection, consider writing a letter to your local American Cancer Society chapter as followup. Here are some points you may wish to include:

1. Lung cancer is the largest cause of cancer death in the United States for both men and women, with 170,000 people dying each year.

2. At stage 1, the treatment is generally easy and straightforward, a surgical resection. However, the more the cancer spreads, the harder the disease is to treat and cure. Thus, early detection is critical.

3. Unlikely other diseases whose cause is unknown, we know that smoking is the primary risk factor. Thus, it is easy to identify those persons primarily at risk.

4. The American Cancer Society contributes to the setting of standards in cancer treatment in the United States. Thus, if the organization advocated early detection, many hospitals and physicians would follow.

5. Telling people not to smoke, while important, is not a program of early detection. We must develop early detection programs along with anti-smoking programs. Indeed, it is the combination of smoking and delayed detection which is the most frequent cause of death for lung cancer.

6. Other countries are employing programs of early detection. Japan has a program which identified smokers with cancer at early staging leading to five year survival rates about 75% in one study.

7. A recent study in New York found excellent results with early detection and CT Scan. Groups like Alcase, the leading non-

profit group devoted to Lung Cancer, are recommending early detection programs. Early detection was recommended at the Cuneo World Lung Cancer conference in Italy in 1998.

You may get a form letter back or an invitation to participate in the chapter. Follow-up, be aggressive. While the ACS is an excellent organization which has helped many people, it clearly lags behind in this important area.

REFERENCES

1. Devita, *Cancer Principles and Practice of Oncology*, 607 (3d Ed. 1989).
2. Aisner, et. at., *Comprehensive Textbook of Thoracic Oncology* (Williams & Wilkins 1996).
3. Henschke. Et. al., *Early Lung Cancer Action Project: Overall Design and Findings from Baseline Screening*, Lancet (1999).
4. www.health.state.mn.us/htacctdr.htm Helical Computed Tomography (CT) for Lung Cancer Screening for Asymptomatic Patients."
5. *Computed tomography screening for lung carcinoma in Japan*, Cancer 2000 Dec 1;89(11 Suppl):2485-8.
6. Kusonoki, *Diagnosis of small peripheral lung cancers using spiral computed tomography lung cancer screening*, Nippon Geka Gakkai Zasshi 1999 Nov;100(11):705-11.
7. Dominioni, *Screening for Lung Cancer*, Chest Surg Clin N Am 2000 Nov;10(4):729-36.
8 Marshall, *Potential Cost-Effectiveness of One-Time Screening for Lung Cancer (LC) in a high risk Cohort*, Lung Cancer32 (2001) 227-236.
9. Editoria, *Lung Cancer Detection: A New Challenge for Irish Medicine*, Irish Medical Journal, February 2001, 94 num. 2.
10. Pass, et. al, Lung Cancer: Principles and Practice (Lippincott Williams & Wilkins 2000).

CHAPTER 33

EXPERIMENTAL AND OVERSEAS TREATMENTS FOR LUNG CANCER

33.1 DEFINING EXPERIMENTAL TREATMENT

Much of lung cancer treatment is uncertain since no established cure exists other than surgery for stage 1 patient which is about 70% successful. Chemotherapy is experimental in the sense that the precise mix of drugs remains the subject of investigation and clinical trial. Different oncologists will recommend varying mixes of anti-cancer drugs. An oncologist could rely on certain studies which found the chemotherapy drug Vinorelbine to be effective, while another would recommend different drugs. Thus, there is a fair amount of choice and discretion for the oncologist and probably the patient. Likewise, treatment for advanced lung cancer is experimental because it is not curative; until a reliable and safe treatment has been established, some would say other possibilities must be considered. However, I use "experimental" to signify treatments for lung cancer which are not FDA approved and are outside the medical mainstream.

33.11 The Rationale Behind Experimental Treatment

Certainly those who can be capably treated by conventional therapy should do exactly that. There are impressive five year survival rates for stage one localized cancer, and it would be sad and foolhardy for a patient to jettison treatments with a proven effectiveness for those which are at best speculative. The only area where alternative treatments should be advanced or stage 4 lung cancer where conventional medical science has not succeeded in creating a cure in most cases.

Even there we must be careful, we have initial response rates of about 25% percent for certain advanced cancers, with a significant percentage of relapse. Thus while cure is not probable, there are a statistically significant number of patients who will benefit from and have their lives extended from conventional treatment, and a certain percentage, albeit small, who will be cured.

33.2 BEWARE OF CHARLATANS AND SCAMS

33.20 The Problem

Sadly there are those who pray about the seriously ill and those families desperately seeking life-saving treatment. Consider these words of caution:

1. Many alternative practitioners, especially those who are not U.S. physicians, have little or no regulation or way of verifying their claims of success. Someone could say, for example, a combination of tree bark and vitamin c, taken in quadruple doses, will kill the carcinogens which comprise cancer, and we would have no way of verifying the claim. For established medical science, one can review a published study in a medical journal, which not only chronicles favorable findings, but explains the methodology and procedure of the study. Medline, the world medical database, (www.healthgate.com) contains over a half a million articles, many dealing with treatments for cancer, and the intelligent patient will want to rely on science, rather than unverifiable, and self-serving claims of certain clinics and facilities.

2. Some alternative practitioners will suggest that the "medical establishment", presented as a monolithic profit-making entity, is preventing discovery and dissemination of life-saving treatment. Words like these are frequently echoed: "Of course, the FDA has not approved our treatment. Don't you understand that we present a direct threat to the pharmaceutical companies who earn millions from cancer; that cancer is a multi-billion dollar

industry and our treatment threatens their wealth and influence and that is why it has been suppressed." The message is that anyone who is skeptical about doctors or pharmaceutical companies should accept their remedy.

3. Brash and arrogant statements are used to justify expensive and questionable treatments. While life is undoubtedly precious, those with cancer must be careful about risking their life savings for unproven and unsubstantiated cures. See also quackwatch (1) for a similar analysis.

There is a saying in medicine-first do no harm. Thus your first task in assessing alternative treatment is exactly that. Substituting an alternative treatment for the proven benefits of chemotherapy is life-threatening; on the other hand, supplementing existing therapy with a nutritional or other plan which your oncologist approves should do no harm and might conceivably help.

33.21 Try to Assess the Scientific Basis for the Treatment

Experimental treatments vary in their medical basis from a drug which many believe is effective in treating the disease but which has not been accepted by the FDA, to an obscure drug or process touted by a little known organization. Consider the following in your assessment:

1. Does your own doctor approve of, or at least not strongly condemn the proposed treatment? Biofeedback and other treatment fall in this category.

2. What is the medical basis for the drug or treatment? Has it been shown to provide beneficial results in lung cancer patients? For example, if product A has been shown to help stage 1 and 2 patients, but not have a proven efficacy with stage 3 and 4, it could still make some sense.

3. Has the product been shown to have beneficial results with cancer generally, even if its efficacy has not been shown with respect to this organ?

4. Does the logical basis for the treatment make sense? For example, if beta carotene has been shown to reduce the incidence of cancer,

one could argue that it might have some positive impact upon the creation of new cancer cells. Thus, adopting a diet for example, rich in beta carotene could make some sense.

The website quackwatch.com reviews and critiques new drugs.

33.3 PARTICULAR EXPERIMENTAL PROGRAMS

33.31 The Gerson and Burzynski Programs

Max Gerson suggested that an imbalance between potassium and sodium contributed to tumor growth and he suggested an unusual diet to combat it. A clinic was established in Tiajuana where promising results were self-reported. (Devita 7). While diet undoubtedly plays a role in the development of tumors including those in the lung, scientists have not shown that diet can reverse results once a cancer has arisen. For example, a diet with fruit including beta carotene will tend to reduce cancers including lung; however, giving patients large amounts of beta carotene once they developed cancer did not help and indeed appeared to increase the severity of the disease. Gerson failed to demonstrate through established clinical trials that his proposal worked and most scientists believe it is speculative.

The Burzynski program suggests that antineoplastons can help prevent cancer. While there was initially some evidence to support his approach, again clinical trials failed to prove the validity of his approach. Devita (7), Barrett (14). Indeed, both approaches have not been shown effective for cancer generally, beyond demonstrating effectiveness for non-small or small cell lung cancer.

33.32 Cancer Treatment Centers of America

If Burzynski and Gerson have been largely discredited, the Cancer Treatment Centers have their mainline adherents. This center offers conventional treatment, with an overall support system, and consideration of alternatives. Conventional chemotherapy may be given in a pretty room with soft music, or radiation combined with relaxation techniques. A whole body approach applies, with the patient's mental as well as physical well-being examined.

33.321 Cost Considerations

Its tough to criticize their approach, but the basic problem is cost. If a whole-body approach makes sense, many insurance companies are unwilling to pay for it. If a back massage is needed, don't send us a bill for $300.00 from a cancer center, have your doctor explain why it is needed, and have it done at a local health club for $45.00. Fractionated radiation treatments may be innovative, but what clear evidence supports their extra cost, an insurer may ask.

The Centers provide individualized treatment and assessment, precisely because they circumvent the many cost-cutting procedures present at the average hospital. Many HMO's negotiate with local hospitals for reduced rates in exchange for the insurance carrier's approval of the hospital. It appears the Center does not participate in these cost-cutting measures. The Center treads gingerly upon these issues.

"Unfortunately, we may not always be able to obtain prompt or full payment from your insurance company. If that happens, you will be expected to assist in expediting the claim and resolving any balances due. Some insurance companies base payment on the average charges for all hospitals in a given area. This practice does not take into consideration the specialized nature of care at certain facilities managed by Cancer Treatment Centers of America and may not cover the full cost of the care you receive. You may be responsible for any balances. You are encouraged to discuss your coverage with your insurance company prior to treatment."

Where innovative but needed treatment is required, an insurer may be required to pay for specialized treatment or diagnosis. A combined CT and PET scanning machine may now represent the standard of care but be unavailable at some local hospitals. However, music and a whole body approach are unlikely to be considered the type of specialized treatment that is unavailable at other hospitals. Indeed, while it touts specialized treatments, relatively few major treatment developments have been uncovered at these centers. Instead, major teaching hospitals like MD Anderson and Sloan-Kettering are the centers for new treatments.

33.33 Chinese Herbal Medicine

Anecdotally, many report benefits from some Chinese medicine. In the last few years, there is a promising tendency to scientifically evaluate these herbs and treatments, with results reported in foreign medical journals.

33.331 Methyl Protoneodioscin

Methyl protoneodioscin is a Chinese herbal remedy for the treatment of various cancers. One study found it was cytotoxic against test cell lines from leukemia and solid tumors including non-small cell lung cancer (NSCLC), with a novel anti-cancer method. While cell studies show some promise, they are a far cry from clinical trial success. Translating laboratory success into a method of delivering the drug to cancer cells without substantial side effects has proven to be difficult with lung cancer. Side effects are unclear.

33.4 TREATMENT IN OTHER COUNTRIES

The United States has many of the best hospitals in the world. Some countries have impressive medical systems, but those are rarely mentioned for alternative treatments. Thus, Japan has an impressive record of treating small cell lung cancer (5), but strange treatments in Mexico are what is generally mentioned.

There is virtually no evidence that treatment in Mexico would improve survival and programs which jettison chemotherapy for natural foods, nutrition therapy, or laetrile may actually cause some harm.

33.41 Particular Overseas Treatments

Some of the most forward-looking material comes from Japan, and is supported by clinical studies and reports in recognized scientific journals. For example, the above discussion by Ohkubo about surgery for small cell patients has solid scientific support and another article found 75-80% five year survival of squamous cell patients through cancer screening also is documented in a recognized journal. (The success is based upon screening high risk smokers and detecting cancers at very early stages, something not done in the United States).

Likewise, the Cuneo Lung Cancer Group in Italy has intensively examined many issues with lung cancer treatment and related hospitals would presumably provide very good care. Mesothelioma is an unusual cancer which has generated a number of clinical studies in France and reporting results superior to those with standard treatment in the United States. The patient who decided to travel to another country to use the services of a world-renowned expert in a particular area or a hospital using a treatment which has shown some success may be making a wise choice-*if* one is to travel to another country, go to a leading cancer center there, not an expensive and obscure facility which touts conspiracy theories and unusual treatments.

33.5 TISSUE TYPING

A promising new treatment is tissue-typing. Chemotherapy response rates are approximately 20%, with oncologists having little way of knowing who will and won't respond, and to which drugs. There are at least 8 drugs with response rates in the low 20's, and no clear way to select among them. With tissue-typing, part of a tumor is taken from the patient and sent to laboratory, where tests are performed on the actual cells to see how they respond to various drugs:

> "Fresh viable tumor tissue is minced and enzymed to disaggregate the tumor cells. The tumor cells are plated in soft agar which preferentially favors tumor cell proliferation. Cells are exposed to tumor type-specific antineoplastic agents for five days in a carefully controlled environment. Drug exposures in excess of the maximum tolerated are used. Due to the reduced rate of drug metabolism, in vitro tumor exposure is 5 to 80 times greater than in vivo . . . . Treated cells are compared to untreated controls. If malignant cells proliferate in vitro under such extreme chemotherapeutic exposure conditions, then in vivo exposures will be ineffective." Oncotech (9).

"Cell culture drug resistance testing" ("CCDRT") is a generic, descriptive term which refers to testing fresh human tumors in cell culture to determine whether they are more resistant or less resistant to individual chemotherapy drugs and drug combinations. Human Assay Journal (9). Indeed, we use cell studies to predict response and determine what drugs should be tested on humans.

Some suggest the technology remains unproven:

> "The rationale for assay-directed therapy is that specific information on an individual patient's in vitro response to a chemotherapeutic regimen may increase the likelihood of selecting a regimen that will be effective for that individual, and thereby avoid one that will be ineffective. However, given the many complex factors that determine the outcomes of chemotherapy, this rationale alone is not sufficient to make the case that assay-directed chemotherapy is superior to empiric chemotherapy. For example, the tissue sample tested might not be representative of the behavior of the patient's tumor. Also, a laboratory finding of "sensitive" or "resistant" may not accurately predict the patient's actual response to treatment. Additionally, there is an imperfect relationship between tumor response and survival, freedom from symptoms or occurrence of treatment-associated adverse events, which are the results most important to patients. Thus, evidence from well-designed trials is needed to determine whether assay-directed chemotherapy actually improves health outcomes." Blue Shield Blue Cross position paper (11).

The technology is sufficiently new to be given various names including human tumor clonogenic assay, histo drug response assay, and in vitro drug sensitivity test.

33.52 Testing Parameters

At this point, testing is more negative than positive, indicating which drugs will be ineffective. However, that is tremendously important if true, improving the chance that the right drug will be prescribed, and reducing discomfort from the use of an ineffective one.

33.53 Clinical Trials

Clinical trial evidence has been encouraging, though not completely convincing. A study of tissue typing on small cell lung cancer found, "Several parameters of in vitro drug sensitivity were significantly associated with clinical response to primary therapy and also with response to the IVBR and were marginally associated with length of survival." Gazdar (12). In a small study, Cortezar found Athe mean response rate for patients treated with in vitroBselected therapy was 27% compared with 18% (range, 0% to 100%; n = 7 studies) for patients treated with empiric therapy." Nonetheless that did not translate into increased survival. A recent study found:

> "Sensitivity was determined in 20 of the esophageal cancer patients and 8 of the gastric cancer patients, accounting for 80% of all the patients. Of the 11 patients judged to have sensitivity by the histoculture drug response assay (HDRA), 7 had a partial response, and of the 17 judged to have no sensitivity, 16 had a minor response or no change (NC). It was thus demonstrated that predictions of the effect of anticancer agents could be made with considerable accuracy using HDRA." Suda (12)

In short, the tests have been able to predict response with some accuracy. That has not yet been shown to translate into better survival.

33.54 Insurance Reimbursement

Blue Cross Blue Shield considers the program experimental at this time. (11).

REFERENCES

1. www.quackwatch.com They list these characteristics of quackery:

    1. **The discoverer pitches the claim directly to the media.** The integrity of science rests on the willingness of scientists to expose new ideas and

findings to the scrutiny of other scientists. Thus, scientists expect their colleagues to reveal new findings to them initially. An attempt to bypass peer review by taking a new result directly to the media, and thence to the public, suggests that the work is unlikely to stand up to close examination by other scientists . . . .

2. **The discoverer says that a powerful establishment is trying to suppress his or her work.** The idea is that the establishment will presumably stop at nothing to suppress discoveries that might shift the balance of wealth and power in society. Often, the discoverer describes mainstream science as part of a larger conspiracy that includes industry and government.

3. **The scientific effect involved is always at the very limit of detection.** Alas, there is never a clear photograph of a flying saucer, or the Loch Ness monster. All scientific measurements must contend with some level of background noise or statistical fluctuation. But if the signal-to-noise ratio cannot be improved, even in principle, the effect is probably not real and the work is not science. Thousands of published papers in parapsychology, for example, claim to report verified instances of telepathy, psychokinesis, or precognition. But those effects show up only in tortured analyses of statistics. The researchers can find no way to boost the signal, which suggests that it isn't really there.

4. **Evidence for a discovery is anecdotal.** If modern science has learned anything in the past century, it is to distrust anecdotal evidence. Because anecdotes have a very strong emotional impact, they serve to keep superstitious beliefs alive in an age of science. The most important discovery of modern medicine is not vaccines or antibiotics, it is the randomized double-blind test, by means of which we know what

works and what doesn't. Contrary to the saying, "data" is not the plural of "anecdote."

5. **The discoverer says a belief is credible because it has endured for centuries.** There is a persistent myth that hundreds or even thousands of years ago, long before anyone knew that blood circulates throughout the body, or that germs cause disease, our ancestors possessed miraculous remedies that modern science cannot understand. Much of what is termed "alternative medicine" is part of that myth. Ancient folk wisdom, rediscovered or repackaged, is unlikely to match the output of modern scientific laboratories.

6. **The discovery has worked in isolation** The image of a lone genius who struggles in secrecy in an attic laboratory and ends up making a revolutionary breakthrough is a staple of Hollywood's science-fiction films, but it is hard to find examples in real life. Scientific breakthroughs nowadays are almost always syntheses of the work of many scientists.

7. **The discoverer must propose new laws of nature to explain an observation.** A new law of nature, invoked to explain some extraordinary result, must not conflict with what is already known. If we must change existing laws of nature or propose new laws to account for an observation, it is almost certainly wrong.1

2. *Some Biological Actions of Alkylglycerols from Shark Liver Oil.* J Altern Complement Med, 1998 Spr, 4:1, 87-99.

3. American Cancer Society, *Informed Decisions* (1999). 4. Ardizoni (4) *Drug Therapy of Non-Small Cell Lung Cancer: News from the Lab*, Cuneo Lung Cancer Conference.

5. Ohkubo, *Surgical Analysis for Small Cell Lung Cancer of the Lung*, Kyobu Geka, 1999 Dec, 52 (13): 1061-6.

6. Lee, et. al., *Gene Therapy 323*, in Pass, Lung Cancer Principles and Practice (Lippincott 2000).

7. Devita, *Cancer Principles and Practice of Oncology* (2002).

8. Hu, *The cytotoxicity of methyl protoneodioscin (NSC-698791)*

against human cancer cell lines in vitro, Anticancer Res. 2002 Mar-Apr;22(2A):1001-59.

9. www.oncotech.com.

10. Human Tissue Assay Journal, http://www.htaj.com/faq.htm.

11. http://bcbs.com/tec/vol17/17_12.html.

12. Gazdar, *Correlation of in vitro drug-sensitivity testing results with response to chemotherapy and survival in extensive-stage small cell lung cancer: a prospective clinical trial,* Journal Of The National Cancer Institute, Vol 82, 117-124.

13. Suda, *Evaluation of the histoculture drug response assay as a sensitivity test for anticancer agents,* Surg Today. 2002;32(6): 477-81.

14. Barrett, Questionable Cancer Therapies, www.quackwatch.com

CHAPTER 34

IMPROVING THE STANDARD OF CARE FOR DIAGNOSIS OF LUNG CANCER

34.1 DEFICIENCIES IN THE STANDARD OF CARE

Over half of lung cancers are diagnosed when the patients have significant symptomotogy indicating advanced cancer. Some could have been saved had they been diagnosed earlier and we need to do a better job of diagnosing lung cancer in the United States. If the notion of saving people has not done the trick, perhaps the threat of legal claims may induce physicians to look at high-risk groups and do the necessary diagnostic work. Thus this chapter deals with improving the standard of care and the filing of malpractice claims for errors.

We can acknowledge that the physician is caught between two conflicting pressures, HMO's who demand that each test be medically justified, and patients who may sue if they perceive a mistake. While we can sympathize with the physician's plight, we can say that the goal of saving lives is more important and that if claims bring the medical community closer to seeing matters from the patient's perspective they have accomplished an important goal. Perhaps such suits will accomplish the goal of establishing that certain diagnostic tests should be performed as a matter of course with high-risk smokers, and eliminate the uncertainty that exposes patients to unnecessary risks and physicians to legal liability. Having a health care system where the number 1 cancer and the second largest cause of death is diagnosed too late is 60% to 70% of cases is not satisfactory.

34.2 ARGUMENTS AGAINST THE BRINGING OF CLAIMS

34.21 Are the Deficiencies in the Standard of Care Rather than the Physicians?

A 55 year old man who smoked a pack a day for 30 years year sees a doctor for a yearly physical. While blood pressure and various other tests are performed, no chest x-ray or other diagnostic test to detect lung cancer is performed. Eighteen months later, he is diagnosed with stage 3B non-small lung cancer. The tumor would probably have been revealed on a chest x-ray, certainly on a CT Scan, with the patient's prognosis significantly improved in both cases. Should the patient and family suffer for the doctor's neglect?

In the example above, the doctor is not negligent. There is no standard of care requiring a doctor to arrange a chest x-ray, Ct Scan, or any other diagnostic test even for a smoker at high risk for lung cancer. Thus, the problem is the standard of care not the treatment, and our focus should be to improve the standard, not punish an individual physician.

34.3 TYPES OF CLAIMS

Failure to diagnose lung cancer claims generally involves these scenarios:

1. Failure to take a chest x-ray or Ct Scan when the patients complaints and prior smoking history indicated the test was warranted.
2. Inaccurate interpretations of a chest x-ray—a difficult diagnostic tool.
3. A chest x-ray notes an abnormality, but nothing is done, no follow-up. Sometimes, there is confusion over whose responsibility it was to take action.

34.31 Failure to Take an X-ray

Again we start with the proposition that no physician is required to take an x-ray as part of a yearly or periodic physical, notwithstanding the patient's smoking history. However, in many cases, the patient will complain of symptoms indicative of lung cancer such as chest pain, shortness of breath, fatigue, or loss of weight. Where the patient's smoking history and symptomology indicate the possibility of a tumor, it may be a breach of the standard of care for the physician to fail to take or follow up with appropriate diagnostic tests.

Some legal terms to know. *Standard of care* is that degree of care that a reasonably competent physician would exercise in the same circumstances. The physician is not required to be the best in his area of specialization; he is only required to do what the average or reasonably competent physician would have done. A breach or violation of the standard of care is negligence. Another somewhat more acerbic word for negligence is malpractice.

While it is clear that screening is not required, what exactly is can be a matter of opinion or even surmise. For example, with some complaint of chest pain, is a chest x-ray required? How about fatigue? It is possible in this area for physicians to reach differing conclusions.

34.311 Misinterpretation of a Chest X-ray

This type of claim is relatively common. Indeed, some studies have shown that one quarter of chest x-rays are misinterpreted. We can separate two problems. First, given the difficulty of interpretation and the frequency of error, it is somewhat unfair to impose liability upon the doctor. We think of malpractice as a substantial error but here, one in four physicians could make the same mistake. The solution is clear. Radiologists should be strongly encouraged to take Ct Scans instead of x-rays. The frequency of Ct Scan error is far lower, as the tumor is readily identifiable on a Ct Scan, whereas it is a faint shadow on some x-rays. Where an x-ray is taken particularly of a smoker, the radiologist should recommend a Ct Scan where there is any ambiguity. Trying to ascertain the difference between a shadow due to emphysema as opposed to a lung tumor is a task far too demanding for many radiologists, the stakes too high. and the consequence of delay too significant for an educated guess.

Most attorneys would consider a missed x-ray a solid case. Some physicians would argue that reading chest x-rays is a matter of interpretation that involves not only the x-ray itself, but the patient's background and complaints, and is an art as much as a science. They would argue that a physician should not be sued for his exercise of discretion and judgment. Nonetheless, in many of these cases, the radiologists not only made an error in reading the x-ray, but missed the chance to recommend Ct Scan followup.

Indeed some clinical studies have examined prior x-rays and found the small shadows which later became serious tumors. These claims are examined in further detail below.

34.32 Follow-up Failures

While chest x-rays are not done for screening, they are frequently done as a part of surgical screening. Going in for an appendectomy, a 60 year old smoker undergoes an x-ray where a small growth is detected. Medically this is an asymptomatic pulmonary nodule. Given the absence of symptomology, it is most likely stage 1 and treatable. Sometimes no followup is done.

The surgeon for the appendicitis is not responsible for his overall care, a general physician may not get the report, and frequently there is no overall doctor. In a time of high-volume medical practice, our diagnostic tools are far more astute, our routine work far worse and records more frequently misplaced. Again, these situations frequently turn into claims.

34.33 Considerations for the Patient

Here are some things you may wish to consider in evaluating whether to pursue a claim:

1. What is your relationship to the physician? Do you believe he did his best notwithstanding the adverse result?
2. How will that affect your treatment? Will you become preoccupied with a claim or feel that you are taking action to right a wrong?
3. Do you see a need to change physician's perspectives in favor of early detection and screening programs?

4. Will you be required to pay any money initially?
5. Is a significant verdict or settlement likely? Will that help pay for any needed treatment or help support your family?

34.4 AVOIDING CLAIMS: ADVICE FOR THE PHYSICIAN

Since some within the medical community may have the opportunity to read this, let me offer some suggestions as to how to avoid claims.

1. On occasion a smoker will avoid a checkup or test for fear of the results. The physician should document that refusal, so the records are clear the test was recommended and even that follow-up was requested and any decision not to undergo tests was by the patient.
2. Given the uncertainty as to the standard of care and the need for early detection, do the maximum. If a chest-xray shows any abnormaltiy, recommend a Ct Scan. You should suggest a Ct Scan if you have a middle-aged smoker with any pulmonary complaints and indeed, discuss the pro-s and cons of screening even for smokers without complaints. Some insurance carriers may not cover the test, but the patient should be given the opportunity to pay for a test on his own.
3. Given the difficulty of interpreting chest x-rays, especially as regard to smaller tumors, have a radiologist interpret the slides and provide a written report. A general physician should not attempt to interpret chest x-rays.

34.5 RADIOLOGICAL MALPRACTICE CLAIMS

An informative study by medical insurers found that radiologists are the chief defendants in medical malpractice cases. Many patients had x-rays taken long before the cancer was diagnosed and a spot or shadow can be seen which at least retrospectively shows the films were not properly read. Since the gap between x-ray and eventual diagnosis may be a number of years, there is a reasonable inference that the patient's opportunity for long-term survival was adversely affected by the delayed diagnosis.

An x-ray is by its very nature an imprecise instrument—"reading x-ray films, therefore, involves considerable interpretation of the patterns of density of shadows on the film and changes that may have occurred." Meyer (2). In one study,

> "Eighteen radiologists failed to detect 27 potentially resectable bronchogenic carcinomas revealed retrospectively on serial chest radiographs . . . Six consultant radiologists, who were biased by knowledge that the cases were of missed bronchogenic carcinoma, were individually shown the radiographs in 22 of the cases. Each consultant missed a mean of 26% (5.8 +/-1.7) of the lesions. At least one of the six consultants missed the lesion in 16 (73%) of the cases." Radiology (3).

While some tumors are relatively clear, in many instances, trying to devine the difference between pulmonary fibrosis or pneumonia and a small tumor can be difficult.

34.51 What Follow-up is Needed

First, where ambiguities are seen on an x-ray, there should be a clear bias toward recommending further testing. This increases the possibility of early diagnosis, as well as limiting the individual radiologist's potential liability. If a tumor is misinterpreted as probable scarring from pneumonia, but the radiologist recommends a follow-up CT Scan to make the determination, he has probably eliminated liability notwithstanding the error. Given the large percentage of lung cancer patients whose disease is diagnosed too late, we need to emphasize more frequent use of the available tools to detect the disease. One radiologist routinely adds to his reports, follow-up with additional tests is recommended if the results are inconsistent with other physician and diagnostic findings. While the language is self-protective, it emphasizes the need for continuing inquiry until the cause of disease is clearly identified.

The radiologist may make a life and death determination. He should do that with as much information as possible. The radiologist may want to contact the referring physician. One article states:

"Double reading of radiographs increases the likelihood of detecting pulmonary disease and, accordingly, physicians have an obligation to view the radiographic examinations performed on their patients, either with the radiologist or independently. It is also essential that the radiologist be proved with the clinical findings before he interprets the radiographs, a practice which will result in significant improvement in the accuracy of radiologic reports." Primary Care (4).

34.52 Referral for CT Scan

There also needs to be a recognition of the inaccuracy of the chest-ray compared with the CT Scan. Using a chest-xray to make or support a diagnosis is a questionable endeavor, as a recent article explained:

"Conventional chest radiography (CXR) is a poor diagnostic tool for detecting lung cancers at a surgically curable stage. To determine the visibility of peripheral small lung cancers on CXR, we retrospectively examined the usefulness of CXR using a consecutive series of 44 cases detected on CT screening and later confirmed by histopathology. All cases had been detected by low dose CT during a population based screening trial for lung cancer . . . . Of the 42 lung cancers < or = 20 mm, 74% (31/42) were located in the well penetrated lung zones and 71% (22/31) of these were missed on CXR. 26% (11/42) were concealed by hilar vessels, mediastinum, heart or diaphragm, and all (11/11) of these were missed on CXR. 93% (39/42) of the lung cancers < or = 20 mm were adenocarcinomas and 79% (31/39) of these were missed on CXR. 7% (3/42) were epidermoid carcinomas or small cell carcinomas and 66% (2/3) of these were missed on CXR. The overall accuracy of interpretation on CXR for lung cancers was 61%, sensitivity was 23% and specificity 96% . . . . Thus, CXR was poor at visualizing CT detectable lung cancers of < or = 20 mm diameter, which are usually of very low density, and cannot be relied upon for detection of surgically curable small lung cancer." British Journal (5).

Thus, chest x-ray failed to detect a number of tumors greater than 20 millimeters. More significantly, it failed in detecting smaller, surgically removable tumors, when timely diagnosis could do the most good. Perhaps, a radiologist cannot recommend a CT Scan in every case referred to him. However, he must recognize that this is a highly imprecise test at best, and using it to base determinations may well cost the patient his life. Where there are smokers, or some type of positive finding on x-ray, Ct Scan should be recommended.

34.6 THE NEED FOR A CLEAR STANDARD AS A WAY TO REDUCE CLAIMS AND SAVE LIVES

Both physicians and patients would benefit from a clear standard regarding diagnostic testing. Today, most patients are diagnosed late, after their cancers have spread, presenting serious questions about long-term survival. Since many of these patients saw physicians before they were diagnosed, we live in a litigious society and the patient's health may have been compromised by the delay, inevitably claims will be brought. Compensating the patient and/or his family does not solve the basic problem.

Ultimately it would reduce claims and benefit physicians were a clear standard enunciated. Thus, if the American Cancer Society determined that CT Scans were warranted for patients with a heavy smoking history, say 30 pack years (packs per day smoked x years smoked), that would establish a benchmark. Doctors could prescribe Ct Scans for such persons at risk, and a clear demarcation would reduce the incidence of claims.

REFERENCES

1. Hamer, *Medical malpractice in diagnostic radiology: claims, compensation and patient injury*, Radiology, 1987 Jul;164(1):263-6
2. Meyer, (2) *Lung Cancer Chronicles* 184 (Rutgers Press 1990).
3. Radiology 1992 Jan;182(1):115-22.
4. Prim Care 1976 Mar;3(1):107-36.
5. Br J Radiol 2000 Feb;73(866):137-45.

CHAPTER 35

ASBESTOS, SILICA AND OTHER OCCUPATIONAL CLAIMS

35.1 WHY SOME LUNG CANCER VICTIMS MAY BE ENTITLED TO COMPENSATION

Exposure to dangerous dusts in the workplace is the second leading cause of lung cancer after smoking. These dusts include silica in its many and varied forms, asbestos, and other carcinogens. Because the cellular changes comprising cancer occur slowly, exposures to dusts of ten and 20 years before may be key in the legal assessment of a claim, and make many victims unaware of their right to compensation.

There are two basic claims, worker's compensation and products liability claims.

35.11 Worker's Compensation Claims

Exposure to dusts such as silica or asbestos can create or contribute to lung cancer. One may present a worker's compensation claim against the employer (s) during which the exposure occurred. See (5) for a description of worker's compensation. For a worker's compensation claim, one need not prove the employer was negligent or that it acted wrongfully. Instead, under most statutes, the employees only burden is to show the exposure contributed to the disease. Disputes about the causative role of carcinogens in the workplace versus smoking are frequent, though many cases are resolved.

35.2 ASBESTOS PRODUCTS LIABILITY CLAIMS

Some cancer victims believe their exposure was due at least in part to exposure to asbestos. Asbestos causes lung cancer, though there are ongoing debates about the nature and extent of exposure needed to cause the disease, how causation is determined, and the relative risks of smoking.

In asbestos claims, the plaintiff argues that there was ample evidence of the dangers of asbestos which were disregarded by the manufacturer and/or distributor of the product. The manufacturer should have placed appropriate warnings, suggested regular pulmonary examinations, encapsulated the asbestos so that it would not become airborne, reduced the concentration of asbestos, or utilized available substitutes. A products liability claim suggests that the product was unsafe and the manufacturer is therefore responsible for any resultant injuries.

35.21 The Nature of Exposure

Asbestos refers to a group of naturally occurring mineral silicates. Although different in chemical composition and physical properties, they share characteristics of heat and chemical resistance. Asbestos has been used for multiple purposes including textiles, asbestos cement, thermal insulation, building materials, and friction products such as brake linings. There have been hundreds of commercial applications of asbestos since the expansion of this industry began in the late 1800's. See Aisner (1).

Asbestos is associated with lung cancer, and asbestosis, a particular type of lung disease involving a reducing in breathing capacity. These occupations may have had significant exposure to asbestos:

1. Pipefitters, steam fitters, insulators, and boilermakers,
2. Construction, carpenters, plumbers, sheet metal workers,
3. Maintenance men, custodians, steam fitters, and
4. Brake mechanics.

These are the considerations a lawyer would use in evaluating a lung cancer asbestos claim:

1. Was there substantial exposure to asbestos? For example, an insulator removing asbestos, or a brake mechanic would have

substantial exposure; in contrast, someone with minor bystander exposure has a tough time arguing asbestos was a causative factor in the disease.

2. Is there accompanying asbestosis or other asbestos disease such as pleural plagues, indicating asbestos fibers penetrated the lung?

3. Was the plaintiff a heavy smoker so that smoking can be regarded as the causative agent?

4. Have there been other claims regarding the particular worksite?

5. Does any pathology of the lung tissue indicate the presence of asbestos fibers?

35.3 OTHER TYPES OF LUNG CANCER CLAIMS

35.31 Silica Claims

The hazards of silica dust have been recognized for decades if not centuries. See Deadly Dust (1). For the last 70 years, inhalation of silica dust has been recognized to cause silicosis, a scaring of the lungs causing reducing breathing capacity. Silica is used in many forms of construction as well as other industries

While the hazards of silica has been noted, many manufacturers and employers continue to fail to use needed precautions to reduce dust inhalation. Manufacturers of products using silica failed to provide warnings, recommend wet methods to reduce dust, use inorganic silica instead of the more toxic crystalline silica, and recommend bi-yearly medical testing. See 3

While silicosis was the first hazard associated with dust inhalation, today scientists are recognizing that silica contributes to lung cancer also. "An excess of lung cancer related to occupational exposure to crystalline silica is reported in many epidemiological studies, regardless of the presence of silicosis." Pairon (2).

REFERENCES

1. See Rosner, *Deadly Dust* (1994).
2. Pairon, *Silica and lung cancer: a controversial issue,* Eur Respir J. 1991 Jun;4(6):730-44.
3. Detailed information regarding potential claims is available on our website, lungcancerclaims.com

4. Soutar, *Epidemiological evidence on the carcinogenicity of silica: factors in scientific judgment,* Ann Occup Hyg. 2000 Jan;44(1):3-14.

5. In the late 1800's and 1900's, employees were injured on the job with no redress. Worker's compensation laws were a product of worker reform. These laws provide compensation to an employee injured as a result of job-related activities. He need not show the employer was at fault or failed to utilize respiratory protection. Compensation is based upon a chart, though most states permit negotiated settlements.

CHAPTER 36

SMOKING CESSATION PROGRAMS

36.1 CAUSES OF SMOKING

36.11 Why Talk About Smoking?

One might conclude that a discussion about smoking is superfluous in a book about lung cancer, since the readers or their families have already contracted the disease. Initially it may be important even for this group to quit smoking. The same disease process which created the initial tumor could theoretically create further tumors with further exposure to carcinogenic smoke. Surgery cannot be performed if breathing function is severely impaired and smoking has the capacity to further damage the lung.

More importantly, since smoking plays such a central role in lung cancer, one must discuss smoking and prevention to discuss the disease. Lung cancer patients may be the most vigorous advocates of educational programs, wanting to teach others how to avoid what they have endured.

36.12 Distinguishing Causation from Personal Worth

Smoking does cause cancer. However, that does make smokers bad people. My father-in-law smoked 2-3 packs a day for 50 years and developed lung cancer. However, he was also an extremely kind and generous man. One could not say he was less worthy of treatment than, for example, non-smokers with other diseases who were less charitable and kind.

36.2 STATISTICS ABOUT SMOKING

"Smoking is a chronic condition that affects more than 46 million Americans. People who smoke are at risk of heart disease, cancer, and other smoking-related illnesses that cost more than $50 billion annually to treat, and an additional $47 billion in indirect costs from lost time at work and disability."

"Smoking is the single greatest preventable cause of death and illness in the United States. An estimated 420,000 people die every year from smoking-related illnesses. Studies show that over 70 percent of adult smokers would like to quit, but only half of them have ever been urged to quit by their health care provider. Smoking with delayed diagnosis is the chief cause of lung cancer."

36.21 The Increase in Lung Cancer Among Women

"Between 1973 and 1995, lung cancer incidence in US women rose by 126% while incidence rates in men rose by only 0.9%. During this period, incidence rates for small cell carcinoma of the lung (SCLC) increased by over 160%, faster than other histologic types in women and 8 times faster than the increase for SCLC in men. Lung cancer now accounts for one of every eight new cancers in women and one of every five lung cancers is SCLC. Small cell carcinoma is diagnosed most frequently in heavy smokers and rarely in non-smokers." Osann (1).

32.22 Particular Risk Factors Associated with Smoking

"All aspects of smoking are associated in a dose-specific fashion with the risk of developing lung cancer. The risk of lung cancer increases with increasing number of cigarettes smoked per day, ranging from 2.5 for those smoking less than one pack per day to 32.8 for those smoking greater than two packs per day. Increased duration of smoking similarly carried proportionately larger risk, going from 3.5 for those smoking up to 29 years to 9.0 for those who smoked >50 years. Starting smoking at an early age also increased the risk; relative risk for those starting before 16 years being 10.3 compared to a relative risk of 6.4 for those who started smoking later." Khuder (3).

36.23 Types of Cancer and Smoking

Khuder discusses the type of cancer in relation to smoking:

> "We found the strongest relationship between smoking and lung cancer for small cell carcinoma. This is consistent with reports in the literature that show a stronger relationship for squamous and small cell carcinomas compared to adenocarcinoma . . . . In this study, the number of cigarettes smoked per day was strongly associated with both squamous cell and small cell cancer of the lung . . . central lesions with more exposure to tobacco smoke particles (squamous cell or small cell carcinoma) may therefore have stronger association than peripheral ones, with less exposure (adenocarcinoma and large cell carcinoma) . . . patients with squamous and small cell carcinomas were heavier smokers compared to patients with adenocarcinoma." Khuder, (3).

36.24 Nicotine as a Risk Factor

Nicotine may be an additional risk factor beyond the various toxins present in cigarette smoke:

> "Although nicotine has been implicated as a potential factor in the pathogenesis of human lung cancer, its mechanism of action in the development of this cancer remains largely unknown. The present study provides evidence that nicotine (a) activates the mitogen-activated protein (MAP) kinase signaling pathway in lung cancer cells, specifically extracellular signal-regulated kinase (ERK2), resulting in increased expression of the bcl-2 protein and inhibition of apoptosis in these cells; and (b) blocks the inhibition of protein kinase C (PKC) and ERK2 activity in lung cancer cells by anti-cancer agents, such as therapeutic opioid drugs, and thus can adversely affect cancer therapy . . . . These effects of nicotine . . . could lead to

disruption of the critical balance between cell death and proliferation, resulting in the unregulated growth of cells. The findings suggest caution in the use of smokeless tobacco products to treat smoking addiction." Heusch (4).

36.25 Pack Years and Risk Factors

Scientists use the term pack years to define risk, number of packs per days smoked x years of usage. One who smokes one pack a day for 20 years has a 20 pack year smoking history. Some people believe that smoking less than a pack a day can reduce one's risk. Von Klaveren suggests the opposite, that the length of usage is the chief risk factor:

> "The lung cancer incidence increases with a power of approximately 4.5 based on duration of smoking, compared with a power of 1.5 based on average daily consumption . . . . The relative risk to develop lung cancer among male smokers with 20 PY's (pack years) is 11.59 when they have smoked 20-29 cigaretts a day (approximately one package) for 20-29 years, but 29.66 when they have smoked 10-19 cigarettes a day (approximately half a package) for 40 years."

36.3 REDUCED BUT CONTINUING RISK FOR SMOKERS WHO HAVE QUIT

Quitting smoking dramatically decreases one's odds of getting lung cancer with the risk decreasing over time. "Cigarette smoking is strongly associated with risk for small cell carcinoma. Odds ratios are nine times higher for current smokers than former smokers." Osann, (1).

> "Even people who stop smoking at 50 or 60 years of age avoid most of their subsequent risk of developing lung cancer, and that those who stop at 30 years of age avoid more than 90% of the risk attributable to tobacco of those who continue to smoke. In the United Kingdom widespread cessation has roughly halved the number of cases of lung cancer that would now be occurring, as by 1990 it had already almost halved the number that would have occurred in the study." British Medical Study (2)

However, it will never be the same risk of a nonsmoker. "The risk of developing lung cancer is 15 fold greater in smokers than in nonsmokers. The relative risk of developing lung cancer decreases from about 15-fold to 1.5 to four fold in former smokers who have quit for 15 years." Mao (7).

When tissue is tested, former smokers have identifiable chromosomal damage. The numerous genetic changes that result in the lungs occur over a period of roughly 15 years. Stopping smoking may eliminate some DNA damage which may contribute to lung cancer; in other circumstances the carcinogenic process may be already in place. In the Cornell study of early detection, a substantial number of lesions and pulmonary abnormalities were associated with former smokers. Thus, former smokers continue to have substantial risks of contracting lung cancer, and systems of early detection must concentrate on them as well as smokers.

36.31 Lung Cancer and Former Smokers

Because of the damage that occurred, lung cancer represents a serious problem for former smokers. Some have estimated that 50% of lung cancer patients are *former smokers*. Dutch Lung Cancer Symposium (11).

36.32 Reduced Tar Cigarettes

Quitting smoking substantially reduces, but does not eliminate lung cancer risk. The question of whether risk is similarly reduced by low tar cigarettes is more difficult. The advent of low tar cigarettes has brought with it an increase in the number of adenocarcinomas, non-small cell cancers which generally arise in the peripheral lung areas. One sensible theory is that low tar smokers breath the smoke more deeply, allowing the carcinogen is reach the smaller pathways of the lung.

Adenocarcinomas are generally more dangerous than squamous cell tumors, since the adeno tumors seem to metastasize more quickly with clinical trials showing a poorer prognosis for patients with adenocarcinoma. Thus, it may be that low tar cigarettes are having a minimal impact. Certainly most researchers would strongly recommend that the patient quit rather than change brand or type.

36.4 PROGRAMS FOR DECREASING SMOKING

A number of articles, books, tapes, and other materials have been compiled dealing with smoking. Here are some of the things which need to be done to reduce smoking rates:

1. **Recognize Our Lack of Success.**

   Lung cancer from smoking is the largest avoidable cause of death in the United States. Lung cancer is responsible for the largest number of cancer deaths in the United States, and is responsible for more deaths among women than breast and cervical cancer combined. Substantial numbers of young people continue to become addicted to smoking. Thus, our starting point must be to recognize that however well-intentioned we have been, our efforts to severely limit smoking have generally been a failure.

2. **School Anti-Smoking Programs Should Candidly and Accurately Describe the Hazards of Smoking.**

   The danger is not frightening a potential smoker but not adequately conveying the serious risks inherent in this habit. We need to spend less time worrying about the sensibilities of teenagers and more time starkly informing them of the hazards of smoking. Anti-smoking programs should include the elements listed. Non-cancer risks such as stroke and heart attack should be discussed.

3. **Personal Testaments from Smokers with Different Types of Cancer Should be a Part of Every Program.**

   It is sad to see someone terminally ill discuss the hazards of smoking, but it is necessary and important to vividly explain what can occur. No lawyer in a personal injury case would rely only on impersonal records; he would want to personalize the injury and give a jury a vivid sense of its impact. Whether the patient is speaking first hand, by videotape or other means, having patients with throat cancer, lung cancer, chronic obstructive pulmonary disease, and other ailments speak is a critical element of any presentation.

4. **Include Slides and Pictures Vividly Showing the Hazards of Smoking.**

   Whether it be a diseased lung, x-ray of a smoker, or the photograph of a family, pictures speak louder than words.

5. **Explain the Difficulty of Curing Metastatic Disease.**
While medical advances continue, metastatic lung cancer continues to be a difficulty disease to confront. Speakers should briefly describe how cancer metastasises and our current difficulties in curing disease once that has occurred.

6. **Include Statistics.**
Some presentations include only statistics, but discussing life expectancies, the difficulties of complete cure, rates of mortality among smokers and other facts can impress the perspective smoker with the hazards of this habit.

7. **Discuss Methods of Quitting.**
Beyond telling people not to smoke, a presentation should discuss the methods of quitting, and how they have worked including the difficulty of quitting.

8. **Discuss other smoking-related hazards** such as stroke and heart attack.

36.5 SMOKING CESSATION PROGRAMS

Genetic and environmental factors combine to prompt smoking and sustain addiction.

36.51 Physical Components of Addiction

There are powerful biological factors at work. One study found smokers who rapidly metabolized nicotine because of a defective gene called CYP2D6 were less likely to quit. Batra (7). Others have looked at dopamine.

> "The role of dopamine D1 receptor gene in nicotine dependence was investigated by Comings et. al., as a part of a study that examined dopamine receptor genes among smokers, Tourette syndrome probands, and pathologic gamblers. In all three groups, there was a significant increase in the frequency of individuals with the 1/1 or 2/2 genotype compared to control subjects, suggesting that there may be an overlap in genetic susceptibility to addictive behaviors, possibly mediated by allelic variants in the D1 gene." Batra (7).

36.52 Social and Environmental Factors

"Social influences such as peer and family smoking, lower educational levels, lack of parental concerns about smoking, and perceptions about smoking that are promoted by tobacco companies also contribute to initiation of smoking." Batra (8).

36.53 Low Tar Cigarettes

Low-tar cigarettes were marketed as a way to substantially reduce cancer risk while still smoking. "Cigarette tar is the condensable residue of cigarette smoke (ie, the total particulate matter from cigarette smoke that is deposited on the filter machine's less the moisture and nicotine). Tar is a complex mixture that includes many chemicals that are cancer initiators and/or promoters." Albert (9).

Study results have been conflicting but overall lower tar appears to only slightly reduce the risk of lung cancer. (9). "Levels of biomarkers were not associated with the yields of tar and nicotine of the current brand that was being smoked." (9). Additionally, smokers adjust; with more frequent and deeper puffs and an increase in the number of cigarettes smoked. (9). The increase in rates of adenocarcinomas in the last 20 years coincided with the use of low tar and filtered cigarettes reflecting deeper inhalation and tumors involving peripheral parts of the lung. (But see footnotes 103-105 in Albert (9) suggesting that better diagnostic tools have also increased the number of peripheral tumors diagnosed).

It is particularly dangerous if people continue to smoke because they view the smoking of lower yield cigarettes as having a more acceptable level of risk. National Cancer Institute (10). The NCI starkly concluded, "compensatory changes in smoking patterns reduce any theoretical benefit of lower yield products . . . changes in cigarette design and manufacturing over the last 50 years had not benefited public health." Instead, the approach over the last decade has been to emphasize smoking cessation.

36.54 NCI Guidelines

The National Cancer Institute provides guidelines and recommendations regarding methods to quit smoking. The guideline found three treatment elements were particularly effective, used either alone or together, in helping smokers quit. They are:

1. Nicotine replacement therapy—either the prescribed nicotine patch or nicotine gum, which doubles the rate of successfully quitting. [Nicotine gum has been approved for over-the-counter (OTC) use by the FDA. The nicotine patch was approved for OTC use by the FDA in July 1996.]
2. Social support—encouragement and support from the clinician.
3. Skills training/problem solving—practical advice and techniques from the clinician that help people adapt to life as a non-smoker.
4. Individual or group counseling programs are also helpful. The guideline panel found a direct relationship between the intensity of treatment and the likelihood for success. The guideline recommends that counseling programs, if chosen, be delivered over 4 to 7 sessions (20 to 30 minutes in length), for at least 2 weeks, but preferably for 8 weeks.

No conclusions were drawn about the effectiveness of the following treatments:

1. Acupuncture or hypnosis. There was insufficient evidence to support the effectiveness of either of these therapies.
2. Clonidine, antidepressants, and anxiolytics/benzodiazepines. Lack of data and/or faulty studies offered little support for their use.

The guideline panel made no recommendations regarding the use of nicotine nasal sprays and nicotine inhalers. There were limited data on these products. At the time of the panel's deliberations, the products were not licensed for prescription in the United States. [As the guideline went to press, the FDA approved the prescription use of nicotine nasal spray.]

These steps are also recommended:

1. Talk with your doctor. Discuss nicotine replacement therapy and strategies to deal with wanting to smoke again. Do everything you can to maximize the chances for success.
2. Be committed. Make sure you're ready to work hard to quit

3. Set a quit date. Don't try to "taper off".
4. Build on past mistakes. If you've tried to quit before, think about what helped and what hurt.
5. Enlist support. Tell your family and friends you're quitting. Create a network you can turn to for help.
6. Learn how to avoid or cope with situations and behavior that make you want to smoke.

36.6 A GUIDE FOR HEALTH CARE

The National Cancer Institute recommends the following for health care facilities:

1. Identify smokers. Ask every patient at every visit if they smoke.
2. Implement a tobacco-user identification system in every clinic.
3. Record smoking status as a vital sign.
4. Ask smokers about their desire to quit and reinforce their intentions.
5. Help motivated smokers set a quit date.
6. Prescribe nicotine replacement therapy.
7. Offer specific, practical advice about how to deal with life as a non-smoker, particularly how to handle situations or emotional states that may cause relapse.
8. Encourage relapsed smokers to try to quit again.

Health care systems face the daily challenge of balancing quality of care and costs for every patient. Health care administrators, insurers (including managed care plans), and purchasers, can play a vital role in tackling the leading preventable cause of illness and death—smoking. (5).

Screening systems that systematically identify and document smoking status result in higher rates of smoking cessation interventions by clinicians and in higher quit rates among patients who smoke. Studies show that smoking cessation interventions involving minimal contact with health care providers-physicians, nurses, social workers, counselors, and others-even in sessions lasting as few as 3 minutes, are more effective at increasing cessation rates than no contact at all. Intensive interventions are more effective and should be used when resources permit.

Implement an office-wide system that ensures that, for every patient, tobacco-use status is queried and documented. Expand vital signs data to include tobacco use. On a regular basis, offer lectures/seminars/ in-services with CME and other credit for smoking cessation treatment. Evaluate the degree to which clinicians are identifying, documenting, and treating patients who smoke, and provide feedback to clinicians about their level of intervention. Include smoking cessation treatments as paid services in all health benefits packages. (5).

36.7 SCREENING TOOLS AND SMOKERS

36.71 The Need for Individualized Assessment

Many smokers quit when diagnosed with lung cancer; by then, the benefits of stopping smoking are limited. Ideally, one would like to see smokers quit early, rather than at diagnosis. For many smokers, disease is an all or nothing proposition, and they assume that the probability is that they will not contract it. While there are numerous warnings and other programs, what is needed is a method of bringing home the dangers of cigarettes for that particular individual.

36.72 CT Scan as an Early diagnosis and Smoking Cessation Tool

We have already discussed the effectiveness of CT Scan in revealing small tumors. Studies have shown CT to be at least five times more effective than x-rays at detecting small, treatable tumors. However, CT does more. In one study of 1,000 asymptomatic smokers, while 26 had tumors, a whopping 233 had some type of serious abnormality short of cancer, such as calcified nodules. Some of the smokers who were diagnosed with cancer had as many as six nodules apparent on CT. Giving smokers a CT alerts them to the fact that serious changes have already taken place in their own body which may lead to cancer, and enable them to quit at a time when some of these changes may be reversible. Additionally, that enables the physician to enable the individual as being in a high-risk category to be intensively followed.

36.73 Molecular Tests

Just as CT may show some serious changes short of cancer, sophisticated molecular tests may do the same. Any test which demonstrated serious changes in chromosomes, genes, or lung tissue, might well lead the smoker to quit.

36.74 P-53 Evaluations

P-53 mutations are one important event in the development of lung cancer. If smokers were advised that they had experienced this specific mutation and that the natural course would be to lead to lung cancer, they might quit.

REFERENCES

1. Osann, *Small cell lung cancer in women: Risk associated with Smoking, Prior Respiratory Disease, and Occupation Lung Cancer,* Vol. 28 (1) (2000) pp. 1-10

2. Smoking, Smoking Cessation, and Lung Cancer in the UK since 1950: Combination of National Statistics with two case-control studies, BMJ 2000;321:323-329 (5 August).

3. Khuder, *Effect of cigarette smoking on major histological types of lung cancer in men,* Lung Cancer, Vol. 22 (1) (1998) pp. 15-21.

4. Heusch, *Signaling pathways involved in nicotine regulation of apoptosis of human lung cancer cells.* Carcinogenesis 1998 Apr;19(4):551-6.

5. Most of the information in this chapter is taken from the National Cancer Institute publication: *Smoking Cessation: A Guide for Primary Care Clinicians*; Smoking Cessation: Quick Reference Guide for Smoking Cessation Specialists; and You Can Quit Smoking, a consumer guide, with a few editorial changes made. Copies of these Guides are available free of charge from the AHCPR Publications Clearinghouse. Call toll-free 800-358-9295, or write to Smoking Cessation, AHCPR Publications Clearinghouse, P.O. Box 8547, Silver Spring, MD 20907-8547, or log on to http://www.ahcpr.gov/clinic/. AHCPR, a part of the U.S. Public Health Service, is the lead agency charged with supporting research designed to improve the quality of health care, reduce its cost, and broaden access to essential services.

6. Von Klaren, *Lung Cancer Screening by Spiral CT: What is the Optimal Target Population for Screening Trials,* Lung Cancer 39 (2002) 243-252.

7. Mao, *Clonal Genetic Alterations in the Lungs of Current and Former Smokers*, Journal of NCI, vol. 89, no. 12, (June 18, 1997).
8. Batra, *The Genetic Determinants of Smoking Chest*. 2003;123:1730-1739.
9. Albert, Epidemiology of Lung Cancer, Chest. 2003;123:21S 49S.
10. US Department of Health, and Human Services (USDHHS). National Cancer Institute. *Risks associated with smoking cigarettes with low machine-measured* yields of tar and nicotine. 2001 National Institutes of Health Bethesda, MD.
11. www.lungcancerfrontiers.org, Highlights from the 5th National Dutch Lung Cancer Symposium, (2003).

CHAPTER 37

RACIAL, GENDER, AND AGE FACTORS IN THE TREATMENT OF LUNG CANCER

37.1 DIFFERENCES BETWEEN WOMEN AND MEN

37.11 Overview

Investigations are finding differences in how men and women respond to smoking. Women appear to be more susceptible to the harmful effects of tobacco-related carcinogens—the odds ratios for major types of lung cancer are consistently higher in women than in men at every level of exposure to cigarette smoke. Furthermore, this gender difference cannot be explained by differences in exposure, smoking history or body size; and is likely due to women's higher susceptibility to tobacco carcinogens.

Men had a significantly higher incidence of precancerous lesions in the large central airways than women. In contrast, women women develop more cancers in the peripheral (outer) parts of the lung which are harder to detect. and sophisticated screening procedures could even take gender into account.

37.12 Adenocarcinoma and Tyrosine Kinase Damage Among Women

Women have a higher incidence of adenocarcinoma and bronchioloalveolar (BAC) cancer, a subtype of adenocarcinoma arising

422

in the small alveolar region of the lung. Women are more likely to have an unusual mollecular presentation involving damage to the tyrosine kinase area of the epidermal growth factor receptor. Hsieh (6).

Research is ongoing. Those with this type of damage tend to be non-smokers or light former smokers, of female gender, have adenocarcinoma or BAC, and be responsive to Iressa or Tarceva. These type of damage can be identified on a sophisticated EGFR tissue test conducted by the Harvard Genetics Lab.

Women with BAC or adenocarcinoma, particularly light or non-smokers will want to have treatment done at regional cancer centers so this recent research is incorporated into their treatments.

37.13 Age at Diagnosis

One study found a higher percentage of women are younger patients. It appears women are more susceptible to smoking-related cancer disease. They develop lung cancer at earlier ages even though the amount of cigarette they smoke is less than men and they generally begin at a later age. Schiller (4).

37.14 Estrogen

One hypothesis for lung cancer development in women is an interaction with estrogen. Lung cancer tissue has higher levels of estrogen substances. Schiller (4). Women may have less effective systems of DNA repair. Schiller (4).

37.15 Prognosis

Performance status and stage of disease continue to be the most important factors in survival. However, female gender status is a favorable indicator in treatment, with women having better survival and response in many studies. Schiller (4).

37.16 Implications for Treatment

Some suggest that clinical trials separate women and men. In the future treatment may be gender related, though one writer on gender differences suggests there is no basis for such separation today. Schiller (4).

37.2 RACIAL DIFFERENCES IN THE TREATMENT OF LUNG CANCER

37.21 The Rate of Lung Cancer in the Afro-American Community

While one is reluctant to ascribe racial motives, studies indicate the following:

1. The percentage of blacks contracting lung cancer is higher percentage wide than whites. This is probably due to higher exposure rates to dangerous dusts such as silica and asbestos in different occupations, higher rates of smoking, residence in cities with poorer air quality and vehicle emissions, and other risk factors.
2. Blacks are diagnosed at later stages and have higher mortality rates than whites.
3. Blacks are less likely to have surgery performed, which is generally the most successful medical alternative.

37.22 Racial and Economic Issues

An article entitled, "The Economics of Surviving Cancer" sets forth some disturbing findings:

> "Disadvantaged Americans are far more likely to die of the most treatable form of lung cancer than average—not because of poor health habits, but because they don't receive the proper treatment for their malignancy. Health care delivery expert Howard P. Greenwald has analyzed more than 5,000 cases of stage-1 non-small cell lung cancer—attempting to explain why cancer mortality rates are higher among racial minorities and the socially disadvantaged than among higher-income Americans and whites. His findings are detailed in "Uneven Odds: Explaining High Cancer Death Rates Among Minorities and the Poor," a paper presented March 28 at an American Cancer Society conference in New Orleans . . . . Greenwald found that surgery may have saved the lives of nearly one in three patients whose cancer was

detected early enough for surgery. But the poorest patients were about a third less likely to receive surgery than the richest patients. Fifty percent of the patients in the bottom 10 percent of income levels received surgical treatment, whereas 72 percent of patients in the top 10 percent of income levels received it. The mortality rates were even more dramatic. Greenwald found that the poorest patients were only half as likely as the richest patients to survive. Only 22 percent of the poorest lived at least five years after diagnosis, compared to 45 percent among the richest patients. As a subset of the study group, African-American patients carried an additional burden. According to Greenwald, they had a one-in-four chance of surviving, compared to a one-in-three chance among white Americans. While 61 percent of whites received surgery, only 51 percent of African Americans did. "In the form of lung cancer studied, lack of appropriate care seems to have contributed strongly to excess mortality among the disadvantaged," Greenwald said. It explains about 50 percent of the excess mortality in poor people and all of the excess mortality in African Americans . . . ." (2).

Greenwald has written extensively about socio-economic factors and cancer. He is the author of Who Survives Cancer (1992) and Social Problems in Cancer Control (1980). A study in the prestigious New England Journal of Medicine said:

"We studied all black patients and white patients 65 years of age or older who were given a diagnosis of resectable nonsmall cell lung cancer (stage I or II) between 1985 and 1993 and who resided in 1 of the 10 study areas of the Surveillance, Epidemiology, and End Results (SEER) program (10,984 patients) . . . . The rate of surgery was 12.7 percentage points lower for black patients than for white patients (64.0 percent vs. 76.7 percent, P<0.001), and the five-year survival rate was also lower for blacks (26.4 percent vs. 34.1 percent, P<0.001). However, among the patients undergoing surgery, survival was similar for the two racial groups, as it was among those who did not undergo surgery. Furthermore, analyses in which adjustments were made for factors that are predictive of either candidacy for surgery or survival did not alter the influence of race on these outcomes . . . Conclusions: Our analyses suggest that the lower survival rate among black patients with early-stage, nonBsmall cell lung cancer, as compared with white patients, is largely explained by the lower rate of surgical treatment among blacks." Beggs (3).

37.23 What Should Be Done

Afro-Americans need to take a more assertive role in their treatment, assess the quality of their hospitals and physicians, and assure themselves that they are receiving the best treatment. Given the extent of risk from lung cancer and its consequences, there needs to be an effective screening program, particularly for Afro-Americans. The message of this book is repeated—lung cancer at early stages is very treatable, the problems occur when the cancer is permitted to spread.

REFERENCES

1. Jon J Cancer Res, 1999 May, 90:5, 490-5.
2. Southern California Chronicle, www.usc.edu.
3. Beggs, *Racial Differences in the Treatment of Early Stage Lung Cancer*, Volume 341:1198-1205, Oct 14, 1999, No. 16.
4. Schiller, *Lung Cancer Outcome: Women versus Men*, Presentation at the 10th World Conference on Lung Cancer, Vancouver, Online at http://www.wclcnetcast2003.com/index.php.
5. Journal of National Cancer Institute, April 21, 1999.
6. Hsieh, *Female Sex and Bronchoalveolar Subtype predicts EGFR Mutations in Non Small Cell Lung Cancer*, Chest, 2005 July 128 (1) 317

CHAPTER 38

FAMILY HISTORY AND DIET

38.1 OVERVIEW

Diet and nutrition is a subject discussed extensively on the Internet though it receives relatively little attention in medical and scientific journals. Pass's 2001 book, *Lung Cancer*, has over 1,100 pages and 66 chapter, but no chapter devoted to diet. Scientists have not been able to identify a diet which cures cancer or develop a clear link between food intake and lung cancer. Anatomically, it is not clear how particular foods would reach the lung tissue.

38.2 DIET AND CAUSES OF CANCER

There is a fair amount of evidence that vegetable and fruit consumption minimize risk, while meat and fat-based diets increase it. "Diet, particularly high fat consumption and low fruit and vegetable consumption, contributes (independent of cigarette smoking) to the excess lung cancer risk in African-American men," one study found. (2).

38.21 Fruit

One European study found, "fruit intake was inversely related to lung cancer mortality. This association was confined to heavy cigarette smokers." (3). A recent British study found, "fish liver oil, vitamin pills, carrots and tomato sauce decreased risk."

38.22 Red Meat

"A significant increase in risk of lung cancer associated with red meat, beef and fried meat was observed. The increase in risk was more evident in squamous cell lung cancer. This association remained after controlling for total energy and saturated fat intake, suggesting a possible role of heterocyclic amines in lung carcinogenesis."

38.23 Vegetables

"12 studies showed a decreased lung cancer risk as vegetable consumption increased." Albert (8).

38.24 Beta-Carotene Supplements

With fruit playing a positive role in cancer prevention, some suggested beta carotene supplements (an important ingredient in certain fruits):

"Beta-carotene and retinoids were the most promising agents against common cancers when the National Cancer Institute mounted a substantial program of population-based trials in the early 1980s. Both major lung cancer chemoprevention trials not only showed no benefit, but had significant increases in lung cancer incidence and in cardiovascular and total mortality. A new generation of laboratory research has been stimulated. Rational public health recommendations at this time include: 1) Five-A-Day servings of fruits and vegetables, a doubling of current mean intake; 2) systematic investigation of the covariates of extremes of fruit and vegetable intake; 3) discouragement of beta-carotene supplement use, due to adverse effects in smokers and no evidence of benefit in non-smokers." Omenn (5) (6).

Indeed, the clinical trial was stopped because of the adverse impact of the Beta Carotene. The reasons are unclear. The author concluded that there must be an important difference between concentrated vitamin supplements and fruit or vegetables which contained that ingredient. Patients should consult knowledgeable physicians and not simply accept theories proposed on the Internet or elsewhere.

38.3 DIET FOR LUNG CANCER PATIENTS

These studies lead to the question of whether tumors can be inhibited through a particular diet.

38.31 Clinical Trials with Vegetable Supplement

In one study, use of a vegetable supplement led to a longer life span for a group of patients with advanced cancer:

> "Daily ingestion of SV (selected vegetables) was associated with objective responses, prolonged survival, and attenuation of the normal pattern of progression of stage IIIB and IV NSCLC. A large randomized phase III clinical trial is needed to confirm the results observed in this pilot study. In the study, the selected vegetable supplement includes Asoybeans, mushrooms, mung beans, red dates, scallion, garlic, lentils, leek, Hawthorn fruit, onion, ginsengs, angelica root, licorice, dandelion root, senegal root, ginger, olive, sesame seeds, and parsley. The mix was blended, boiled, and then stored frozen." (1).

What is the difference between this study and the beta-carotene study? Here, the supplement was simply a group of vegetables given in concentrated form. There, two specific vitamins were given.

38.4 FAMILY HISTORY OF LUNG CANCER AND ITS ROLE

Systems of genetic repair play a role in cancer making some individuals particularly susceptible to gene damage from smoking:

> "The major risk factor for lung cancer is exposure to tobacco smoke. Exposure to radon, heavy metals used in smelting, and asbestos also greatly increases risks for lung cancer. However, only about 11% of tobacco smokers ultimately develop lung cancer, suggesting that genetic factors may influence the risk for lung cancer among those who are exposed to carcinogens . . . . Epidemiological studies show

approximately 14-fold increased risks for lung cancer among average tobacco smokers and approximately 2.5-fold increased risks attributable to a family history of lung cancer after controlling for tobacco smoke . . . common genetic variants or polymorphism are hypothesized to affect lung cancer risk. Environmental carcinogenesis resulting from tobacco smoke exposure is a complex process that can involve activation of procarcinogens that lead to abduct formation and subsequent failure of DNA repair, which should normally remove these abducts. Studies comparing DNA repair capacity among newly diagnosed lung cancer patients and age-matched controls indicate significant differences between the two groups. DNA repair capacity influences risk for lung cancer among individuals."

While tobacco is the primary risk factor, family history plays an important but subsidiary role. Those with a family history of lung cancer may have less of a capacity to repair smoking related DNA damage, therefore leading to increased incident of lung cancer.

REFERENCES

1. Sun, *Study of a Specific Dietary Supplement in Tumor-Bearing Mice and in Stage IIIB and IV Non-Small Cell Lung Cancer Patients*, Nutrition and Cancer 39(1):85-95, 2001.
2. Pillow, *Case-control assessment of diet and lung cancer risk in African Americans and Mexican Americans*, Nutr Cancer 1997;29(2):169-73.
3. Jansen, *Cohort analysis of fruit and vegetable consumption and lung cancer mortality in European men*, Int J Cancer 2001 Jun 15;92(6):913-8.
4. Darby, *Diet, smoking and lung cancer: a case-control study of 1000 cases and 1500 controls in South-West England*, Br J Cancer 2001 Mar 2;84(5):728-35.
5. Omenn, *Chemoprevention of lung cancer: the rise and demise of beta-carotene*, Annu Rev Public Health 1998;19:73-99.
6. Omenn, *Effect of a Combination of Beta Carotene and Vitamin A on Lung Cancer and Cardiovascular Disease*, N Engl J Med 1996 May 2;334(18):1150-5.

7. *Is there a genetic basis for lung cancer susceptibility:* Recent Results Cancer Res, 1999, 151:, 3-12.
8. Albert, *Epidemiology of Lung Cancer*, Chest. 2003;123:21S 49S.

CHAPTER 39

HANDLING LUNG CANCER FOR THE FAMILY

39.1 SOME OVERALL SUGGESTIONS

Family and close friends can play a vital role in helping a cancer patient. Here are some things you can do for a family member with lung cancer:

1. **Do the research.** Some of the information patients will see is hard. It is frequently better for a close family member to cull through medical studies, and help locate the best physician, hospital, and form of treatment.
2. **Support with Chemotherapy or Radiation.** If a patient is undergoing chemotherapy or radiation, make arrangements to accompany him to the physician or hospital or at least pick him up. Dealing with cancers every day, oncologists may not have time to provide the emotional support a family member can.
3. **Handle Medical Bills and HMO Problems.** Dealing with HMO's can be time-consuming and exasperating. Taking this task off the patient's mind can be a welcome relief.
4. **Contact Support Groups** for the Patient and Spouse. Alcase is the national lung cancer support group. Find out about support options, learn about new treatment developments, and learn from others how to deal with the disease.

5. **Keep Track of Records.** Mistakes happen especially as nursing and medical caseloads increase. Keep duplicate material about the patient's medical condition in addition to the hospital. Doctor Smith is the patient's usual doctor, but while on vacation, Dr. Jones orders a test. As a safegap, we want to make sure there is appropriate followup. Likewise, we need to maintain for the hospital a list of medications and the patient's current condition.

39.2 RESEARCH AND DEALING WITH LUNG CANCER

Some patients will want to fully understand their disease and obtaining information about it is helpful in dealing with it. Most however, say they would rather not spend their time thinking about metastasis and disease process. For this group, the family member who can studiously but quietly obtain information about treatment alternatives can provide a great help. For many, simply saying, "Your doctor recommends this particular form of chemotherapy, my research shows he is very well-qualified and this is the best choice!" is sufficient.

39.21 Family Relationships

Here are some suggestions from the online lung cancer support group livingwithit.org.

"Some people exhaust themselves trying to be the same healthy, energetic spouse/partner they were before cancer. Respect your body's signals for rest. Your spouse/partner is probably juggling a lot of responsibilities now—trying to deal with fears of losing you, keeping up with household chores, taking care of children. Let your spouse/partner know it's all right to take a break or to find some quiet, personal time. Talk! Your spouse/partner can love you and still not always know what you want all the time. Honest and open communication can help your spouse/partner feel more comfortable about helping you throughout your illness.

Encourage listening. Your spouse/partner may feel the need to solve problems, make things better, or offer advice. This reaction can be a way of dealing with feeling powerless, but it also can make you feel misunderstood, frustrated, unsupported, or even rejected.

39.22 Patient Feelings

A diagnosis represents a tremendous change and the patient may feel shock, devastation, anger, depression, frustration, and guilt.

39.3 PARTICULAR FAMILY ISSUES

39.31 Men and Cancer

While many women can talk about an illness, many men become uncomfortable. Some are not happy to see large numbers of people come to the door and see them in a weakened position. Discuss feeling but differences and preferences must be respected.

39.4 PRACTICAL TIPS

One support group put together this list of "25 PRACTICAL TIPS TO HELP THOSE FACING A SERIOUS ILLNESS":

1. Don't avoid me. Be the friend . . . the loved one you've always been.
2. Touch me. A simple squeeze of my hand can tell me you still care.
3. Call me to tell me you're bringing my favorite dish and what time you are coming. Bring food in disposable containers, so I won't worry about returns.
4. Take care of my children for me. I need a little time to be alone with my loved one. My children may also need a little vacation away from my illness.
5. Weep with me when I weep. Laugh with me when I laugh. Don't be afraid to share this with me.
6. Take time out for a pleasure trip, but know my limitations.
7. Call for my shopping list and make a "special" delivery to my home.
8. Call me before you visit, but don't be afraid to visit. I need you. I am lonely.

9. Help my family. I am sick, but they may be suffering. Offer to come stay with me to give my loved ones a break. Invite them out. Take them places.

10. Help me celebrate holidays (and life) by decorating my hospital room or home or bringing me tiny gifts of flowers or other natural treasures.

11. Be creative! Bring me a book of thoughts, taped music, a poster for my wall, cookies to share with my family and friends . . . an old friend who hasn't come to visit me.

12. Let's talk about it. Maybe I need to talk about my illness. Find out by asking me: "Do you feel like talking about it?"

13. Don't always feel we have to talk. We can sit silently together.

14. Can you take me or my children somewhere I may need transportation? To a treatment? . . . . To the store? . . . To a doctor?

15. Help me feel good about my looks. Tell me I look good, considering my illness.

16. Please include me in a decision. I've been robbed of so many things. Please don't deny me a chance to make decisions in my family . . . in my life.

17. Talk to me of the future. Tomorrow, next week, next year. Hope is so important to me.

18. Bring me a positive attitude. It's catching!

19. What's in the news? Magazines, photos, newspapers, verbal reports, keep me from feeling the world is passing me by.

20. Could you help me with some cleaning? During my illness, my family and I still face: dirty clothes, dirty dishes, dirty house.

21. Water my flowers.

22. Just send a card to say "I care."

23. Pray for me and share your faith with me.

24. Tell me what you would like to do for me and, when I agree, please do it!

25. Tell me about support groups like Make Today Count, Cancerwise, and American Cancer Society so I can share with others.

From the brochure "25 Tips to Help Those Facing a Serious Illness" from Saint Anthony's Hospital's Make Today Count.

Another cancer survivor provides these suggestions

Educate and empower yourself. **Learn about wellness,** which is making positive choices toward a more balanced and healthy lifestyle. **Maintain a positive attitude.** Attitude is everything! Belief is biology! Humor helps! Lighten-up! Surround yourself with humorous books, movies, videos, and television programs. **Laugh every day!** Connect with your spirit. **Take quiet time for yourself,** meditate, and pray. **Keep a journal.** The rules are date the entries and don't make any other rules. **Practice deep focused relaxed breathing.** Go outdoors and **walk briskly for thirty minutes every day. Use your senses for healing.** Find healing through touch and massage. Use wonderful scents to **sooth your nerves** such as cederwood, patchouli, moss lavender, ylang-ylang and chamomile. These can be found in bath and body products, essential oils and placed in aromatherapy units. Listen to relaxing music. **Drink calming teas.** Chamomile is especially good. Nurture yourself through intimacy with a loving partner. It is an important part of maintaining wellness so **explore acts of love and tenderness.** Remember the most important sexual organ of the body is the brain! Enjoy. Poor concentration and memory loss may be a side effect of cancer treatment so **know that you are not losing your mind.** Be patient with yourself and ask for family and friends to be tolerant. **Don't forget the basics of good health.** Exercise, drink 8-10 glasses of water per day and eat nourishing, well-balanced meals, rest and stay connected with people. Remember every day is a new beginning. **Face each day with a positive outlook. Stop asking "Why me?".** Know that the answer is BECAUSE. **Words of Wisdom to Consider** *"Cancer may rob you of that blissful ignorance that once lead you to believe that tomorrow stretched forever. In exchange, you are granted the vision to see each day as precious, a gift to be used wisely and richly. No one can take that away." Anonymous*

39.41 Sharing Your Feelings

Many patients provide inspiration in online and personal support groups. Some note that sharing feelings helps:

"I feel it easier to on with my normal life people know that is going on with me. I think this is a pretty personal decision, but for me, I feel like I'm hiding something if I spend any significant time with someone and they don't know I have cancer. I've also found everyone to be completely understanding and willing to help out. My side effects have been pretty limited, but they do affect my energy level, . . . (Cancer Survivor's Network (2)

Gender can play a role, with men less able to share their feelings of pain, weakness, or discomfort. For some, drawing out feelings may help, while others would simply prefer to be left alone. Others offer different advice. A wife of a cancer patient notes three points:

1) Learn to accept help.
2) Redefine and accept your new role,

She wrote about her husband:

"I have had to learn to accept Gary the way he is and love him for who he is and for the reasons why I married him. All of this has brought that back around full circle. At this point Gary has his little house out in the backyard. It started out to be a little shed, but it looks like it could be a little efficiency apartment. He has made a Murphy bed in there. It's the size of an efficiency apartment with a big 8-foot porch on it. So he goes out and he stays in his little domain, and he feels as though he is more in control of himself, which I allow. He always asks me to forgive him for going out there, but I let him do what he needs to have his life, too." ACS (American Cancer Society) (2)

Someone with a third with a different type of cancer wrote,

"To enjoy each day. To set your priorities. To not give in to feeling down. To decide you're going to be around for a long time so you better be nice. To help your caregivers by eating and drinking what they give you and just doing your best to recover. To even eat stuff like jello and rice pudding without kvetching. To pray every day for everyone else you know who has cancer. On my computer I tape lift-ups like this "Prayer for the New Year" by St. Francis De Sales."

That prayer says,

> Do not look forward in fear to the changes of life; Rather look to them with full hope that as they arise, God, whose very own you are, will lead you safely through all things; And when you cannot stand, God will carry you in His arms. Do not fear what may happen tomorrow; the same everlasting Father who cares for you today will take care of you today and every day. He will either shield you from suffering or will give you unfailing strength to bear it. (2)

Many find solace in their religion, and religious leaders emphasize that those in need are always welcome.

39.42 Finding Personal Strength

Some find surprising strength in confronting their illness. "Don't Underestimate yourself or the people around you. Nobody knows what they are capable of until faced with challenges. Let people help any way they are able." (2)

Yet others speak of recognizing your limitations. "Don't try to be superheroes. Some People exhaust themselves trying to be the same healthy, energetic spouse/ partner they were before cancer. Respect your body's signals for rest." (2). Others speak of enjoying small pleasures, a pretty flower, or a night out.

39.43 Speaking with Others.

Many find that sharing similar experiences is helpful. "I have met a lot of strong people through my treatments and Drs visits. Always remember you are not alone on this journey."

39.44 Religion

We are given a short time here on earth, and many find solace in their church or synagogue in understanding some of the mysteries of life. A poster on the American Cancer Society website writes,

The two things that have helped me the most are 1) all the prayers and the understanding support from my son and my granddaughter (both of whom flew out to visit me when they learned about the Cancer Monster that had attack my body . . . and my two beloved older brothers (who also flew clear across the country to come visit me when they learned of my plight; and 2) my ability to maintain a DELIGHTFUL sense of humor no matter how depressing or shattering the news was that the doctors were obligated to present me with as the different test were completed. I've always needed laughter in order to survive like most people need air to breath . . . and I still do . . . so a sense of humor is of paramount importance to me! I just thank God that I've been able to maintain mine . . . Amen!

She found this prayer inspirational

Do not look forward in fear to the changes of life; Rather look to them with full hope that as they arise,God, whose very own you are, will lead you safely through all things; And when you cannot stand, God will carry you in His arms. Do not fear what may happen tomorrow; the same everlasting Father who cares for you today will take care of you today and every day. He will either shield you from suffering or will give you unfailing strength to bear it.

Many find solace in their religion, and religious leaders emphasize that those in need are always welcome. Ministers and religious leaders are trained to deal with the mysteries of life and dealing with pain and illness. Even if you were less observant, utilize the resources of your church, mosque, or temple.

39.5 THE ROLE OF THE CAREGIVER

39.51 Rewards of Caregiving

While care-giving is difficult, many find it rewarding. "97% said their roles were important, 81% stated that they wanted to provide care and could not live with themselves if they did not assume caregiving responsibilities. 67% said they enjoyed providing care." Strength for Caring (1).

Yet, care-giving takes its toll. Many care-givers were themselves taking medication, a quarter noted their own physical limitations, about a third found the role demanding, and close to one half noted financial limitations.

39.52 Help for Caregivers

82% of caregivers were married and 71% women. The large number of women in the caregiving role brings up an obvious point, men in the family should be asked for their help, whether in dealing with insurance questions, helping to find information, or assisting with medical visits.

That is not to say men do not play vital roles, "I have a lot of support from my husband and my children." (2). Practical advice can be important too. "Take advantage of community resources. You and your loved one can benefit greatly from resources in your area. Utilize transportation agencies, home care services, support groups and educational programs." (1).

39.53 Leave of Absence from Work

Many married women try to juggle 3 roles, raising a family, working, and caregiving. The first two are demanding in themselves, adding a third is draining. Consider a leave of absence with many companies providing unpaid leaves of absence for caregivers.

39.54 Tasks for Caregivers

Doctors can have limited time and important information can become lost. An astute caregiver can transmit patient information in a clear and well-organized fashion, for example explaining when pain or side effects occur. One needs to be careful that the patient is not put aside, and many older patients talk of the phenomenon where their condition is discussed as if they are not present or are somehow incompetent. Substantial time can be required. Make time for yourself.

For others, helping a close family member continue to enjoy life can be the important contribution: "I do little things to make him smile. He had bad days when we will just sit and talk, others when he feels up to it will go to dinner and a movie like a normal couple."

REFERENCES

1. www.strengthforcaring.com/resource/factsheet.html.
2. American Cancer Society, The Cancer Survivor's Network, www.acscsn.org.
3. www.Livingwithit.org.

CHAPTER 40

DEALING WITH TERMINAL ILLNESS

40.1 DEFINING THE TERM TERMINALLY ILL

Beyond inspiring fear and despair, the phrase terminally ill is not particularly descriptive. It means different things to different people, physician or layman, and is so imprecise to be as misleading as helpful. It can describe someone with a life expectancy ranging from 1 to 18 months. It is misleading because some patients may decide not to utilize treatments which have a fair probability of extending their lives.

Terminally ill is best used for stage 4 non-small cell patients and small cell patients with extensive disease. For many of these patients, science currently has no clear cure, though there are treatments which can extend life and reports of complete remission. Members of support groups surviving advanced cancer 2-5 years after diagnosis counsel optimism. In a typical clinical trial of patients in this group, there will be reports of partial responses, that is, elimination of 50% of disease, and an occasional report of complete response, complete elimination of disease as seen on Ct Scan or other testing.

40.11 When is Hospice Appropriate

Thus, it makes sense for patients to fight; one cannot say there is no hope. Nonetheless, there are times, particularly with older patients, that the burden and stress of fighting the disease, enduring chemotherapy with side effects, may lead a patient to stop fighting. Typically these are situations with substantial loss of weight and fatigue, and diminishing returns from chemotherapy. While other treatments are a legitimate option, after two or more different types of chemotherapy and other treatment, the patient may simply want to die with dignity.

40.2 HOSPICE

Hospice is basically designed to provide a humane way of dying. Advocates explain, "End of life treatments were overly aggressive and too often not in accordance with patients' wishes. Furthermore, 50% of conscious patients dying in the hospital were reported by their surviving family members to have been in moderate to severe pain in the last week of life. Respondents were more likely to be dissatisfied with their treatments for their symptoms than for their cancer." Devita (1).

> "There were several predictors of inadequate pain management, including minorities, female subjects, and the elderly. The reality is inadequate pain relief. For some patients, the physician did not attribute the reported pain to the cancer, perhaps because these patients had a good performance status. The simple message is that pain is being undertreated."   I.

Hospice can improve these results. "Several groups have confirmed significant improvement in symptom control, especially pain during hospice care. Good control of overall symptom distress increased from 64% of patients on admission to a palliative care unit to 84% of the day of death." Devita (1).

40.21 Assessment of Pain

A central part of hospice is maintaining the patient's comfort through the vigorous use of pain relievers. "Assess pain carefully and reassess frequently. Believe the patient and treat pain promptly. Successful analgesia is possible in 85%-95% of cancer patients using basic pain management techniques." Devita (1) at 3081.

40.22 Pain Relief Tools

The use of analgesics and opiates is a part of many hospice programs. For those opposed to opiates, patient's wishes would be respected. Indeed, the goal of Hospice is to provide autonomy at end of life, providing the patient or family members with the ability to dictate the type of treatment when it is clear medical intervention will not substantially extend life.

40.23 Restrictions on Medical Methods/Means of Extending Life

Some may suggest that feeding or intravenous methods of providing nutrition not be used:

> "Intravenous hydration and nutrition may prolong life so that patients die from other less comfortable causes. They may cause prolonged suffering from other symptoms, including increased respiratory and gastrointestinal secretions, . . ." Devita (1).

On the other hand, family members may see a lack of intervention as a sign that an older or severely ill patient is given low priority by hospital staff, particularly if he is on Medicaid or other programs providing the hospital with limited reimbursement. One must distinguish a carefully considered decision to restrict intake to maximize comfort from a decision to pay little attention to a dying patient. While hospitals may wish to prioritize their resources ("overoptimistic prognoses can inappropriately commit the patient to futile intervention, thereby increasing the anguish of the patient and family and also increase the expenditure of valuable time and resources") family members should insist on the best treatment for a beloved father, wife, or mother. Hospice simply says that the best treatment in some cases may be limited medical intervention but careful attention to the patient's needs, particularly relief of pain. "In hospice care, no single approach to provision of fluid by nonoral routes is used. Most caregivers would agree that the patient's choice is paramount." Devita (1).

40.24 Life Support Tools

Similar considerations apply to medical methods of life support. "Among the most difficult of all tasks for caregivers are withdrawal of life support and sedation for refractory symptoms to provide patients with calm and comfort as they die." Devita (1). Patients may provide legal advance directives or living wills indicating how they wish these matters to be handled.

40.25 Insurance, Medicare, and At Home Care

Many insurance programs provide at home care, so a patient can be with family in his home as he dies. Medicare provides various benefits:

> "Medicare beneficiaries, who make up 80% of the hospice clientele, receive noncurative medical and support services that otherwise would not be covered. These include at-home nursing care, physician services, medical appliances, medications, short-term hospitalization, home health aides, homemakers, physical therapy, psychological therapy, speech therapy, and social services." Silvestri (4).

40.3 LIVING WILLS AND ADVANCED DIRECTIVES

Providing intravenous food and nutrition can prolong life for a patient in a poor condition. Likewise, many would prefer that a patient debilitated by cancer not be artificially resuscitated. Most states permit living wills, which advise a hospital of what type of treatment the patient will permit and under what conditions. The goal is to permit the patient to die with dignity and having a living will may frequently be comforting to the patient worrying about being artificially kept alive in a debilitated state. Religious issues may also come into play.

40.4 PERFORMANCE STATUS AND DATE OF DEATH

Lung cancer is generally a progressive process. Few patients die at stage one and the process of death generally involves metastasis and progression to stage four and with that curtailment of body functions, loss of weight, increased fatigue, lack of ambulation and death. Yet the process is not always clear or consistent, presenting difficult issues for patient and family. Go to acor.org, the newsgroup for non-small cell patients, and you find patients with stage 4 who have survived longer than doctors or family anticipated.

Statistically, performance status is the most reliable indicator of poor survival. Being bed ridden, suffering large amounts of weight loss, chronic fatigue, indicates the patient may expire within the near future.

40.41 Incontinence

Lung cancer rarely metastasizes to the colon or adjoining areas, and fecal incontinence is not an acknowledged side effect of lung cancer. Devita and Pass, two well-known writers devote little attention to it and there are few articles on the subject. Nonetheless because incontinence is associated with reduced functioning, it can be a problem for patients and family.

Fecal incontinence is associated with advanced age. "Fecal incontinence is a socially devastating disorder which affects at least 2.2 percent of community dwelling adults and 45 percent of nursing home residents." (2) (3). If it does occur, the problem is likely to arise with advanced disease where the patient's activities have been greatly diminished. Diarrhea is associated with some forms of chemotherapy and may contribute to the problem.

It appears that lung cancer does not directly cause incontinence by, for example, metastasis to the colon. However, the combination of fatigue, weight loss, and occasional diarrhea in older patients may contribute to disruption. Incontinence is defined as a lack of control and may simply involve a sick patient's inability to move quickly from bed to bathroom.

40.42 Who to Consult and What to Do

The first person to consult is your oncologist. Patients may vary as to their willingness to discuss the matter, and a physician's interpersonal skills can improve or inhibit discussion. Because the condition does not impact survival, some physicians may give it limited attention. In such situations, the patient should insist the issue be addressed, try to speak with a nurse or other professional, or change physicians. Gastroenterologists specialize in incontinence problems, so consider a referral, and write for informative publications from the International Foundation for Functional Gastrointestinal Disorders, Inc. and check the internet for www.aboutincontinency.org.

The following can be done to address the problem:

1. Use anti-diarrhea medications. "Diarrhea is the most common aggravating factor for fecal incontinence, and anti-diarrheal medications such as loperamide and diphenoxylate or bile acid binders may help." Incontinence.org (3). Over the counter remedies can also be tried.

2. Incontinence with the lung cancer patient is sometimes a question of not having sufficient time to go to the bathroom once the urge hits. Place a portable facility in the patient's room.

3. Try to arrange for regular bathroom visits.

4. Use protective clothing.

40.5 FAMILY ISSUES

Patients will vary in the extent they wish to confront the possibility of death. For many patients, this can be a time to convey your thoughts to family members, to tell children your love them, to recognize the help of friends and family during a difficult time, and to attempt to put their minds at ease.

The death of a loved one poses many types of difficulties. Organizing one's affairs can help. In particular, consider:

1. Reviewing where various assets are located,

2. Discussing who family members can call upon for advice, and

3. Reviewing religious preferences and funeral arrangements, (if possible funeral arrangements should be examined before a death so that decisions do not have to be made by the family in a heightened emotional state).

A will is a narrow legal document which deals primarily with the disposition of property. A directive or instruction sheet can encompass much more, setting forth suggestions or requests which may not be legally binding but are usually respected.

Family members need to recognize the different approaches people have during this difficult time. While many women will appreciate the opportunity to cry together, some men may not welcome visitors or being seen in a weakened state. There are no rights and wrongs, and care should be taken to respect the wishes of someone seriously ill.

REFERENCES

1. Devita, *Cancer Principles and Practice of Oncology* (Lippincott 2001).
2. Whitehead, *Treatment options for fecal incontinence*, Dis Colon Rec 2001; 44:131-144.
3. www.aboutincontinency.org.
4. Silverstri, *Caring for the dying patient with lung cancer*, Chest, Sept. 2002. www.findarticles.com.

CHAPTER 41

RESOURCE SOURCES

41.0 RESEARCH INTRODUCTION AND OVERVIEW

Hopefully this book has provided some useful information about lung cancer. I also hope that you have heeded some of the cautionary notes, recognizing that new science is being created, some studies may have been missed and the precise application of medical knowledge to a specific condition is for your doctor. However, you may want to obtain some further information so that you can understand the nature of your treatment and medical options.

41.1 GENERAL TEXTS

Some readers may have assimilated a large amount of information while for many others, a good general text can still be helpful. *Informed Decisions* (1997) from the American Cancer Society is a good over all text. You may also want to use a medical dictionary to understand basic concepts.

41.2 SPECIALIZED BOOKS DEALING WITH LUNG CANCER

Currently the best single volume on lung cancer is Pass's book, *Lung Cancer, Principles and Practice* (Lippincott Publishers). Published in 2001 and written by some of the leading medical authorities around the world, this is the authoritative work on lung cancer. Although it is intended for a medical audience, many of the chapters are comprehensible for a patient or family member reading slowly and equipped with a medical dictionary. (Unfortunately, the beginning chapter launches into a tortured description of molecular biology).

The book provides the medical community's view on accepted forms of treatment, at least as of 2001. You may hear about new and unusual treatments from friends. Check the index in Pass and see what is said. If a suggested treatment is not in the book, you will know it is at best experimental and at worst, a fraud. The only exception is that since the book was written in 2001, there may be some treatment developments.

Devita, et. al., *Cancer Principles and Practice of Oncology* is the most well-known general medical text on cancer. Comprising over 2500 pages with contributions from the foremost scientists and oncologists throughout the world, it is the book many medical professionals first consult. While pricey at $260, many patients will find used copies at under $100.

41.3 MEDLINE RESEARCH

The premier search device for information about lung cancer and other medical subjects is Medline. Medline is the search engine to use for specific information about a new form of treatment or a particular area of medicine. The service is free and available on the Internet.

The National Library of Medicine makes Medline available in various ways. First you can go to the National Library of Medicine itself-www.ncbi.nlm.nih.gov/entrez. The site title is complicated; alternatively just use the search terms Medline National Library of Medicine on Yahoo, Google, or other search engines. Some companies which market to physicians have medline. Medscape.com has a good site. A number of different companies offer free Medline courtesy of the National Library of Medicine including www.medscape.com and www.healthgate.com. Medline will give a list of medical abstracts of articles from the last 20 years. Here is the description of Medline furnished by the National Library of Medicine.

- Medline is the National Library of Medicine's (NLM) premier bibliographic database covering the fields of medicine, nursing, dentistry, veterinary medicine, the health care system, and the preclinical sciences.

- It contains bibliographic citations (e.g., authors, title, and journal reference) and author abstracts from over 3,900 biomedical journals published in the United States and 70 foreign countries during the current four years and contains over 9 million records dating back to 1966.

- It has worldwide coverage, but 88% of the citations in current MEDLINE are to English-language sources and 76% have English abstracts.

- It contains the citations that appear in Index Medicus, as well as the citations of "special list" journals. Special list journals include those indexed for the Index to Dental Literature and the International Nursing Index. Citations for MEDLINE are created by the National Library of Medicine, International MEDLARS partners, and cooperating professional organizations.

- An English abstract, if published with the article, is included in MEDLINE.

- Approximately 33,000 new citations are added each month (about 7,300 weekly; 350,000-400,000 yearly).

41.31 Sample MEDLINE Record

Here is what a sample Medline record dealing with heart disease would look like:

TITLE: *Screening for cardiac disease in patients having noncardiac surgery* [comment] [see comments]

AUTHOR: Fleisher LA; Eagle KA

AUTHOR AFFILIATION: Johns Hopkins University School of Medicine, Baltimore, Maryland, USA.

SOURCE: Ann Intern Med 1996 Apr 15;124(8):767-72

CITATION IDS: PMID: 8633839 UI: 96213860

COMMENT: Comment on: Ann Intern Med 1996 Apr 15;124(8):763-6

ABSTRACT: The preoperative evaluation of the cardiac patient having noncardiac surgery offers an opportunity to identify occult and further define known cardiovascular disease to modify both perioperative and long-term care. The baseline probability of cardiovascular disease should initially be assessed using clinical variables and identifying unstable symptoms, including unstable angina and congestive heart failure. The decision about whether to obtain noninvasive testing to further define cardiovascular status should be made on the basis of the testing's potential to modify perioperative care, . . .

41.4 MEDICAL JOURNALS AND MEDICAL ORGANIZATIONS DEALING WITH LUNG CANCER

You can obtain relevant medical articles through your Medline search. However, you may wish to order or review the many medical journals which deal with cancer. Recognize that some of the material may be technical, but you have the opportunity to obtain detailed information on critical issues at your local medical or hospital library. The International Association for the Study of Lung Cancer prepares a journal called lung cancer which is published by Elsevier Publishing Co. There are other journals which deal generally with lung cancer:

American Journal of Respiratory and Critical Care Medicine
   (from the American Thoracic Society
Annals of Thoracic (chest) Surgery-
CA Cancer Journal for Clinicians (published by the American
   Cancer Society) A peer-reviewed journal for physicians. An
   article which is peer-reviewed generally will have greater
   credibility and impact than one which is not.
Cancer (also published by the American Cancer Society) (published
   detailed information about cancer cause and treatments).
Cancer Control, Journal of the Moffit Cancer Center

41.5 ORGANIZATIONS DEALING WITH LUNG CANCER

Founded in 1972, International Association for the Study of Lung Cancer (IASLC) is an international organization of 1150 members in 53 countries. The purpose of the Association is to promote the study of the etiology, the epidemiology, the prevention, the diagnosis, the treatment, and all other aspects of lung cancer and to disseminate information about lung cancer to the members of the Association, to the medical community at large, and to the public. They publish a journal devoted exclusively to lung cancer, which while somewhat technical in nature, is worthwhile reading to learn about new developments in this area.

41.6 SUPPORT AND INFORMATION GROUPS

41.61 Alcase

A group called Alcase, (Alliance Against Lung Cancer) has been active in promoting early detection programs, and increasing funding for lung cancer. They have excellent materials and are accessible on the web.

41.62 American Cancer Online Resources Acor.org

This is an excellent online group where people exchange experiences about cancer. Categorized by disease type and moderated by Lorraine Johnson, author of an excellent book on lung cancer, the quality of information is usually far better than on other internet sites. People discuss side effects from various drugs, family issues, and how they have responded to new drugs. Search archives for specific topics, post questions, or review other materials. While the site is good, getting on can take a little time and knowledge. Ask for help if needed.

41.63 Support for Caregivers

The Well Spouse Foundation, Care Pathways.com provide online support resources.

41.7 WEBSITES DEALING WITH LUNG CANCER

41.71 www.Lungcanceronline.org

The leading online site is www.lungcanceronline.org, a comprehensive site written by a former patient.

41.72 Oncolink

This University of Pennsylvania site provides a comprehensive search tool for locating information about cancer.

41.73 Acor.Org

Acor.org has four separate online support groups dealing with different types of lung cancer. Beyond providing support, they are an excellent source of information with Lorraine Johnson, author of a book on lung cancer, and the creator of lungcanceronline serving as moderators.

41.8 PLACES TO GET BOOKS AND OTHER INFORMATION

Many hospitals and medical schools have detailed libraries which are open to the general public for reading. Occasionally, you may need an introductory letter from your local library to use another library. Generally you cannot take out books from another library but your own library may be able to arrange to borrow the book for you. Amazon.com, and Barnes & Noble.com have extensive lists of books including those in specialized areas available for purchase.

REFERENCES

1. www.carepathways.com
2. www.wellspouse.org

CHAPTER 42

DIRECTIONS IN LUNG CANCER TREATMENT

42.0 OVERVIEW

New discoveries are being performed each day. I will try to provide an overview of some of the directions for lung cancer treatment in the future. Treatment will become increasingly sophisticated with the large teaching hospitals leading the way.

42.1 COMBINING CHEMOTHERAPY WITH GENE THERAPY

Today's patient has the option of chemotherapy or experimental treatments like Iressa. These treatments will be FDA approved and integrated into a treatment regimen for the stage 3 and 4 patient in otherwise good health, prolonging their life expectancy and holding out the promise of cure for some.

Epidermal growth factor receptor therapy, such as Iressa, will become a standard part of therapies for advanced stage patients, and even early stage patients displaying certain risk factors. Cox-2 inhibitors like Celebrex will also become accepted and multi-pronged attacks on tumors will delay metastases, improve the rate of overall cures, and extend lives.

42.2 MONITORING THE STAGE 1 PATIENT

Approximately 35% of stage 1 patients have a recurrence. Tumors are removed and an x-ray or Ct each year or 6 months is the extent of treatment until a metastasis is detected. The modern physician will use available tools before the cancer spreads. Blood work will detect microvessel density, epidermal growth factors or other molecular markers which indicate a particular patient is at risk. Those patients will be given different types of gene therapy such as Iressa and watched more closely.

42.3 MONITORING SMOKERS

We know that approximately 1 in 10 smokers contract lung cancer; today most are diagnosed at advanced stages. In the future, we will utilize screening tools such as the CT Scan to detect early stage tumors along with various molecular methods of detection. Today, we tell smokers that might get cancer in the future, years from now, we will provide that with Ct Scanning report, and pathology, demonstrating how their risk factors have increased, pushing them to stop smoking before a tumor develops.

42.4 CELL TESTING IN A LABORATORY

We may recognize that lung tumors are a group of similar tumors with distinct microscopic differences. Tumor cells from a patient may be removed and tested in a laboratory with various forms of drugs and gene therapies. See Gazdar (2) and Suda (3). With the aid of such testing on the patient's actual cells, a treatment plan would be developed. A company called Oncotech explains its procedures:

> "Fresh viable tumor tissue is minced and enzymed to disaggregate the tumor cells . . . . Cells are exposed to tumor type-specific antineoplastic agents for five days in a carefully controlled environment. Drug exposures in excess of the maximum tolerated are used. Due to the reduced rate of drug metabolism, in vitro tumor exposure is 5 to 80 times greater than in vivo. Treated cells are compared to untreated controls . . . . If malignant

cells proliferate in vitro under such extreme chemotherapeutic exposure conditions, then in vivo exposures will be ineffective." Oncotech (1).

There is some evidence of negative success, that is, excluding drugs which are likely to show no impact upon cancer cells. However, these tests have not yet reliably shown which drugs will work and translate that into longer life. For that reason, most insurers though still reject reimbursement for the process.

A variety of studies have reported a correlation between in vitro prediction or response and clinical response. While these studies may have internal validity, they cannot answer the question of whether patients given assay-guided therapy or empiric therapy have different outcomes . . . . The TEC assessment concluded that decision analysis would not be a useful tool for assessing the relative effectiveness of assay-guided and empiric treatment . . . . A total of 7 studies were identified, none of which provided strong evidence to validate the clinical role of chemosensitivity or chemoresistance assays . . . No studies were identified that provided direct evidence comparing outcomes for patients treated either by assay-guided therapy or contemporaneous empiric therapy. Therefore, the policy statement is unchanged. In 2004, the American Society of Clinical Oncology (ASCO) published a technology assessment of chemotherapy sensitivity and resistance assays (CSRA) (18) along with a systematic review of the literature. (19) The assessment concluded that "review of the literature does not identify any CSRAs for which the evidence base is sufficient to support use in oncology practice." Regence Group (4)

REFERENCES

1. www.oncotech.com.
2. Cazdar, *Correlation of in vitro drug-sensitivity testing results with response to chemotherapy and survival in extensive-stage small cell lung cancer: a prospective clinical trial,* Journal Of The National Cancer Institute, Vol 82, 117-124.

3. Suda, *Evaluation of the histoculture drug response assay as a sensitivity test for anticancer agents*, Surg Today. 2002;32(6):477-81.
4. Regence Group, Laboratory Section—*In Vitro Chemoresistance and Chemosensitivity Assays*, www.regence.com/trgmedpol/lab/lab06.html
5. *Yoshimasu, Histoculture Drug Response Assay on non-small cell lung cancer*, GanTo Kagaku Ryoho. 2000 May;27(5):717-22.

APPENDIX

I. ONLINE INFORMATION

Medline

Medline is the world database of medical literature and contains abstracts of over 500,000 articles about treatment, diagnosis, chemotherapy, and a host of other issues. Medline is the source cancer researchers use to review recent studies and medical literature. Abstracts of articles are available with some full-text articles and books available online. Go to the official site, www.ncbi.nlm.nih.gov/entrez/query.fcgi or commercial sites like ng medscape.com carry medline.

Acor.org

Acor provides three support groups devoted specifically to different types of lung cancer. Its non-small cell and small cell lung cancergroups discuss treatments, chemotherapy side effects, and the psychological impact of cancer.

EGFR-Info.com

This site if devoted to epidermal growth factor research. The journal Signal is available on-line along with a host of references. Some of the material is technical but this is a valuable resource.

Cancer.gov

Comprehensive information about treatments, clinical trials, chemotherapy and much more are contained on this official government site.

Lungcanceronline.com

This comprehensive sits written by a lung cancer patient continually updates and reviews studies, medical, literature, and other materials.

Asco. Org The American Society for Clinical Oncology has important abstracts, presentations, and other material on its website. Designed for medical professionals, the material is technical but valuable. Many important findings come up first as abstracts on this site.

Lungcancerclaims.com A continually updated version of this book and newsletter are among the items on our website.

II. BIBLIOGRAPHY

General Books on Lung Cancer

Johnson, *Lung Cancer Making Sense of Diagnosis Treatment & Options* (2001) A well-done book designed for layman, good discussion of side effects and the psychological issues of lung cancer.

Alcase *Lung Cancer Manual*, (2000) (available on-line at alcase.org as of this date) a good compilation of materials from the leading lung cancer advocacy group.

Hentshke, *Lung Cancer*, Myths, Facts, Choices (2002) written by the leading authority on lung cancer screening, the book is designed for patients and family and summarizes treatment options.

Parless, *Hundred Questions and Answers about Lung Cancer* Written by a patient and creator of Lung Cancer Online, the book answers many basic question about lung cancer.

General Books on Cancer

1. Buchman, *What You Really Need to Know About Cancer* (Johns Hopkins Press an excellent overview of the cancer process, but not specifically devoted to lung cancer. Read this first, and then try to specialized medical books.

2. Coleman, *Understanding Cancer* (Johns Hopkins Press, 1997) A good book which explains medical terms in easy to understand language. Read this book, and What you Really need to Know about Cancer, and try the specialized medical books.

3. American Cancer Society *Informed Decisions, The Complete Book of Cancer Diagnosis*, Treatment, and Recovery (Viking Press 1997)

MEDICAL BOOKS ON LUNG CANCER

1. *Pass, et. al., Lung Cancer* Principles and Practice Lippincott Publishing Co) (2004), an excellent, but detailed examination of lung cancer, designed for medical professionals

2. Devita, *Cancer, Principles and Practice of Oncology (2001)* The leading source of cancer overall, designed for physicians, this comprehensive text covers everything you would need to know, but the reading is not always easy.

GOVERNMENTAL AGENCIES

The National Cancer Institute publishes a wide range of materials, oversees clinical trials, and answers questions. Call 1-800 4Cancer, or check, www.nci.gov.

III. LUNG CANCER ORGANIZATIONS

Alliance for Lung Cancer Advocacy, Alcase

Founded by a former patient, Alcase (The Alliance for Lung Cancer

Advocacy) is the leading lung cancer advocacy organization in the world. Their services include an online manual, advocacy problems, and an informative website. Additionally, The ALCASE Phone Buddy program matches lung cancer survivors or family members who have similar circumstances, such as disease type, treatment regimens, or caregiving situations. Once the match is made, participants can phone each other for support, encouragement, and above all, hope.

Contact: ALCASE www.alcase.org, 1601 Lincoln Avenue, P.O. Box 849 Vancouver, WA 98666 USA Tel: (800) 298-2436

American Cancer Online Resources Acor.Org.

Acor has online support groups devoted specifically to non-small lung cancer, small cell, and even mesothelioma. Moderated by Lorraine Johnson, author of a book on lung cancer, the group provides information and support, ranging from reports of new clinical trials, to discussion of side effects, to discussion of family issues.

International Association for the Study of Lung Cancer (IASLC)

The IASLC is an international organization of 1150 members in 53 countries and holds conferences each year, where new data and findings relating to lung cancer are disseminated. Founded in 1972, IASLC is the leading medical group devoted to lung cancer and publishes the respected publication called Lung Cancer. While the journal is intended for physicians, it has important information about new forms of treatment and diagnosis of the disease. Abstracts from the publication are available on-line, though full text access requires a subscription.

Cuneo Lung Cancer Study Group

This Italian medical group investigate the cause and treatment of lung cancer. Its website, www.culcasg.org. contains the text of recent studies, presentations, and other important information.

European Lung Cancer Working Party

This is a group of European physicians whose focus is the diagnosis and treatment of lung cancer. Their website is unfortunately limited though some information is available online.

Lung Cancer Frontiers

This Arizona group compiles information about lung cancer available online, puts out a journal dealing with lung screening and other issues. Www.Lungcancerfrontiers.org 899 Logan, Suite 203 Denver, CO 80203,e-mail to tlpdoc@aol.com

Cancer Care, Inc.

While not devoted specifically to lung cancer, this organization had taken a leading role in many areas to enlighten people about lung cancer, and bring more public resources to the problem. National Office, 275 7th Ave $ New York, NY 10001 Services: 212 302 2400 $ 1 800 813 HOPE (4673) info@cancercare.org Administration: 212 221 3300 $ Fax: 212 719 0263.

National Cancer Institute

This United States government entity conducts research on all forms of cancer and approves clinical trials. Information about standard forms of treatment, experimental therapies, clinical trials, and virtually anything about cancer is available from either their website or their offices themselves. Www.cancer.gov, and www.NCI.net.

American Cancer Society

The American Cancer Society may be the important cancer-fighting organization in the world. It has locations across the United States where volunteers provide assistance and programs are held. The American Cancer Society has played a leading role in smoking cessation programs but has lagged in the equally important area of early diagnosis of lung cancer. ACS does not simply help patients; it sets policies. Thus, if ACS embraced the idea of lung cancer screening for high-risk patients, it would likely be adopted.

American Society for Clinical Oncology *(ASCO)*

Many important studies are presented at ASCO annual meetings prior to publication. The discovery that certain adenocarcinoma patients respond particularly well to Iresaa was highlighted at the 2004 ASCO meeting. Since the site is designed for oncologists, the materials can be technical. Nonetheless, it is far more worthwhile to try to slowly go through reliable materials here than use newspaper articles and obscure internet sites as a basis for treatment decisions. www. asco.org has both print and video seminars available at no charge.

IV. CONFERENCES AND SEMINARS ON LUNG CANCER

Many of these conferences will be rather technical. Nonetheless, a family member may want to attend to learn who are the leading authorities on lung cancer and what new developments are being discussed. Some conferences will charge a fee, and others may restrict attendance, but some may permit the public or interested patients or families to observe. To check for further conference, look at these sites: www.docguide.com, a site which provides a list of many medical conferences throughout the world.

Conference Listing

2005 Asco Annual Meeting, May 13-17, 2005

The 11th World Conference on Lung Cancer—International Association for the Study of Lung Cancer July 03, 2005—July 06, 2005 Barcelona, Spain.
6th European Conference: Perspectives in Lung Cancer, November, 2005 Athens, Greece

V. JOURNALS

Lung Cancer The leading journal devoted to this disease is Lung Cancer, put out by the International Association for the Study of

Lung Cancer. Membership in the organization is $165.00 which includes complete access to present and past journals on-line. The organization is designed for physician and oncologists in the area, and it is unclear whether membership for patients or family members would be accepted.

New England Journal of Medicine. Quite graciously, this premier journal permits free access to the complete text of all issues, excepting articles published in the last six months. The Journal also allows 24 hour access to all articles for the cost of $29.00

VI. NATIONAL CANCER INSTITUTE COMPREHENSIVE CANCER CENTERS AND CANCER CENTERS.

ALABAMA

Albert F. LoBuglio, M.D. UAB Comprehensive Cancer CenterUniversity of Alabama at Birmingham1824 Sixth Avenue South, Room 237 Birmingham, Alabama 35293-3300 Tel: 205/934-5077 Fax: 205/ 975-7428 **ARIZONA**

Daniel D. Von Hoff, M.D.Director, Arizona Cancer CenterUniversity of Arizona 1501 North Campbell Avenue Tucson, Arizona 85724 Tel: 520/ 626-7925 Fax: 520/626-2284 **CALIFORNIA**

Theodore G. Krontiris, M.D., Ph.D.Director, City of Hope National Medical Center &Beckman Research Institute 1500 East Duarte RoadDuarte, California 91010-3000Tel: 626/395-8111 X64297 Fax: 626/930-5394(Comprehensive Cancer Center)

Walter Eckhart, Ph.D.Director Cancer CenterSalk Institute 10010 North Torrey Pines RoadLa Jolla, California 92037Tel: 858/453-4100 X1386, Fax: 858/457-4765(Cancer Center)

Erkki Ruoslahti, M.D., Ph.D.President & CEOThe Burnham Institute 10901 North Torrey Pines RoadLa Jolla, California 92037Tel: 858/ 455-6480 X3209, Fax: 858/646-3198(Cancer Center)

David Tarin, M.D., Ph.D.Director UCSD Cancer CenterUniversity of California at San Diego 9500 Gilman DriveLa Jolla, California 92093-0658Tel: 858/822-1222 Fax: 858/822-0207(Comprehensive Cancer Center)

Judith C. Gasson, Ph.D.Director, Jonsson Comprehensive Cancer CenterUniversity of California Los Angeles Factor Building, Room 8-68410833 Le Conte AvenueLos Angeles, California 90095-1781Tel: 310/825-5268 Fax: 310/206-5553(Comprehensive Cancer Center)

Peter A. Jones, Ph.D. Director USC/Norris Comprehensive Cancer CenterUniversity of Southern California 1441 Eastlake Avenue, NOR 8302LLos Angeles, California 90033Tel: 323/865-0816 Fax: 323/865-0102(Comprehensive Cancer Center) Frank L. Meyskens, Jr., M.D.

DirectorChao Family Comprehensive Cancer CenterUniversity of California at Irvine 101 The City Drive Building. 23, Rt. 81, Room 406Orange, California 92868Tel: 714/456-6310 Fax: 714/456-2240(Comprehensive Cancer Center)

Frank McCormick, Ph.D.Director UCSF Cancer Center & Cancer Research Institute University of California San Francisco 2340 Sutter Street, Box 0128San Francisco, California 94115-0128Tel: 415/502-1710 Fax: 415/502-1712(Comprehensive Cancer Center)

COLORADO

Paul A. Bunn, Jr., M.D. Director University of Colorado Cancer CenterUniversity of Colorado Health Science Center 4200 East 9th Avenue, Box Bl88Denver, Colorado 80262Tel: 303/315-3007 Fax: 303/315-3304(Comprehensive Cancer Center)

CONNECTICUT

Vincent T. DeVita, Jr., M.D.Director Yale Cancer Center Yale University School of Medicine 333 Cedar Street, Box 208028New Haven, Connecticut 06520-8028Tel: 203/785-4371 Fax: 203/785-4116(Comprehensive Cancer Center)

DISTRICT OF COLUMBIA

Kevin J. Cullen, M.D. Interim DirectorLombardi Cancer Research CenterGeorgetown University Medical Center 3800 Reservoir Road, N.W.Washington, DC 20007Tel: 202/687-2110 Fax: 202/687-6402(Comprehensive Cancer Center)

FLORIDA

John C. Ruckdeschel, M.D. Center Director & CEO H. Lee Moffitt Cancer Center & Research Institute at the University of South Florida 12902 Magnolia DriveTampa, Florida 33612-9497Tel: 813/979-7265 Fax: 813/979-3919(Comprehensive Cancer Center)

HAWAII

Carl-Wilhelm Vogel, M.D., Ph.D. Director Cancer Research Center of Hawaii University of Hawaii at Manoa 1236 Lauhala Street Honolulu, Hawaii 96813Tel: 808/586-3013 Fax: 808/586-3052(Clinical Cancer Center)

ILLINOIS

Nicholas J. Vogelzang, M.D.Director University of Chicago Cancer Research Center5841 South Maryland Avenue, MC 1140Chicago, Illinois 60637-1470Tel: 773/702-6180 Fax: 773/702-9311(Comprehensive Cancer Center)

Steven Rosen, M.D.Director Robert H. Lurie Cancer Center Northwestern University 303 East Chicago AvenueOlson Pavilion 8250 Chicago, Illinois 60611Tel: 312/908-5250 Fax: 312/908-1372 (Comprehensive Cancer Center)

INDIANA

Richard F. Borch, M.D., Ph.D.Director Purdue University Cancer Center Hansen Life Sciences Research Building South University Street West Lafayette, Indiana 47907-1524 Tel: 765/494-9129 Fax: 765/494-9193 (Cancer Center)

Stephen D. Williams, M.D.Director Indiana University Cancer Center Indiana Cancer Pavilion535 Barnhill Drive, Room 455Indianapolis, Indiana 46202-5289Tel: 317/278-0070 Fax: 317/278-0074(Clinical Cancer Center)

IOWA

George J. Weiner, M.D. Director Holden Comprehensive Cancer Center at The University of Iowa5970 "Z" JPP 200 Hawkins Drive Iowa City, Iowa 52242 Tel: 319/353-8620 Fax: 319/353-8988 (Comprehensive Cancer Center)

MAINE

Kenneth Paigen, Ph.D.Director The Jackson Laboratory 600 Main StreetBar Harbor, Maine 04609-0800Tel: 207/288-6041 Fax: 207/288-6044(Cancer Center)

MARYLAND

Martin D. Abeloff, M.D. DirectorThe Sidney Kimmel Comprehensive Cancer Center at Johns Hopkins North Wolfe Street, Room157Baltimore, Maryland 21287-8943Tel: 410/955-8822 Fax: 410/955-6787(Comprehensive Cancer Center)

MASSACHUSETTS

Edward J. Benz, Jr., M.D. DirectorDana-Farber/Harvard Cancer Center Dana-Farber Cancer Institute 44 Binney Street, Rm. 1628Boston, Massachusetts 02115Tel: 617/632-4266 Fax: 617/632-2161 (Comprehensive Cancer Center)

Richard O. Hynes, Ph.D. Director & Professor of Biology Center for Cancer Research Massachusetts Institute of Technology 77 Massachusetts Avenue, Room E17-110Cambridge, Massachusetts 02139-4307Tel: 617/253-6422 Fax: 617/253-8357(Cancer Center)

MICHIGAN

Max S. Wicha, M.D. Director Comprehensive Cancer CenterUniversity of Michigan 6302 CGC/09421500 East Medical Center Drive Ann Arbor, Michigan 48109-0942Tel: 734/936-1831 Fax: 734/615-3947(Comprehensive Cancer Center)

John D. Crissman, M.D. Interim Director Barbara Ann Karmanos Cancer Institute Wayne State University Operating the Meyer L. Prentis Comprehensive Cancer Center of Metropolitan Detroit 540 East Canfield, Room 1241Detroit, Michigan 48201 Tel: 313/577-1335 Fax: 313/577-8777 (Comprehensive Cancer Center)

MINNESOTA

John H. Kersey, M.D.Director University of Minnesota Cancer Center MMC 806, 420 Delaware Street, S.E. Minneapolis, Minnesota 55455 Tel: 612/624-8484 Fax: 612/626-3069 (Comprehensive Cancer Center)

Franklyn G. Prendergast, M.D., Ph.D.Director Mayo Clinic Cancer Center Mayo Foundation

200 First Street, S.W. Rochester, Minnesota 55905 Tel: 507/284-3753 Fax: 507/284-9349 (Comprehensive Cancer Center)

MISSOURI

Timothy J. Eberlein, M.D.Director Siteman Cancer Center Washington University School of Medicine 660 South Euclid Avenue, Box 8100 St. Louis, MO 63110-1093 Tel: 314/747-7222 Fax: 314/454-5300 (Clinical Cancer Center)

NEBRASKA

Kenneth H. Cowan, M.D., Ph.D.Director University of Nebraska Medical Center/Eppley Cancer Center 600 South 42nd Street Omaha, Nebraska 68198-6805 Tel: 402/559-4238 Fax: 402/559-4652 (Clinical Cancer Center)

NEW HAMPSHIRE

Mark A. Israel, M.D. Director Norris Cotton Cancer Cente rDartmouth-Hitchcock Medical Center One Medical Center Drive, Hinman Box 7920Lebanon, New Hampshire 03756-0001Tel: 603/650-6300 Fax: 603/650-6333(Comprehensive Cancer Center)

NEW JERSEY

William N. Hait, M.D., Ph.D.Director The Cancer Institute of New JerseyRobert Wood Johnson Medical School 195 Little Albany Street, Room 2002BNew Brunswick, New Jersey 08901Tel: 732/235-8064 Fax: 732/235-8094(Clinical Cancer Center)

NEW YORK

I. David Goldman, M.D. Director Cancer Research CenterAlbert Einstein College of Medicine Chanin Building, Room 2091300 Morris Park AvenueBronx, New York 10461Tel: 718/430-2302 Fax: 718/430-8550(Comprehensive Cancer Center)

David C. Hohn, M.D.President & CEO Roswell Park Cancer InstituteElm & Carlton StreetsBuffalo, New York 14263-0001Tel: 716/845-5772 Fax: 716/845-8261(Comprehensive Cancer Center)

Bruce W. Stillman, Ph.D.Director Cold Spring Harbor LaboratoryP.O. Box 100Cold Spring Harbor, New York 11724Tel: 516/367-8383 Fax: 516/367-8879(Cancer Center)

Steven J. Burakoff, M.D.Director Kaplan Cancer Center New York University Medical Center 550 First Avenue New York, New York 10016Tel: 212/263-8950 Fax: 212/263-8210(Comprehensive Cancer Center)

Harold E. Varmus, M.D. President & CEO Memorial Sloan-Kettering Cancer Center 1275 York Avenue New York, New York 10021Tel: 212/639-6561 Fax: 212/717-3299(Comprehensive Cancer Center)

Daniel W. Nixon, M.D.President, American Health Foundation300 East 42nd Street New York, New York 10017Tel: 212/551-2500 Fax: 212/ 687-2339(Cancer Center)

Karen H. Antman, M.D.Director Herbert Irving Comprehensive Cancer Center College of Physicians & SurgeonsColumbia University 177 Fort Washington Avenue6th Floor, Room 435New York, New York 10032Tel: 212/305-8602 Fax: 212/305-3035(Comprehensive Cancer Center)

NORTH CAROLINA

H. Shelton Earp, M.D.Lineberger Professor of Cancer Research& Director UNC Lineberger Comprehensive Cancer CenterUniversity of North Carolina Chapel Hill School of Medicine, CB-7295102 West Drive Chapel Hill, North Carolina 27599-7295Tel: 919/966-3036 Fax: 919/966-3015(Comprehensive Cancer Center)

O. Michael Colvin, M.D.Director Duke Comprehensive Cancer Cente Duke University Medical Center Box 3843Durham, North Carolina 27710Tel: 919/684-5613 Fax: 919/684-5653(Comprehensive Cancer Center)

Frank M. Torti, M.D.Director Comprehensive Cancer Center Wake Forest University Medical Center Boulevard Winston-Salem, North Carolina 27157-1082Tel: 336/716-7971 Fax: 336/716-0293(Comprehensive Cancer Center)

OHIO

James K. V. Willson, M.D.Director Ireland Cancer Center Case Western Reserve University andUniversity Hospitals of Cleveland 11100 Euclid Ave., Wearn 151Cleveland, Ohio 44106-5065Tel: 216/844-8562 Fax: 216/844-4975(Comprehensive Cancer Center)

Clara D. Bloomfield, M.D. Director Comprehensive Cancer Center Arthur G. James Cancer Hospital &Richard J. Solove Research Institute

Ohio State University A455 Staring Loving Hall300 West 10th AvenueColumbus, Ohio 43210-1240Tel: 614/293-7518 Fax: 614/293-7520(Comprehensive Cancer Center)

OREGON

Grover C. Bagby, Jr., M.D.Director Oregon Cancer Center Oregon Health Sciences University 3181 S.W. Sam Jackson Park Rd., CR145Portland, Oregon 97201-3098Tel: 503/494-1617Fax: 503/494-7086(Clinical Cancer Center)

PENNSYLVANIA

John H. Glick, M.D.Director University of Pennsylvania Cancer Center16th Floor Penn Tower, 3400 Spruce Street Philadelphia, Pennsylvania 19104-4283Tel: 215/662-6065 Fax: 215/349-5325(Comprehensive Cancer Center)

Clayton A. Buck, Ph.D. Interim DirectorThe Wistar Institute 3601 Spruce Street Philadelphia, Pennsylvania 19104-4268Tel: 215/898-3926 Fax: 215/573-2097(Cancer Center)

Robert C. Young, M.D.President Fox Chase Cancer Center7701 Burholme Avenue Philadelphia, Pennsylvania 19111Tel: 215/728-2781 Fax: 215/728-2571(Comprehensive Cancer Center)

Carlo M. Croce, M.D.Director Kimmel Cancer Center Thomas Jefferson University 233 South 10th Street BLSB, Room 1050Philadelphia, Pennsylvania 19107-5799Tel: 215/503-4645 Fax: 215/923-3528(Clinical Cancer Center)

Ronald B. Herberman, M.D.Director University of Pittsburgh Cancer Institute 3550 Terrace Street, Suite 401Pittsburgh, Pennsylvania 15213 Tel: 412/648-2255 Fax: 412/648-2741(Comprehensive Cancer Center)

TENNESSEE

Arthur W. Nienhuis, M.D.DirectorSt. Jude Children's Research Hospital

332 North LauderdaleP.O. Box 318Memphis, Tennessee 38105-2794Tel: 901/495-3301Fax: 901/525-2720(Clinical Cancer Center)

Harold L. Moses, M.D.Director Vanderbilt-Ingram Cancer CenterVanderbilt University Medical Research Building IINashville, Tennessee 37232-6838Tel: 615/936-1782, Fax: 615/936-1790(Comprehensive Cancer Center)

TEXAS

John Mendelsohn, M.D.President University of TexasM.D. Anderson Cancer Center 1515 Holcombe Boulevard, Box 91Houston, Texas 77030Tel: 713/792-6000 Fax: 713/799-2210(Comprehensive Cancer Center)

Charles A. Coltman, Jr., M.D. DirectorSan Antonio Cancer Institute 7979 Wurzbach Dr.Urscel Tower, 6th FloorSan Antonio, Texas 78229-3264Tel: 210/616-5580 Fax: 210/692-9823(Comprehensive Cancer Center)

UTAH

Stephen M. Prescott, M.D.Director Huntsman Cancer InstituteUniversity of Utah 2000 Circle of HopeSalt Lake City, Utah 84112-5550Tel: 801/585-3401Fax: 801/585-6345(Clinical Cancer Center)

VERMONT

David W. Yandell, Sc.D.Director Vermont Cancer CenterUniversity of Vermont 149 Beaumont Ave., HRSF326Burlington, Vermont 05405Tel: 802/656-4414 Fax: 802/656-8788(Comprehensive Cancer Center)

VIRGINIA

Michael J. Weber, Ph.D.Director Cancer CenterUniversity of Virginia, Health Sciences Center Jefferson Park Ave., Room 4015Charlottesville, Virginia 22908Tel: 804/924-5022 Fax: 804/982-0918(Clinical Cancer Center)

Gordon D. Ginder, M.D. Professor of Medicine & DirectorMassey Cancer CenterVirginia Commonwealth University P.O. Box 980037Richmond, Virginia 23298-0037Tel: 804/828-0450 Fax: 804/828-8453(Clinical Cancer Center)

WASHINGTON

Leland H. Hartwell, Ph.D. President & DirectorFred Hutchinson Cancer Research Center 1100 Fairview Avenue, NorthP.O. Box 19024, D1060Seattle, Washington 98104-1024Tel: 206/667-4305 Fax: 206/667-5268(Comprehensive Cancer Center)

WISCONSIN

John E. Niederhuber, M.D.DirectorComprehensive Cancer CenterUniversity of Wisconsin 600 Highland Ave., Rm. K4/610Madison, Wisconsin 53792-0001Tel: 608/263-8610 Fax: 608/263-8613(Comprehensive Cancer Center)

INDEX

Printed in the United States
38057LVS00003B/59